THE
HERBAL
DRUGSTORE

Linda B. White, M.D., holds B.S. and M.S. degrees from Stanford University and an M.D. from the University of California, San Diego. She is the author of *Kids, Herbs, & Health* and *The Grandparent Book.* She has written for many health publications, including *Herbs for Health, Mothering, Nutrition Science News,* and *Natural Pharmacy.*

Steven Foster, technical consultant to *The Herbal Drugstore,* is one of the most respected names in herbal health. He has written nine books on the subject including *101 Medicinal Herbs* and *Field Guide to Medicinal Plants* (co-authored with James A. Duke, Ph.D.). A photographer and consultant specializing in medicinal plants, Foster lectures worldwide and serves on the advisory board of *Herbs for Health* magazine.

THE
HERBAL
DRUGSTORE

THE <u>BEST</u> NATURAL ALTERNATIVES
TO OVER-THE-COUNTER
AND PRESCRIPTION MEDICINES!

LINDA B. WHITE, M.D., STEVEN FOSTER

and the staff of **Herbs for Health**™

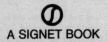

A SIGNET BOOK

SIGNET
Published by New American Library, a division of
Penguin Putnam Inc., 375 Hudson Street, New York, New York 10014, U.S.A.
Penguin Books Ltd, 80 Strand, London WC2R 0RL, England
Penguin Books Australia Ltd, Ringwood, Victoria, Australia
Penguin Books Canada Ltd, 10 Alcorn Avenue, Toronto, Ontario, Canada M4V 3B2
Penguin Books (N.Z.) Ltd, 182–190 Wairau Road, Auckland 10, New Zealand

Penguin Books Ltd, Registered Offices: Harmondsworth, Middlesex, England

Published by Signet, an imprint of New American Library,
a division of Penguin Putnam Inc. This is an authorized reprint of a hardcover edition published by Rodale.

First Signet Printing, April 2002
10 9 8 7 6 5 4 3 2 1

The Herbal Drugstore Editorial Staff

Project Editor	Susan Clotfelter
Editorial Consultants	Jody Berman
	Cindy L.A. Jones, Ph.D.
	Pat A. Meller, M.S.
Technical Consultant	Steven Foster
Contributing Writers	Paul Barney, M.D.
	Michael Castleman
	Logan Chamberlain, Ph.D.
	Christopher Hobbs, L.Ac.
	Lois Johnson, M.D.
	Cindy L.A. Jones, Ph.D.
	Erika Lenz
	Robert Rountree, M.D.
	Linda B. White, M.D.
	Victor Zeines, D.D.S.
Copy Editors	Jean Scorgie
	Chris Roerden, M.A.
Cover Designer	Bren Frisch
Design Specialist	Dean Howes
Illustrators	Susan Strawn Bailey
	Gayle Ford
Editorial Coordinator	Vicki Yost

Rodale Healthy Living Books

Editor	Susan G. Berg
Art Director	Darlene Schneck
Vice President and Publisher	Brian Carnahan
Editorial Director	Michael Ward
Vice President and Marketing Director	Karen Arbegast
Product Marketing Director	Denyse Corelli

CONTENTS

PART IV: HERB PROFILES

A Close-up Look at the Most Common Herbs 549

RESOURCES

FOREWORD

T HE HERBAL DRUGSTORE—in particular, one medicinal herb—
changed my life and my career.

More than 20 years ago, in the late 1970s, I was a young medical
writer. At the time, "medical writing" meant mainstream, high-tech
medicine, because in the American news media, that was pretty
much all that existed. The alternative therapies, such as acupuncture, yoga, and meditation, were still in their infancy in this country,
while herbal medicine was at the dawn of a renaissance after
decades of neglect.

I felt open to medical alternatives, thanks in part to my grandmother, who was a big believer in the folk medicine of her native
Ukraine. I learned to meditate, and enjoyed it. But professionally, I
focused pretty much on mainstream medicine: heart bypass surgery,
organ transplantation, and new drugs.

Meanwhile, for vacations, my wife and I headed to the
Caribbean, where we fell in love with snorkeling, and in 1981, became certified scuba divers. We adored diving and went on week-
long dive trips whenever we could. My wife had no problem on the
small boats that ferried us out to the reefs, walls, and shipwrecks,
but I became deathly seasick if the water was the least bit choppy.
If you've ever been seasick, you know how horrible it can be. If you
haven't, pray that you never find out.

I tried everything to settle my stomach: looking at the horizon,
positioning myself amidships (the middle of a boat rocks the least),
munching crackers, and taking mainstream antinausea drugs such
as Dramamine, Bonine, and scopolamine. All these approaches
helped to some degree, but I still felt queasy. Even worse, I started
to develop a conditioned reflex: Just looking at a dive boat made me
nauseous.

Then in 1982, in a dive publication, I came across a report of a
study published in the British medical journal *Lancet*. Daniel
Mowrey, Ph.D., then a researcher at Brigham Young University in
Salt Lake City, had tested ginger, an herb traditionally used to prevent nausea, head-to-head against Dramamine. Dr. Mowrey motor-
ized a chair, rigging it to rock in a way guaranteed to produce

motion sickness in anyone who was susceptible. The chair was also fitted with a "kill" switch so its occupants could turn it off at will.

Dr. Mowrey gave 36 volunteers either a standard dose of Dramamine or 940 milligrams of ginger powder (about a teaspoon) 30 minutes before they got in the chair. He told them to hit the "kill" switch when they became uncomfortably nauseated. Compared with the people taking Dramamine, those taking ginger were able to ride in the chair 57 percent longer.

I was amazed that an herb I'd had on my spice rack forever prevented motion sickness better than a standard pharmaceutical. At the time, my wife and I were planning a dive trip to Tortola, one of the British Virgin Islands. Before we left, I picked up a bottle of ginger capsules at my local health food store, and took 1,000 milligrams a half-hour before boarding the boat. As fate would have it, the water was quite choppy that day, and several passengers became seasick. But not me—the ginger completely conquered my nausea.

Fascinated, I returned home and did some research on ginger. Ancient Chinese sailors chewed the root to prevent seasickness. Ancient Indians adopted the practice and introduced it to Arab traders, who took the fleshy root (actually a rhizome) to ancient Greece. The Greeks ate slivers of ginger wrapped in sweetened bread after big meals to settle their stomachs. Eventually, they began baking the herb into sweet bread, inventing the world's first cookie, gingerbread. In Elizabethan England, ginger beer was a popular stomachsettler. That beverage evolved into ginger ale, which my grandmother always recommended for indigestion and nausea.

If I'd had this book then, I could have turned to one resource to find out if there was anything that worked as well or better than the pharmaceutical motion-sickness cures.

My experience with ginger turned me into an avid student of herbal medicine, and eventually spurred me to specialize in writing about herbs and the many other alternative therapies. In the 20-plus years that I've been studying alternative healing, herbal remedies have moved steadily from the fringes of medicine into the mainstream.

On my last dive trip, I explored the magnificent reefs surrounding Roatan, a Caribbean island off the coast of Honduras. As always, I had my trusty bottle of ginger capsules with me, and on the first morning, I took 1,000 milligrams a half-hour before boarding the boat.

Our dive master, Dave, was a big, burly, expatriate Texan, about

30, who looked more like a pirate than an alternative medicine aficionado. As people boarded the boat, Dave helped them set up their tanks and stow their gear and joked that whoever dropped their equipment once we were underwater would have to buy beer for the whole boat that evening. But before we shoved off, Dave got serious. He pulled out a plastic bag and held it aloft for all to see. It contained translucent yellow wafers.

"Hey, y'all, listen up," he said. "I don't want anyone getting seasick, so I brought along some candied ginger. Forget the drugs. If you chew a piece of this stuff between here and the reef, I guarantee you won't get sick."

Welcome to the herbal drugstore. I wish you good health, and good adventures.

Michael Castleman (signature)

Michael Castleman
Author of *Nature's Cures* and *Blended Medicine: The Best Choices in Healing*

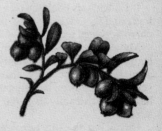

PART I

FINDING YOUR WAY AROUND THE HERBAL DRUGSTORE

WELCOME TO THE HERBAL DRUGSTORE

REMEMBER YOUR LAST TRIP to your local pharmacy for a nonprescription medicine? How long did you stare at the shelves, reading the tiny print on dozens of product labels, comparing doses and side effects, and wondering about price differences between drugs that seemed to contain the same ingredients?

Worse yet, have you ever have a bad experience with a prescription medicine? If you regularly take medications for high blood pressure, allergies, diabetes, or another chronic condition, you may have experienced side effects as your doctor adjusted the dosage or tried different pharmaceutical formulas to find just the right one for you.

The good news is that there are alternatives to such experiences. Alternatives that cost less, work just as well or better, and promote overall health with fewer side effects. You can find them in a place that we like to call the herbal drugstore.

WHAT IS THE HERBAL DRUGSTORE?

Isn't herbal drugstore an oxymoron, you might ask? Like jumbo shrimp? Not exactly. As you'll learn in the first chapters of this book, herbs and drugs have some similarities. But more important, they have differences that sometimes make herbs a better choice than the drugs people commonly take. We hope that this book will help you weigh those differences and assess the pros and cons of taking herbs for any health problems you may have.

Calling it an herbal drugstore isn't an exaggeration. Just as a conventional drugstore carries hundreds of over-the-counter and prescription drugs for almost any health problem you can think of, more and more herbal remedies are becoming available for an ever-expanding number of conditions. Just as a conventional drugstore sells products for skin care, hair care, and even pet care, manufacturers are developing herbal alternatives for such needs. And just as a conventional drugstore can be a bewildering place, competing herbal products can leave you confused as to what to buy. We created this book to be your guide to an ever-growing herbal marketplace.

NEW CHOICES FOR YOUR HEALTH

Why are so many people flocking to the herbal drugstore? Twenty years ago, most doctors would have said that patients who used herbs were poorly educated and were being bamboozled by charlatans posing as healers. But a study by Stanford University researchers revealed that consumers of alternative therapies tend to be highly educated. These consumers use herbs, vitamins and minerals, essential oils, and other techniques, first, because they work, and second, because they dovetail with people's values about health and life.

Herb sales have exploded in recent years, with consumers spending more than $3 billion annually on herbal remedies. And consumers are not the only ones increasingly interested in herbal medicine. Many of today's physicians and medical students are using herbs as well, with good results. Not long ago, only a handful of medical schools even broached the subject of alternative therapies. Today, at least 75 medical schools offer courses in various alternative healing techniques.

So these days, if you catch a cold virus; your family physician may advise you to take echinacea, zinc gluconate lozenges, and vitamin C—all of which have been proven to shorten the duration of a cold—rather than antibiotics, which don't kill cold viruses, or over-the-counter pharmaceuticals, which research shows can actually prolong cold symptoms. If your doctor does a thorough evaluation of your health and lifestyle, he may tell you stress is compromising your immune system, making you more susceptible to infection. But for a view of how taking a few simple, inexpensive herbs can help repair and strengthen that immune system, you'd need to turn to a qualified herbalist—or to this book.

MAKING INFORMED CHOICES

In the pages that follow, a top-notch team of medical doctors and herbal practitioners pool their knowledge to provide the information you need to compare and choose between conventional drugs and their herbal alternatives. For each of 98 conditions, these experts summarize the most common drug treatments, their functions (what they do), and their potential side effects. That's followed by profiles of the available herbal treatments as the experts review the scientific research, assess each herb's effectiveness, and describe typical dosage and potential side effects. They also explain when *not* to take a certain herb.

Besides drugs and their herbal alternatives, you'll find supplement recommendations, dietary strategies, and other lifestyle changes that may help treat or prevent certain conditions. There's discussion of other alternative therapies as well. To date, no other resource provides such a breadth of information in one comprehensive package.

Why did we—the writers and editors of *The Herbal Drugstore*—commit to such an undertaking? Because we want to help you make intelligent, informed decisions about what's best for your health. The fact is, despite the abundance of herbal products, there just aren't very many places that you can find accurate, impartial information about these herbs—places that will tell you the risks as well as the benefits. That's what *Herbs for Health* magazine has been doing for the past five years. It's the first magazine dedicated to reporting the most accurate research and recommendations from the field of herbal medicine.

Several of the magazine's top herbal experts have contributed to the creation of this book. In many cases, they've written books of their own about herbal medicines. You can count on these women and men to tell you the plain truth about using herbs to fight disease, promote longevity and vitality, and boost overall health. You can also count on them to tell you when you need to consult your doctor.

It's true that you can get lost in the maze of information about herbal remedies. But in *The Herbal Drugstore*, you have a reliable expert guide. We hope that it helps you reclaim your health if you're sick, and preserves your good health for a long time to come.

HOW TO USE THIS BOOK

If you have a particular health problem for which you'd like to try herbal remedies, you're probably eager to turn to part 3 of this book. But we recommend reading all of the introductory chapters first, especially if you are new to herbal medicine. These chapters explain key terms and principles and may help you decide the best way to take herbs. They also tell you how to read the labels of herbal products and how to choose the best product for you.

Once you've become informed about the basics of herbal medicine, you can look up information about your particular condition in three places. "The Remedies at a Glance," a chart beginning on page 48, gives a quick rundown of the drug and herb treatments most often recommended.

The chapters in part 3 provide more specific information about treatments for various conditions, including the potential side effects of each drug, as well as dosage information and safe-use guidelines for each herb. The herbs are listed in order of their importance to each condition, based on their effectiveness, safety, and how easy they are to obtain.

For example, if you develop nausea but also have gallbladder disease, you shouldn't take ginger, but may want to try some other antinausea herbs. Likewise, if you have diabetes, heartburn, or are already taking a certain drug, there are herbs that you should not take.

Part 4, Herb Profiles, offers a more in-depth look at selected popular herbs: where they originated, the conditions they're used to treat, which parts are used, and other important consumer information—for example, whether they are endangered in the wild. It also compiles all the appropriate cautions for each herb in one place. So if you're thinking about taking a certain herb for a condition that isn't covered in this book, you may want to look the herb up in this section before buying or taking it. Better yet, consult your doctor or other qualified health practitioner. The majority of serious reactions to herbs or herbal products stem from misinformation.

One final note: The rapid pace of research involving both drugs and herbs isn't likely to slow down at any time soon. If a drug that you're taking isn't mentioned in this book, that may be because it was developed after the book was produced. Likewise, new herbal remedies are being discovered every year. So if you can't find an answer in this book, your best bet is to ask your doctor or other qualified health practitioner.

CHAPTER 1

WHAT IS HERBAL MEDICINE?

HERBS WERE THE FIRST DRUGS that we humans had at our disposal.

Our ancestors learned over time which plants harmed them and which plants seemed to help them. They developed ways to preserve and extract the healing compounds from these plants. The world over, most cultures have some knowledge about local plants that can do them good.

In some cases, what ancient civilizations learned about treating illnesses with herbs has been proven correct by modern researchers. Echinacea, for example, has been shown to increase the activity of immune cells and help fend off infection by viruses and bacteria—attributes that help explain the herb's cold-fighting power. Italian cooks of centuries ago added fennel seeds to sausage recipes; it turns out that the seeds help digestion and dispel gas.

The first herbal drugstore, then, encompassed all of nature, with its amazing array of medicinal plants. By comparison, the modern drugstore seems far removed from its natural roots. You can take herbs as capsules or liquids or sprays that bear little resemblance to living plants. You can use products that contain combinations of herbs or compounds that have been chemically isolated from herbs and highly concentrated. And you can buy these products just about anywhere—in health food stores and conventional pharmacies as well as in supermarkets, from mail-order catalogs, and over the Internet.

DEFINING THE LANGUAGE

To choose wisely among the many remedies available to you, it's best to have a basic knowledge of what herbs are, how they work, and what they can do for you.

First of all, what's an herb? For the purpose of this book, an herb is any plant material that's used to alleviate unwanted symptoms or boost overall health. So in this context, garlic (a bulb), cayenne (a spice), and ginkgo extract (from the leaves of a tree) can all properly be called herbs. So can reishi, a mushroom, even though you're most likely to take it in the form of a liquid or tablet. One of the few herbs that you might still take in its fresh, green form is feverfew, used to relieve headaches.

Herbal medicine, then, is the use of plants, plant extracts, or plant preparations to improve health. It is one of a number of healing techniques that fall into the category of alternative medicine. (For information about other healing disciplines, see "'Alternative' Medicine: What Is It Really?")

There are two fundamental principles that herbal medicine shares with other alternative therapies. One is the concept of working with the body instead of against a disease, as mainstream medicine does. Rather than killing germs, alternative therapies seek to enhance the body's innate ability to fight disease and return itself to health. That's why practitioners of many alternative therapies, including herbal medicine, put an emphasis on diet, exercise, deep relaxation, and massage.

The other principle common to many alternative therapies is the use of medicinal plants instead of pharmaceutical drugs. Medicinal plants are the basis of not only herbal medicine but also aromatherapy and flower therapies. Herbs play central roles in homeopathy, Traditional Chinese Medicine, Ayurvedic medicine, and naturopathy. In addition, medicinal plants are connected to nutritional therapies because some herbs, such as onions and apples, are foods.

This book focuses mainly on herbal medicine, a discipline that offers remedies for most health problems. For some conditions, it will also touch on vitamins and supplements, dietary changes, and other ways you can support your own health.

HOW HERBS AND DRUGS ARE ALIKE

While medicinal plants and pharmaceutical drugs are often viewed as opposites, they actually have a good deal in common.

One little-known similarity is that an estimated 25 percent of all pharmaceuticals are still derived directly from plants. The world's first "wonder drug," the malaria treatment quinine, was extracted

"ALTERNATIVE" MEDICINE: WHAT IS IT REALLY?

Alternative medicine, natural medicine, holistic medicine, and complementary medicine are all loose umbrella terms for an enormous number of healing arts, including the following:

◆ Nutritional therapies, notably low-fat eating, vegetarianism, and elimination diets

◆ Supplementation, the therapeutic use of vitamins, minerals, and compounds such as coenzyme Q_{10}, sometimes in large doses

◆ Relaxation therapies, among them: meditation, biofeedback, hypnotherapy, and visualization therapy

◆ Exercise, notably walking and the meditative disciplines: yoga, tai chi, and qi gong

◆ Manipulative therapies, including massage, chiropractic, osteopathy, and the many schools of bodywork

◆ Herbal medicine, the therapeutic use of medicinal plants as substitutes for or in combination with pharmaceutical drugs

◆ Aromatherapy, the therapeutic use of the essential oils found in medicinal plants, notably to enhance relaxation

◆ Flower therapies, the use of essences that deliver minute to infinitesimal amounts of therapeutic substances, or even vaguely described "energies," from medicinal plants

◆ Homeopathy, a healing system whose medicines are microdoses of medicinal plants and other substances

◆ Traditional Chinese Medicine, which combines herbal medicine, nutritional approaches, and acupuncture

◆ Ayurvedic medicine, the ancient Indian discipline that combines herbal medicine, nutritional approaches, massage, and exercise, specifically yoga

◆ Naturopathy, which focused on nutrition a century ago, but today encompasses all of the above therapies

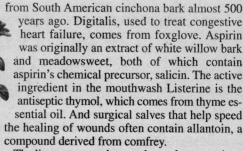

Thyme

from South American cinchona bark almost 500 years ago. Digitalis, used to treat congestive heart failure, comes from foxglove. Aspirin was originally an extract of white willow bark and meadowsweet, both of which contain aspirin's chemical precursor, salicin. The active ingredient in the mouthwash Listerine is the antiseptic thymol, which comes from thyme essential oil. And surgical salves that help speed the healing of wounds often contain allantoin, a compound derived from comfrey.

The list goes on and on, and new drugs continue to be derived from plant sources. One of the biggest breakthroughs in recent years is the discovery of taxol, a compound derived from the yew tree and used in the treatment of breast and ovarian cancer.

Another similarity is that both medicinal plants and synthetic drugs contain compounds that alter body processes. That's the whole point of using them to treat illness—to change things from bad to better. When you have an infection, you might take a pharmaceutical antibiotic or the natural antibiotics contained in garlic or goldenseal. In either case, compounds from the drug or the herb enter the bloodstream and help the immune system eliminate the micro-organism that's causing the problem.

What's more, scientists study herbs and drugs in much the same way, using what they call randomized, placebo-controlled, double-blind trials. "Randomized" means that the subjects are not specially preselected, which might bias the results. Instead, they may be all the residents of a certain nursing home, or the next 250 patients to visit a particular clinic.

"Placebo-controlled" means that some of the participants take the active herb or drug, while others receive an inactive substance, or placebo. Because of the ability of the mind to stimulate the immune system, placebos typically provide significant relief for around one-third of those who take them. To be judged effective, the drug or herb being tested must significantly outperform the placebo.

Finally, "double-blind" means that neither the participants nor the researchers know in advance who took the test compound and who got the placebo. This prevents the researchers from treating subjects differently, which might bias the results.

Researchers at Albert Einstein College of Medicine in New York

City used a randomized, placebo-controlled, double-blind study to test an extract of ginkgo as a treatment for Alzheimer's disease. They recruited 309 people newly diagnosed with Alzheimer's and gave them either ginkgo extract or a placebo for a year. Compared with the placebo, the ginkgo significantly slowed the participants' mental deterioration. Several previous studies had hinted that ginkgo might be an effective Alzheimer's treatment. But because this study was large and scientifically rigorous (that is, randomized, placebo-controlled, and double-blind), it got published in the *Journal of the American Medical Association*, made headlines, and established ginkgo as a viable treatment for Alzheimer's.

How Herbs and Drugs Differ

As you can see, medicinal herbs and pharmaceutical drugs have quite a bit in common. But they also have several key differences.

Dose for dose, most herbs are less potent than drugs. While this may sound like a disadvantage, it actually makes herbs safer to take.

To make conventional pharmaceuticals, manufacturers extract unique chemical constituents from plants or create synthetic versions in the laboratory, then pack the substances into pills or capsules that can hold large quantities. With most herb products, however, the plant material itself limits how much of the medicinal compounds you get.

Sometimes, you want drug-level potency—even at the risk of experiencing side effects. If you're in severe pain from rheumatoid arthritis, then you may opt to take strong anti-inflammatory drugs, even if they cause abdominal distress. But if you have a run-of-the-mill tension headache, you probably don't need such strong medication. You probably don't even need two aspirin. A cup of chamomile tea might be enough to soothe your nerves—with a substantially lower risk of side effects. (Some products concentrate herbal ingredients for greater potency. However, such products usually come at a premium price.)

Reduced risk of side effects is a big reason why medicinal herbs have become so popular. Just check out the potential side effects of any over-the-counter cold remedy—or, if you really want to read a lot of small print, the side effects of any blood-pressure medication. They may make you feel worse than the condition itself! For this book, we list only common side effects of the most commonly prescribed drugs.

HOW HERBS ARE REGULATED

Herbs are classified by the United States government not as drugs but as dietary supplements. This broad category also includes vitamins, minerals, enzymes, and other nutritional products.

What this means for you is that you don't have to wait years for costly research to be done on the herbs you want to take. But it also means that the manufacturers of herbal products are limited in the claims they can make on the labels—even when those claims have research to support them.

Specifically, manufacturers are permitted to make what's called structure and function claims—in other words, they can say only that a product affects the structure and function of a body part or system. So a product label for a standardized ginkgo extract can say, "increases microcirculation to the brain." But it cannot say "cures early-stage Alzheimer's" or "alleviates tinnitus"—even though there is research to support the ability of ginkgo extracts to do just that.

When any manufacturer puts a product on the market that bears a structure and/or function claim, the company must also create a file of research evidence that supports that claim. Then the Food and Drug Administration (FDA) has 30 days in which to investigate and challenge this evidence. Whether or not the agency chooses to do so, the file must remain available for inspection indefinitely at the

By comparison, many medicinal herbs have no known side effects for people who are otherwise healthy and are not taking other prescription or over-the-counter drugs. Many are safe for everyone except pregnant or nursing mothers and infants. Some are even safe enough for babies.

But just like any medicine, herbal remedies must be used with care. One of the worst mistakes people can make is to assume that because medicinal plants are natural, they're completely harmless. Cascara sagrada, for example, is a potent laxative that can help manufacturer's place of business. If credible research exists, the FDA may not prohibit the manufacturer from making reasonable claims—as long as they are stated in terms of structure and function rather than curing disease.

The herb and supplements industry has its own organizations that informally regulate against harmful products or outright fraud. For example, the American Herbal Products Association—a group of herbalists, researchers, and manufacturers—has created a Code of Ethics that members are expected to abide by. It also releases product safety alerts regarding adulteration—that is, contamination with an unlabeled substance—of herbal products and it publishes an important reference work, the *Botanical Safety Handbook.*

There's also the Natural Nutritional Foods Association (NNFA), a group of manufacturers and retailers devoted to product quality and truth in packaging and advertising. Among its many activities, the NNFA supports a True Label Program intended to ensure that the products put out by its members actually contain what their labels claim.

Other countries take different approaches in regulating herbs. In Germany, herbal remedies are overseen by a specific body, known as the Commission E. This government panel evaluates the available research on an herb's effectiveness for an ailment, its tradition of use, and its safety. Panel members then approve the sale of some herbs and combination products for specific conditions. German doctors can prescribe herbs or herbal products just as they would drugs.

relieve constipation. But in large doses, it causes abdominal distress, intestinal cramping, and diarrhea. Licorice root is a scientifically proven treatment for ulcers. But if you take unusually large amounts or take it for extended periods, you may experience water retention that raises your blood pressure to possibly hazardous levels. That's why there's a form of licorice that has certain compounds removed, developed especially for people with ulcers who need to take licorice for a period of months.

The point is this: Just like drugs, herbs and herbal products have the potential to do good when used responsibly. But they may cause harm when used carelessly.

In addition to being less potent than drugs, herbs are usually cheaper. As an example, consider the "statin" drugs now widely prescribed to reduce cholesterol. Garlic also reduces cholesterol—not as dramatically, but a lot more economically. If your cholesterol is sky high, a statin-type drug might be the most medically advisable treatment. But if your cholesterol is only mildly elevated—as is the case for millions of Americans—garlic from the grocery store may well be all you need.

A big reason why drugs are so much more expensive than herbs is that drugs must be approved by the Food and Drug Administration (FDA) before they're made available to the public. Pharma-

ESSENTIAL HERB SAFETY TIPS

While herbal medicines generally have far fewer and far milder side effects than pharmaceuticals, they may still cause problems if used improperly. Here's how to take herbs safely.

◆ Become well-informed. Read up on herbs before you use them. This book is a good place to start. Don't follow a friend's advice about dosage (unless that friend is a practitioner with years of clinical experience). Get your information from a reliable source that includes safety warnings.

◆ Start with a low dose. Herb dosages are typically presented as ranges; for example, 1 to 2 teaspoons of herb per cup of just-boiled water, steeped for 10 to 20 minutes and taken two or three times a day. Begin at the low end of the recommended range—with 1 teaspoon steeped 10 minutes twice a day. If a low dose does not provide sufficient relief, gradually move toward the top of the recommended range. If you still do not experience noticeable benefit, consult an herbalist, a naturopath, or your physician.

ceutical companies spend millions of dollars to prove that their drugs are safe when taken as directed (though sometimes hazardous side effects are discovered only after FDA approval, as was the case with the diet drug Fen-phen). They also have to prove that their drugs actually work for each disorder they're prescribed for.

Herbs do not face such costly regulatory hurdles, so manufacturers can get their products to market quicker and more cheaply and pass their savings along to consumers. Some experts are concerned that this lack of regulation puts the public at risk for wasting money on worthless products—or worse, experiencing serious side effects. That's why it's so important to find out which herbs are effective and safe—perhaps by referring to a book like this one—before starting an herbal regimen.

- ◆ If you buy commercial preparations (teas, tinctures, pills, capsules, combination products, and so on), follow the label directions. These preparations may vary in strength; some are concentrated. So if the label and this book disagree, go by the manufacturer's dosage recommendations.

- ◆ If you experience any unusual symptoms within eight hours of taking an herbal medicine, discontinue use. Everyone reacts to herbs differently. If you're unusually sensitive, you may experience side effects and allergic reactions even at low doses.

- ◆ Do not give herbal medicines to children younger than age 2 without the approval of the child's doctor.

- ◆ If you are over age 65, stick with dosages at the low end of the recommended ranges. Sensitivity to drugs and the medicinal compounds in herbs increases with age. So does the risk of side effects.

- ◆ If you are pregnant or nursing, or if you have a chronic illness and/or are taking any medication, do not take medicinal herbs without consulting your physician.

- ◆ If you consult an herbal practitioner, follow that person's instructions, and promptly report any unusual symptoms to them or to your doctor.

Finally, some herbs are what herbalists call tonics. Rather than treating specific conditions, as drugs are designed to do, tonics exert a gentle health-promoting effect on the whole body over time. The best example is ginseng. Many studies show that ginsenosides, the medicinal compounds in ginseng, help defend the body against the harmful effects of stress, enhance mental sharpness, and improve physical stamina. Siberian ginseng and astragalus are two other tonic herbs. No known drugs have similar tonic effects.

HOW TO USE HERBS SAFELY

When discussing medicinal herbs, the news media often quote skeptical doctors who warn ominously that if you fool around with herbs, you're playing with fire. With herbs, they say, it's impossible to guarantee good dose control. Dose control means knowing exactly how much of the active ingredient—the chemical that exerts the healing effect—you're getting per dose.

To a certain extent, those skeptics are right. Drugs offer a precise amount of chemical, usually measured in milligrams. With herbs, potency can vary with the health of the individual plant, how much time the product spent in storage, and other factors. But warnings about dose control obscure a larger truth. When used as recommended by reputable herbalists, medicinal herbs are almost always less potent than their pharmaceutical counterparts. So with most herbal remedies, the risk of overdose is tiny. In fact, it's virtually nonexistent, according to the latest research.

The Washington, D.C.–based American Association of Poison Control Centers compiles annual statistics on accidental poisonings around the country, including statistics on accidental poisonings from pharmaceutical side effects and plants. In 1996, the most recent year for which complete statistics were available, there were more than 600 deaths associated with various classes of pharmaceuticals, including pain relievers, antidepressants, cardiovascular medications, sedatives, and anticonvulsants. Guess how many deaths were reported to poison control centers as being caused by herbal medicines? None.

Granted, many more Americans use pharmaceuticals than herbs, so you'd expect more problems with drugs. But these figures clearly show that most herbs are not a public health hazard.

That's not to say you can buy anything that claims to be natural or herbal, use it in any way, and expect absolute safety and effectiveness. Extremely high doses of ephedra, a stimulant herb, have caused deaths. Some essential oils are very dangerous when taken internally, even in small amounts. That's why their labels will warn you not to ingest them. Some herbs have interactions with drugs or other herbs that can range from uncomfortable to life-threatening. Some even interact with food substances as common as caffeine.

As with any product, the most important thing to do before using an herb is to read the label carefully and completely. Don't take an herbal product simply because a friend says that it works—unless that friend is a medical doctor or an experienced clinical herbalist. Take the right amount of the right herb at the right time for the correct number of days. And if you do have an ongoing health problem or are taking a prescription drug, it's essential to consult your doctor before launching an herbal regimen.

CHAPTER 2

UNDERSTANDING HERBAL REMEDIES

THERE'S A LOT OF confusion on the subject of herbal medicine. While it's wonderful to have so many herbal products available in pharmacies and health food stores, it's frustrating not to have easy access to information that will help you make the right choices. Which herb is best, say, for a sinus infection? Should you buy a capsule or a liquid? Do standardized extracts offer more for your money? Can you take an herb if you're also taking antibiotics? Can you take an herb if you're on blood pressure medication?

That's a lot of questions. But before you answer any of them, you need to know for certain what condition or symptom you're trying to treat.

WHAT'S WRONG—AND WHY IT MATTERS

Sometimes you *can* diagnose your own symptoms. For example, you can certainly tell when your stomach is upset—and often you'll also know why. It's fine, in such instances, to treat yourself with peppermint or chamomile or fennel tea.

But if such digestive upsets occur frequently, they could well be caused by something other than food that disagrees with you. They could be a sign of a serious condition. In such cases, some herbs can be exactly the wrong things to take. After all, peppermint is one of the safest, most widely used herbs, but people with heartburn or esophageal reflux disease should avoid it because it relaxes the valve between the stomach and esophagus, actually worsening symptoms.

If your symptoms are serious, recur, or persist, see your doctor or health care practitioner. If you don't know what's causing a minor symptom, it can't hurt to consult your doctor for an accurate diagnosis. If you have already been diagnosed and are under a doctor's care, or if you're taking over-the-counter or prescription drugs for any chronic health problem, you must consult your doctor before adding any herbs to your treatment regimen. Some herbs interact with drugs in dangerous ways. *Do not discontinue routine medication and substitute herbs without your doctor's consent and supervision.*

In many ways, herbal treatment is still self-treatment because many people don't have access to an herbal expert. But doctors, whether or not they know natural remedies, do know disease; it's what they see day in and day out. Enlist their help in determining what you have, then go about researching the best way to heal it. Many medical doctors are becoming better informed about the effectiveness and safety of medicinal herbs, nutritional supplements, dietary changes, and other natural therapies.

TYPES OF HERBS

Herbalists have developed a set of categories to describe what herbs do. While you won't see these terms very often in this book, they tend to crop up in health publications, advertisements, and manufacturers' literature as well as on herb product labels. These categories are sometimes called action-types.

Many herbs fit into more than one category because they have more than one specific effect on the body. For example, ginkgo enhances circulation in the microscopic blood vessels of the body, including those in the eyes and the brain. But it's also a potent antioxidant, meaning that it cleans up free radicals, a type of cellular waste product that attacks body tissues.

It's helpful to understand a few of these action-type categories in choosing an herbal remedy.

Specifics and Tonics

These two broad terms refer to whether an herb targets a particular symptom or enhances the health and efficient operation of a whole organ or body system. Valerian, for example, is a specific for insomnia. Chemical compounds in the herb are sedating and promote sleep. Astragalus, on the other hand, is a tonic. When repeated illness or stress weakens the immune system, astragalus slowly rebuilds immune strength.

Specifics are taken for brief periods or only when symptoms are present. Tonics, on the other hand, are taken long-term, sometimes with short breaks. Some herbs have several uses; they may function as a specific for one symptom and have a tonic use as well.

The "Anti's"

The prefix "anti" means against. Herbs that fall into this category are used to combat whatever follows the prefix. So antiviral herbs fight viruses, antifungals fight funguses, and so on. A few of the "anti" action-types bear further explanation.

Antispasmodics relieve spasms or cramps in muscles, whether it's the skeletal muscles that hurt when they're cramped or the smooth muscles that encircle the airways and intestines. Some antispasmodic herbs that act on smooth muscles can help ease coughs or diarrhea.

Antioxidants inhibit oxidation. These herbs contain certain compounds that help prevent a particular set of chemical reactions implicated in diseases such as arthritis and macular degeneration. These chemical reactions are called oxidation reactions. They're set off by free radicals, unstable molecules that grab electrons from stable ones. Free radicals are neutralized by antioxidants, which can give up their electrons without becoming unstable themselves.

Anti-inflammatories counteract or suppress the body's production of chemicals that inflame tissues, such as histamine. In an inflammatory response, whether it's caused by a bee sting or hay fever, small blood vessels dilate and leak fluid into the surrounding tissue. What you experience is swelling—of a stung foot or your airways.

Other Action-Types

Adaptogens are a particular type of tonic. They enhance the body's ability to deal with stress, strengthening the disease-fighting immune system and the hormone-producing endocrine system, which includes the adrenal glands. The adrenal glands are important because they're responsible for releasing hormones in response to stressful situations. When you experience a lot of stress, these glands can become overworked. Adaptogens help repair the adrenal and other glands of the endocrine system and help them work together with the immune system.

Bitters are bitter-tasting herbs such as dandelion and gentian that stimulate the stomach's production of digestive fluids. These digestive fluids help your body absorb nutrients from the food you eat. Bitters are often a component of a nutritional healing plan.

Carminatives help dispel gas from the intestines, relieving the cramps that often accompany such gas.

Demulcents soothe inflamed mucous membranes or digestive tissues. These herbs contain mucilage, sticky or slippery substances that coat body tissues and help protect them from irritation.

Expectorants help the body expel mucus from the respiratory tract. They do this either by stimulating bronchial secretions that thin the mucus, or by making the mucus itself less sticky.

CHOOSING AN HERB FORM

Unless you have a trained herbalist whom you trust and depend on for advice or your doctor is knowledgeable about herbal medicine, you'll have to educate yourself about which herbs to take, how much, and how often. Part 3 of this book discusses which herbs may be appropriate for specific conditions. Here we'll discuss the various forms in which herbs are available, how to choose among them, and how to read an herb or dietary supplement label.

Not only are hundreds of different herbs available in the marketplace, they come in many different forms. Understanding the different preparations and how they're made will help you decide which one is best for you.

Capsules

Eighty percent of all herbal supplements are sold in capsule form. They're not necessarily better than other forms. They are, however, convenient, palatable, and portable. Some are made from gelatin, while others are made from vegetable sources.

But capsules do have some disadvantages. They contain dried, ground herbs, and when herbs are that finely chopped, they can lose their potency more quickly. If you're taking whole herb capsules, not a concentrated extract, you may have to take quite a few capsules to get enough of the herb.

If you choose capsules, it's important to buy them from a reputable manufacturer, for the bottle to be safety sealed, and for the label to contain a future expiration date.

Fresh vs. Dry

If you garden or harvest wild herbs (which you shouldn't do unless you're certain of your ability to identify a particular species), then you have ready access to fresh herbs. Some herbs just taste better fresh; others are more effective that way, whether the herb is cut from your garden, grown in commercial farm fields, or plucked from a wild hillside (a practice known as wildcrafting).

Fresh herbs are wonderful to add to foods, make into teas, or mash up and apply topically to a minor skin irritation such as an insect bite (plantain) or a minor sunburn (aloe vera). But for most people, dried herbs are more convenient to use, and if they haven't outlived their shelf life, they're effective. You can check the freshness of some dried herbs by their scent. If they have a smell when fresh, they should still retain some of that smell when dried.

Teas, Infusions, and Decoctions

Teas are the most familiar, most traditional herbal preparation. To make them, you buy dried plant material—leaves, flowers, bark, roots, seeds, or berries. Then you add hot water, which extracts some of the plant material's active components.

Some herbs lend themselves very well to this process. Peppermint, chamomile, and sage are examples of herbs whose aerial, or above-ground, parts readily release their volatile oils in near-boiling water. Herbalists call this process infusing and the product it yields an infusion.

Barks, roots, seeds, and berries tend to require a little more heat and time to release their medicinal compounds. They usually need to be simmered on low heat for anywhere from 10 to 30 minutes. Herbalists call this process decocting and the product it yields a decoction.

What do you do if your tea contains both types of plant parts? You can simmer the tough parts, strain the liquid, reheat it to boiling, remove it from the heat and then steep the more fragile herbs in the hot liquid. If you're using finely chopped roots, bark, or berries, you may be able to get away with just steeping the tea for a longer time—say, 10 to 20 minutes. Follow the tea recipes in part 3 (or the manufacturer's instructions on the tea you've purchased).

Of course, one of the most familiar ways to buy tea is in tea bags. These prefilled and premeasured bags make tea a simple and portable remedy. Generally speaking, however, the dried herbs in

MEDICINAL TEA TECHNIQUES

Medicinal teas are simple to prepare. What's more, they can be used in several ways. Teas can be drunk from a cup, poured into a bath, or used as a compress for rashes, minor burns, and mild sprains.

Medicinal teas are made by either steeping or simmering. To steep an herb, you soak it in water that has been brought just to a rolling boil, then removed from the heat. Use a timer; the few minutes necessary for soaking a regular tea bag are not quite enough time for medicinal teas.

To simmer an herb, on the other hand, you need to leave it over the heat, but with the mixture of herbs and water gently but barely boiling.

tea bags have been chopped finer, which means the herbs lose their freshness more quickly. So if you're buying tea bags, make sure the manufacturer has a reputation for freshness, store them away from heat and light, and pitch unused bags after a year has passed.

Tinctures and Glycerites

Sometimes herbs (either fresh or dried) are soaked in a liquid other than water to release the medicinal compounds. For tinctures, that liquid is alcohol; glycerites use glycerin.

With some herbs, the chemicals that do the healing work don't extract well into certain liquids. Alcohol is able to extract more chemical components from more plants than glycerin, so we recommend using tinctures if you're able to consume alcohol.

Standardized Extracts

The concentration of medicinal compounds in herbs varies a great deal from one kind of plant to another. For instance, a teaspoon of dried peppermint leaves is powerful enough to make a tea that's very effective in calming an upset stomach. But a tea made from a teaspoon of ginkgo leaves would have no value at all in restoring your memory. It takes many, many pounds of ginkgo leaves to make a single effective dose, and the doses must be repeated regularly over time.

HERBS COMMONLY SOLD AS STANDARDIZED EXTRACTS

The chart below lists several widely used herbs and the compounds to which they're usually standardized. As research on herbs continues, you may see products standardized to different compounds.

Bilberry	25% anthocyanocides
Garlic	5.4 milligrams of allicin per dose
Ginkgo biloba	24% ginkgo flavone glycosides
Grapeseed	95% proanthocyanidins
Hawthorn	19% oligomeric procyanidins
Kava-kava	29% kavalactones
Licorice	2% glycyrrhizin
Milk thistle	70% silymarin
Saw palmetto	95% free fatty acids
St.-John's-wort	0.3–0.5% hypericin

So how do you know if the ginkgo product you're thinking about buying is concentrated enough to do any good? By checking to see whether it's standardized. For ginkgo, standardization means that a product contains approximately 24 percent flavone glycosides, a compound found in the herb. (In some standardized herbal products, the compound that's measured is not one of the herb's "active ingredients." But for various reasons—ease of measuring or uniqueness to that particular herb—the compound has been designated a marker of a product's potency.)

Most herbs that are standardized don't require the extreme concentration that ginkgo does, and, in fact, may be standardized for other reasons. Perhaps a single compound has been isolated for research, and the manufacturer wants to be sure the amount that was found to be effective on actual patients is found in the product.

Does this mean that standardized products are superior to others that are not standardized? Not necessarily. But standardization does

give some assurance of potency and benefit.
Standardized products are available as capsules, tablets, and liquids.

Those who advocate whole-herb
preparations argue that there are many,
many compounds in any given herb, and
that these compounds act synergistically
to provide the maximum benefit to the
user. Those who favor standardized preparations contend that without a rigorous
process of concentrating and measuring
one or more compounds in the product, you
don't really know what you're getting. Both sides
are correct.

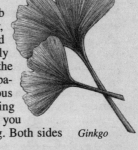

Ginkgo

For example, most St.-John's-wort products are standardized to
contain a certain amount of hypericin, one of the compounds that
researchers believe is responsible for the plant's ability to ease mild
and moderate depression. At the time of this writing, however, new
research suggests that another of the herb's compounds, hyperforin,
might have therapeutic effects. It's possible that right now, new
studies of St.-John's-wort are identifying other compounds with
health benefits.

"Herbs Commonly Sold as Standardized Extracts" lists other
often-used herbs that are usually standardized, the component that
is identified for standardization, and the amount of that component
you'll find in most products.

Infused and Essential Oils

These two similar-sounding forms of herbs are actually very different. Infused oils are oils in which herbs have been steeped, usually for several weeks, over low heat or at room temperature. They
are most often used topically for skin irritations (calendula oil) and
muscle aches (arnica oil and/or St.-John's-wort oil). They're also
easy to make yourself.

Essential oils, on the other hand, are chemical concentrations of
a plant's volatile, or easily evaporated, oils. Most often produced by
distillation, essential oils are very, very strong and in most cases
should not be used on the skin in their undiluted form. The great
majority of them should not be taken internally. Some are even
toxic.

The use of essential oils in healing is known as aromatherapy—

SINGLE HERB, OR FORMULA?

A century ago, preparations of single herbs were called simples, and the skill of making them, simpling. These days, you can still get simples. But you can also choose from a host of products that combine several herbs to treat specific conditions such as colds or premenstrual syndrome. (You'll see these products referred to as formulas or as combination products.) There's a place for both simples and herbal formulas.

If you're sure of what's causing your illness, it's relatively minor, and you have no allergies or sensitivities to herbs, you may wish to purchase a formula product. Read its label carefully, however, and check the quantities of the herbs to make sure you're getting enough of the ones that you need the most.

Formula products have their drawbacks. They may or may not contain an adequate amount of the most important, or most well-researched, herb for your condition. They may also contain herbs that you don't want to take or that are not well-researched.

What's more, it's often hard to tell the difference between the various formulas. The only solid advice is to buy a brand you know you can trust, and make sure to check the product's expiration date. If it doesn't have one, don't buy it.

On the other hand, formula products can be a very convenient way to take herbs. Just as whole herbs offer you chemical compounds that work together, not in isolation, formula products may offer benefits that come from combinations of herbs. They can also be a lot cheaper than buying several different bottles of capsules!

Single herbs, however, offer you greater control. You decide how much of each herb you're going to take; if you do wind up with a reaction or sensitivity to one of them, you simply discontinue using it. If you buy from a reputable manufacturer, you're sure of what's in those capsules or that bottle of liquid extract.

whether or not they smell good! Some of the best-known essential oils are tea tree oil, which doesn't smell pretty but is a potent anti-fungal, and lavender oil, which smells wonderful and also heals burns.

Other Forms of Herbs

Sprays. A relatively new form of herbal supplement, a spray is a liquid that is taken under the tongue. The active ingredients enter the bloodstream quickly, bypassing the gastrointestinal tract where they might be damaged by stomach acids. Sprays are useful for people who have difficulty swallowing tablets or capsules.

Tablets. A carefully controlled quantity of finely milled herbal material is compressed into the chosen shape and given a thin coating. One type of coating, called an enteric coating, is formulated in such a way that it doesn't dissolve until the tablet reaches the small intestine, where the active ingredient can be absorbed without being affected by stomach acids. Some tablets are made to dissolve under the tongue, where absorption of the active ingredient into the bloodstream is rapid.

BUYING AND USING HERBAL PRODUCTS

EVEN THOUGH THERE ARE more and more herbal products for sale, and more and more people buying them, choosing and using herbs isn't easy for the typical shopper. Federal laws won't allow manufacturers to provide straightforward benefit statements on their product labels.

Why is this so? For an answer, you have to go back several years to about 1993. That's when the U.S. Food and Drug Administration (FDA) presented Congress with an initiative to control and limit consumer access to dietary supplements such as herbs, vitamins, and minerals.

There was a huge public outcry against such limitations. During the months that the FDA proposal was being considered, congressional representatives received more mail from concerned constituents than they had received on any issue in history except for the Vietnam War. It was one of the strongest grassroots campaigns this country had ever witnessed.

The resulting law—the Dietary Supplement Health and Education Act (DSHEA) of 1994—bowed to the will of the people. It permits the unrestricted sale of herbs, vitamins, minerals, and other substances such as hormones and amino acids—as long as their manufacturers make no medical claims for them. In other words, a manufacturer may sell a product such as echinacea, which is useful against colds and flu, as long as the package doesn't say it will cure colds and flu.

So what can a manufacturer say about the usefulness of a product? It can describe how the product affects a body's structure—its various parts such as nerves, blood vessels, organs, and organ systems—and the function of those structures. For example, a product label for hawthorn can say, "Promotes heart health." It cannot say, "Cures angina pectoris." A product label for echinacea

COMMON HERB/DRUG INTERACTIONS

This list isn't exhaustive, but it provides some examples of how certain herbs can alter the activity of certain drugs.

Herb	Effect
Bromelain	Increases risk of bleeding when taken with blood thinners
Echinacea	May counteract immune-suppressive drugs
Ephedra	May worsen the side effects of other stimulants (including caffeine)
Garlic	May increase the effects of blood thinners
Ginkgo	May increase the effects of blood thinners
Ginseng	May worsen the side effects of stimulants
Hawthorn	May increase the action of some heart medicines and decrease their side effects
High-tannin herbs such as black or green tea, white oak bark, bearberry, witch hazel, black walnut husk, and raspberry leaves	Reduce the absorption of most drugs
High-berberine herbs such as goldenseal, Oregon graperoot, and barberry	Counteract short-acting blood thinners
High-fiber herbs such as fennel seed, psyllium husk, marshmallow root, Icelandic moss, apple pectin, flaxseed, aloe gel, and slippery elm	May delay the absorption of most drugs taken at the same time
Licorice	May worsen the effects of drugs that cause potassium loss
Siberian ginseng	Increases the effects of antibiotics
St.-John's-wort	May increase the effects of narcotics and some antidepressants
Valerian	Increases the effects of sedatives

can say, "Supports the health of the immune system during cold and flu season." It cannot say, "Cures the common cold."

CHOOSING AMONG SEVERAL BRANDS

If three or four different brands or varieties of an herb are available, how do you choose which to buy?

Here are some issues to consider when making your decision.

◆ Whole plant or standardized extract? Let's say that you want a whole-plant product because it contains multiple compounds that may work together therapeutically or because standardization doesn't seem to offer many benefits for that particular herb. Then look for a product made from the correct part of the plant. For example, if you want to use echinacea, go for products made from echinacea root rather than the above-ground parts, because most herbalists believe the root has higher concentrations of the useful compounds. The root is also less likely to be adulterated with other plants that look the same when dried. Products made from echinacea root tend to be more expensive, though, because the plant has to be destroyed to get it. (If you see labels that list an ingredient as "echinacea herb" or "horsetail herb," that means the product contains the above-ground or aerial parts of the plant.)

◆ Organically grown or custom wildcrafted? People who are concerned about pesticides, whether because of their own health or the impact on the environment, tend to choose organically grown products. In addition, some herbs are endangered in the wild, so you may want to avoid the wildcrafted versions. (To find out which herbs fall into this category, see part 4, the Herb Profiles.) In either case, plant matter grown on the same continent where it will be processed (for example, the United States or Canada) is likely to be fresher.

◆ How much active ingredient? When you're comparing products, compare the amounts of active ingredients in each one. Ask yourself how many capsules you'll have to take per day, and how many times. This allows you to compare cost per day among products.

◆ Is the package safely sealed? This is one of the few reliable ways to address concerns about product tampering.

◆ Is there an expiration date on the product, and is it in the future? If there's no expiration date, you're taking your chances on whether the product is still effective.
◆ Is there a batch number on the product in case you want to ask the manufacturer about it? Does the manufacturer provide an address, telephone number, or Web site address so you can get more information?

How Much to Take

When trying a new herbal remedy, start out with the lowest recommended dose—from this book, a doctor or trained herbal practitioner, or the product label—and monitor your response carefully. If you have any unpleasant side effects such as rashes, dizziness, nausea, or headaches, stop taking the herb immediately.

Dosage advice includes how long you should take an herb. As with drugs, there are some herbs that may do harm if taken for more than a specific number of weeks. Others take several months to produce benefits; still others can be taken long-term with no ill effects.

Some people have allergic reactions to certain plant foods or airborne plant substances. Since herbs are both plants and food, and since herbal supplements may be very concentrated, it's not unheard of for allergic reactions to occur. There are some commonsense predictors. If you're allergic to ragweed, for example, you will want to be cautious about using chamomile, which is in the same plant family as ragweed.

It is also known that some herbs can interact in negative ways with certain foods, pharmaceutical drugs, caffeine, or alcohol. If you're using any of these substances, be careful about taking an herb that could cause a critical interaction. Always check for cautions on the labels of herbal products you buy. Even if you're using fresh herbs, do your homework.

Herbal supplement manufacturers tend to be very careful and conservative in making dosage recommendations. It's wise to follow label instructions, especially at first, unless they are contradicted by your health practitioner or another information source that you trust. One thing product labels won't tell you, though, is that most herbal supplements are formulated for the needs of a 150-pound man. If you're much heavier or lighter than that, consider adjusting your dose accordingly. For example, divide your weight by 150; multiply the result by the dosage on the product label. If you weigh only 100 pounds, you'd take two-thirds the recommended dose.

Quality Counts

Make sure that you're buying your herbs from a reputable manufacturer or another herbal provider whom you can trust. Be wary of products that are unusually inexpensive or promoted by companies that make excessive claims. It's also good to buy herbs from a store or mail-order company that stands behind its products. Most retailers do a good job of researching the manufacturers whose products they sell.

Most herb and supplement manufacturers are very concerned about quality, but more and more mass merchandisers are jumping into the sale of herbal products. There are good and bad buys available everywhere. Use the information in this book to read labels knowledgeably and become a good herbal shopper.

Customizing Your Own Herbal Regimen

As a society, the United States is beginning to focus more on wellness than illness. This shift is partly a result of the changing healthcare industry and the emergence of managed-care organizations. But more important, it's because people want to live well as they age. More of us are focusing on diet, exercise, and general fitness. Using herbs to build and sustain good health is as logical as it is smart.

To feel well, to age gracefully, to correct minor health problems—these are some of the best reasons to use herbs in your day-to-day life. You can learn enough about herbs on your own to make a real difference in your level of health. Just remember that for serious or chronic health problems, you need to be under the care of a qualified medical professional.

But if you're generally healthy now, you can use herbs in a conservative, responsible way to fight disease and improve your physical and emotional well-being. There are health problems that can be avoided—or treated, if they already exist—with herbal remedies.

COMMON HERBS IN HERBAL REGIMENS

These two charts list a few of the herbs you might find in an herbal regimen, both to support overall health and to prevent specific illnesses.

HERBS FOR GENERAL WELLNESS

American ginseng	General tonic, adaptogen
Astragalus	General tonic, boosts energy
Bilberry	Improves circulation, repairs veins
Chinese ginseng	General tonic, boosts energy
Garlic	Lowers cholesterol, helps prevent cancer
Ginkgo biloba	Antioxidant, improves circulation and memory
Gotu kola	Improves circulation, healing, and memory
Green tea	Antioxidant and tonic, helps prevent cancer
Milk thistle	Repairs liver cells, liver tonic
Reishi	Adaptogen, tonic, immune stimulant
Siberian ginseng	Adaptogen, tonic, boosts energy
Turmeric	Antioxidant

HERBS FOR DISEASE PREVENTION

Bilberry	Hardening of the arteries, hemorrhoids, poor night vision
Cranberry	Urinary tract infections
Evening primrose oil	Essential fatty acid deficiencies
Feverfew	Migraines
Garlic	Hardening of the arteries, high cholesterol, high blood pressure
Ginkgo biloba	Memory loss, tinnitus, macular degeneration
Hawthorn	Angina pectoris, congestive heart failure
Licorice	Ulcers
Milk thistle	Liver problems
Saw palmetto	Prostate enlargement (benign prostatic hyperplasia)
St.-John's-wort	Mild depression

As an example, let's consider a 50-year-old man who has some family history of liver and heart disease, and who wants to stay well and boost his mental and physical energy. His regimen might include ginkgo biloba for memory and vision, saw palmetto for his prostate, garlic to keep his cholesterol low, Siberian ginseng for energy and overall well-being, bilberry for eyesight and circulation,

FINDING AN HERBAL PRACTITIONER

So, who are these folks who practice herbal medicine? Some of them are the same doctors, physician assistants, nurse practitioners, and nurses that you're already seeing. It's becoming more and more common to find medical doctors who know herbal medicine, and that trend is likely to continue because the demand exists and will probably grow.

On the other hand, what if none of your health practitioners knows about herbs and other botanical medicines?

There is no nationwide, government-approved certification for herbalists. But there are professional designations that indicate certain levels and types of training. Here's a brief overview of them.

◆ N.D. (naturopathic doctor). A practitioner with this degree trains for four years at an accredited naturopathic medical school instead of a regular medical school. At this time, only 11 states in the United States recognize N.D. degrees. Some other states may allow the use of this title through correspondence study. You should ask where your naturopathic doctor has studied and whether it is an accredited school.

◆ M.N.I.M.H. or F.N.I.M.H. This designation means that the herbalist has studied at the National Institute for Medical Herbalism in England, where clinical herbalists are nationally registered (the "M" stands for "member"; the "F" stands for "fellow"). A few practitioners in the United States have completed this course of study.

milk thistle to protect his liver, and kelp to stimulate his thyroid. This typical man might also want to take an iron-free multivitamin, coenzyme Q_{10}, and three key antioxidants—vitamin C, vitamin E, and selenium.

A typical woman of the same age might also want to take the ginkgo biloba, garlic, Siberian ginseng, and bilberry. She might add

- ◆ A.H.G. The American Herbalists Guild confers this level of certification on herbal practitioners. Each applicant is peer-reviewed by a panel. If the applicant has not attended a three- to four-year herbal training program, he must have a similar depth of training and three letters of recommendation from other professional herbalists or health professionals, or extensive experience in a native healing tradition.

- ◆ L.Ac. This abbreviation stands for licensed acupuncturist. Why include it in a list of herbal certifications? Because some acupuncturists, though not all, are also trained in the use of herbs, particularly Chinese herbs. Acupuncturists train for three to four years; they are usually licensed by the state, and requirements vary from one state to another.

Just because an herbalist doesn't have one of the titles you see above doesn't mean he can't help you. Many herbalists are self-taught, simply because the training they need has not been widely available. You should be aware, however, that some herbal education programs give their students titles that have no legal standing beyond the completion of that particular course of study at that school.

When you're looking for a qualified herbal practitioner, a recommendation from someone you know and trust is often valuable. So is a referral from other health-care professionals who have certifications themselves. Whomever you choose, be ready to ask questions. If their promises seem too good, or they cost too much, don't use them.

black cohosh and red clover for their beneficial phytoestrogens, compounds capable of evening out the hormonal fluctuations that often precede menopause. Or, if the women in her family have great eyesight into their nineties, but she has a problem with anemia right now, she might want to leave out the bilberry and add yellow dock. She'll also want to take the three antioxidants, get a little bit of iron in her multivitamin, and add a big dose of calcium to prevent osteoporosis.

When crafting your own herbal regimen, you'll want to take these five factors into account.

1. Any improvements you want to make in your health now
2. Any health problems for which you may be at risk
3. Your age, size, gender, fitness level, and lifestyle
4. Any health problems you may have now, especially if you are taking other drugs or herbs for them (in which case, you'll want to consult your doctor before you begin taking the herbs)
5. Any allergies or sensitivities that you may have

After you research the conditions you want to treat or prevent and the improvements in your health you want to make, list the herbs you've chosen, along with the recommended dosages you've found. Double-check the caution statements in the appropriate condition chapters in part 3 and in the Herb Profiles in part 4. Check your list with your doctor if have any pre-existing conditions or are taking any prescription drugs. Finally, shop for herbal products with the guidelines from this chapter in mind.

You may find combination products that contain most of the herbs you want to take. Follow the manufacturer's dosage recommendations on the product labels. If you don't find a combination product that you trust, choose the most important health issue that you want to address. Purchase and begin taking the herb on your list that addresses that condition or risk. Watch for a few weeks for any negative reactions. If you experience side effects, discontinue the herb and try a different one for that condition or risk. Then pick the next most important herb on your list and try it for a few weeks. If you find an herb effective, add the next one to your regimen, and so on.

CHAPTER 4

MAKING YOUR OWN PRODUCTS

WHAT IF THERE'S NO GOOD HERB STORE in your area—or you're simply interested in making your own herbal remedies? Or what if no available product contains all the herbs you need and you want to customize your own preparation?

While few people actually have the time to customize their herbal regimens in this way, it can be easy, affordable, and enjoyable. Plus, knowing a few simple techniques can make you a more educated consumer of the products that you buy.

With that in mind, here are some instructions for making and using your own herbal remedies.

TEAS

These are among the simplest products to purchase and prepare. You can buy an already-blended herbal tea, or purchase individual herbs and combine them at home. And if a medicinal tea you've purchased has a taste you dislike, you can add herbs of your own choosing to make it sweeter or spicier.

Remember to steep your tea longer if some of the plant matter is bark, roots, or seeds. If your tea consists completely of bark, roots, or seeds, you'll need to simmer them, because these tough plant parts need a bit more time to release their medicinal compounds.

When you're buying herbs in bulk for tea, check for freshness first. Also make sure you're buying the right part of the plant. You may see some bulk herbs labeled with the name of the plant and then simply "herb." What this means to an herbalist is that the product in the bin is dried above-ground parts—stems, leaves, and flowers if the plant produces blooms. In other words, you might see licorice root and horsetail herb.

If tea bags are the only convenient way for you to drink your medicine, don't despair. Many health food stores carry tea bags that you can fill yourself and seal with an iron. Such bags are also available from some of the sources in the Resource Directory.

Always store dried tea blends in airtight containers away from heat and light. Keep brewed tea in the refrigerator for no more than three days.

Capsules

Rarely will you be unable to find an herb in capsule form, especially if you consult mail-order sources. If, however, a trusted herbal practitioner advises that you encapsulate your own custom blend of herbs, it isn't difficult to do. You'll need a coffee grinder, empty capsules, and preferably a capsule block (a small stand that holds empty capsule halves, making them much faster and easier to assemble). You can buy empty capsules and a capsule block at your local health food store, or from the mail-order sources listed in the Resource Directory.

Begin by cleaning any coffee residue off the grinder blades with any drinking alcohol or a cloth dampened in hot, soapy water. Grind the herbs very fine in short bursts (you want to avoid allowing the grinder blades to become too hot because this causes the medicinal compounds to evaporate). Then fill your capsules, either by hand or using the capsule block.

Tinctures

Sometimes you may wish to customize a blend of herbs for your own condition and make them into a tincture, or alcohol-based extract. If you're taking a lot of different herbs or have trouble swallowing capsules, this can be more convenient for you.

Making a tincture isn't difficult, though the mixture does take several weeks to mature. The ratio of alcohol to water, and the ratio of herbs to liquid, varies from herb to herb. A few custom tincture recipes are included in this book. With some of them, all you have to do is blend purchased tinctures. The rest of the recipes include instructions on ingredients and steeping times.

INFUSED OILS

Infused oils are easy to make and good to have on hand for many minor injuries and illnesses. Simply combine herbs, chosen for the condition they'll treat, in a heavy, nonreactive (not aluminum or cast iron) pan. Cover the herbs with extra-virgin olive oil and heat on the lowest possible setting for 30 minutes. Then pour the oil and plant matter into a jar that seals tightly, and steep for two weeks, shaking daily. Strain the oil and put it into clean jars.

SALVES

These solid preparations are handy for travel, and they can soothe many skin irritations, bug bites, and minor bumps and bruises. If you can make an infused oil and have access to beeswax, you can make a salve.

Simply grate about ¾ ounce of beeswax for each half cup of infused oil that you have. In a heavy, nonreactive pan, warm the infused oil over low heat. Add the beeswax and stir it until it melts. Remove the pan from the heat and allow to cool slightly; pour the mixture into jars while still warm. Once the mixture has cooled completely, close the jars tightly.

POULTICES, PLASTERS, AND COMPRESSES

These old-fashioned preparations are time-honored ways to use herbs externally. If you've ever smeared eucalyptus balm on a child's chest, you've used a modern version of them.

Each of these preparations requires fresh or dried whole herbs. With poultices and plasters, the herbs are mashed or dissolved into a paste, which can be applied directly to the skin or wrapped in a cloth before application. Heat may be applied as well. Compresses involve dipping a cloth into a tea, then applying it to the affected area; they can be used cold or hot.

GROWING AND WILDCRAFTING HERBS

There are many resources that can give you much more detailed information on growing and wildcrafting medicinal herbs. Either technique can provide you with quality fresh herbs and the satisfaction of knowing their source.

To get you started, here is an overview of five medicinal herbs that are easy to grow in many climates, and five herbs that are easy to harvest from the wild. Naturally there are many more.

FIVE HERBS TO GROW

Calendula (*Calendula officinalis*)

Also known as pot marigold, this edible annual flower is easily grown from seed in a sunny spot. The fresh flowers are marvelous to add to salads or cooked foods. Dried, they can be used in teas or gargles for sore throat or inflammations of the mouth or in infused oils for minor skin injuries or irritations. In Germany, doctors apply preparations of the herb to surgical incisions and other wounds that are slow to heal.

Calendula

Chamomile (*Matricaria recutita*)

This cheery, daisylike flower comes in two varieties: German chamomile (*Matricaria recutita*) is an annual, and Roman chamomile (*Chamaemelum nobile*), a perennial. The German variety is the one usually used in tea and herbal medicines. A tea made from fresh chamomile flowers is a taste not to be forgotten. Both varieties like full sun to partial shade and a light, well-drained soil; they're difficult to start from seed, so you may want to purchase plants.

Lemon Balm (*Melissa officinalis*)

Mild sedative, herpes remedy, bee magnet: You can call lemon balm all of these and more. This bushy, somewhat weedy-looking plant, with its large, lemon-scented leaves, has a long tradition as a medicinal herb. Research has verified that it contains antiviral compounds, and clinical studies show that a lemon-balm cream can help cold sores and genital herpes lesions heal more quickly.

Peppermint (*Mentha* × *piperita*)

Many gardeners will tell you that this herb is easier to grow than to get rid of! A spreading, even invasive, perennial, mint is probably the most common ingredient in herb teas. It can be used dried or fresh, added to foods, made into

Lemon balm

syrups or jellies, and used in homemade cosmetics; it can ease gastrointestinal spasms, nausea, and congestion. Contain it in a pot or confined garden bed unless you want it to spread out of control.

Sage (*Salvia officinalis*)

This common culinary herb has many home health care applications and is easily preserved by drying bundled sprigs. Plant it in well-drained, moderately rich soil and full sun, and sage will bloom around June and draw clusters of bees. In shade, it tends to pout. Sage tea can be used as a gargle for sore throats, mouth ulcers, and gingivitis, and it has a high mineral content. Sage often figures in formulas for premenstrual syndrome.

FIVE HERBS TO WILDCRAFT

Unscrupulous entrepreneurs have given wildcrafting a bad name by overharvesting some wild-growing herbs to the point of endangerment. Such is the case with arnica (*Arnica montana*), goldenseal (*Hydrastis canadensis*), and some ginsengs. Some of these endangered plants are now being cultivated; that's why we've included such information in the Herb Profiles at the back of this book, under "Conscientious Consumer Information."

Those who harvest herbs from the wild must be careful for the sake of more than the plants. We don't advise wildcrafting herbs unless you are absolutely, positively, rock-solid sure of three things.

1. You can with absolute certainty identify the plant you seek. Consult resources in addition to this book if you want to gather herbs from the wild. Best of all, take a locally sponsored course in wildcrafting. It can be difficult to identify plant species merely from photographs, drawings, and descriptions.

2. You have permission to gather the plant. National, state, and county properties tend to have different rules. Ask. If the land is private, ask the landowner. When you do have permission to harvest, proceed prudently; take no more than 10 percent of the plants you see around you.

3. You know the plants have not been sprayed with chemicals. Avoid plants near roadsides, especially busy ones.

That said, here are five medicinal plants that are easily recognized, fairly widespread, plentiful in the wild, and good to use fresh.

Dandelion (*Taraxacum officinale*)

This familiar weed, the bane of lawns, yields more than dandelion wine. The young spring leaves are often eaten in salads as an herbal diuretic. Interestingly, the compounds in the leaves act differently on the body than pharmaceutical diuretics: They restore the potassium lost through increased urination. The root can be roasted and used as a coffee substitute. Even dandelion, however, can be mistaken when it first comes up in the spring. To make sure you have the right plant, look for the white, milky sap in the central vein of the leaves. Or you may wish to wait to take the leaves until the plant sends up its characteristic flower shoot, though they taste more bitter by then.

Mullein (*Verbascum thapsus*)

This common Western weed grows its soft, furry leaves in a rosette pattern during its first year, then sends up a tall, yellow-flowering spike in its second year. Both the leaves and the flowers are used for respiratory irritations of various kinds, including coughs and asthma. The dried leaves are easily made into a tea; an infused oil of the flowers has sometimes been used for earaches. Mullein has shown an ability to fight some viruses in the laboratory; it's not yet known whether it can do so in the human body.

Plantain (*Plantago major, P. lanceolata*)

Another common lawn weed, plantain is a handy first-aid herb for bug bites, stings, scrapes, and other minor skin irritations. Once you've seen the round clusters of leaves of the plantain, with its characteristic flower spike, it isn't hard to spot again. Plantain tends to pop up almost anywhere in disturbed earth. Instead of removing it from your yard with weed killers, you might consider just leaving it where it's handy.

St.-John's-Wort (*Hypericum perforatum*)

To use this herb for mild depression, you'll want to buy a standardized extract. But you'll want the fresh plant for making infused oil to apply to minor burns, cuts, abrasions, and ear infections. This shrubby blooming plant can be found in shady cool woods. Harvest the

Plantain

flowering tops in June when they are in bloom (legend has it the plant is most potent on St. John's Day, or June 24). St-John's-wort also happily adapts to the garden, but don't uproot a healthy wild plant; this herb is so easy to grow from seed that transplanting it is unnecessary.

Stinging Nettle (*Urtica dioica*)

The fine hairs on this plant do sting, so wear gloves, long sleeves, and long pants when you gather it. Drying the leaves takes the sting out of them, after which they can be used in tea for anemia or prostate enlargement (benign prostatic hyperplasia) or as a mild diuretic. Nettle has also been used for allergies such as hay fever.

Stinging nettle

PART II

DRUGS AND THEIR HERBAL ALTERNATIVES

THE REMEDIES AT A GLANCE

IF YOU HAVE BEEN DIAGNOSED with a certain disease or disorder, scan the available herbal remedies outlined on the following pages, then turn to the complete chapter for that condition. Herbal medicine has much to offer for some disorders; for others there are only a few herbs that are effective. For some conditions, there are separate internal and external herbal treatments, and for some there are herbs that can be used both internally and externally.

But for many conditions, such as heart disease, asthma, and depression, it's critical that you don't discontinue your medication, substitute herbs, or begin taking herbs without the direct supervision of your doctor. Both herbs and pharmaceutical drugs act on the body; both can have side effects. Some herbs interact with pharmaceutical drugs or other herbs in dangerous ways. For ailments that are serious, continuing, or both, you should not attempt to treat yourself with herbs. Your best place to begin is with a medical professional who respects your desire to try the safest, most non-invasive treatment first.

Even with very minor conditions, such as sunburns, stomach upsets, or headaches, remember that recurring or severe symptoms call for the attention of a professional.

Finally, be aware that it would be impossible to include all of the rare side effects of drugs in a book of this size, just as it is impossible to predict what miraculous herbal treatments may be discovered in the future. The best strategy for your health is to stay informed and stay safe.

Condition	Commonly Used Drugs	Herbal Alternatives
ACNE (page 69)	**External:** Benzoyl peroxide (Clearasil, Oxy-10); keratolytics (Propa pH, StriDex); topical retinoids (Retin-A)	**External:** Calendula tea, lavender essential oil, tea tree essential oil
	Internal: Antibiotics; isotretinoin (Accutane); oral contraceptives	**Internal:** Burdock, dandelion
ALTITUDE SICKNESS (page 74)	Acetazolamide (Diamox, Acetazolam); dexamethasone (Deronil, Dexone)	**Internal:** Ginger, ginkgo, ginseng, Siberian ginseng
ANGINA (page 79)	Aspirin; beta blockers: labetalol (Normodyne, Trandate), metroprolol (Lopressor), propranolol (Inderal); calcium channel blockers: diltiazem (Cardizem, Dilacor), nifedipine (Adalat, Procardia), verapamil (Calan, Covera); nitrates: isorbide dinitrate (Dilatrate-SR, Isordil), isorbide monoitrate (Imdur, Ismo), nitroglycerine ointment (Nitrobid), sublingual nitroglycerine	**Internal:** Coleus, forskohlii or the extract, forskolin, khella, garlic, ginkgo, hawthorn, khella, onion
ANXIETY (page 84)	Benzodiazepines: alprazolam (Xanax), chlordiazepoxide (Librium), clonazepam (Klonipin), diazepam (Valium); beta blockers: propranolol (Inderal); buspirone (Buspar); selective serotonin reuptake inhibitors (SSRIs): fluoxetine (Prozac),	**Internal:** Chamomile, kava-kava, oats, Siberian ginseng, valerian **External:** Lavender essential oil

Condition	Commonly Used Drugs	Herbal Alternatives
	fluvoxamine (Luvox), paroxetine (Paxil), sertraline (Zoloft); trycyclic antidepressants: amitriptyline (Elavil, Limbitrol), doxepin (Adapin, Sinequan), imipramine (Tofranil)	
ARTHRITIS (page 92)	Analgesics (aspirin, acetaminophen with codeine); cortisone (Cortone Acetate); cox-2 inhibitors (Celebrex); cyclosporine (Sandimmune); methotrexate (Rheumatrex); newer nonsteroidal anti-inflammatories (Indocin, Feldene)	**Internal**: Evening primrose, yucca **External**: Cayenne, yucca
ASTHMA (page 102)	Anticholinergics (Atrovent); beta-agonists (Proventil, Maxair, Tornalate); cromolyn sodium (Intal, Fivent); inhaled corticosteroids (Azmacort, Pulmicort); leukotriene antagonists (Accolate, Xyflo); oral corticosteroids (Deltasone, Medrol); theophylline (Slo-Bid, Theobid)	**Internal**: Ephedra, garlic, ginkgo, licorice, onion, turmeric
BLADDER INFECTIONS (page 108)	Antibiotics (Bactrim, Septra, Cipro)	**Internal**:Bearberry, cranberry, goldenrod, goldenseal, Oregon graperoot

Condition	Commonly Used Drugs	Herbal Alternatives
BLISTERS (page 113)	Over-the-counter remedies are recommended if a blister has torn, exposing skin underneath; antibacterial creams and ointments can be applied with adhesive bandages to keep the wound clean	**External**: Calendula, comfrey, lavender essential oil, St.-John's-wort, tea tree essential oil
BODY ODOR (page 116)	Over-the-counter deodorants and antiperspirants	**Internal**: Fennel, parsley, rosemary, sage **External**: Rosemary, sage
BREAST CYSTS (page 118)	Birth control pills (Norinyl, Ortho-Novum); danazol (Danocrine)	**Internal**: Black cohosh, butcher's broom, evening primrose oil, saw palmetto, vitex **External**: Wild yam
BREAST PAIN (page 122)	Analgesics (aspirin, acetaminophen, ibuprofen); birth control pills (estrogen and progesterone); danazol (Danocrine)	**Internal**: Evening primrose oil, vitex
BREAST-FEEDING PROBLEMS (page 126)	No drugs exist for mothers whose milk supply is not adequate	**Internal**:Aniseed, fennel, fenugreek
BRONCHITIS (page 129)	Cough suppressants, with or without codeine and with or without antihistamines and decongestants (Comtrex, Contac, Actifed);	**Internal**: Horehound, licorice, marsh-mallow, mullein, wild cherry bark

Condition	Commonly Used Drugs	Herbal Alternatives
	expectorants (Dimetane, Robitussin); inhaled bronchodilators (Proventil, Brethaire)	
BRUISES (page 134)	Analgesics (aspirin, acetaminophen, ibuprofen)	**External**: Arnica, calendula, chamomile, comfrey, St.-John's-wort
BURNS (page 138)	Analgesics (aspirin, acetaminophen, ibuprofen); topical anesthetics (Bactine, Solarcaine, Lanacane)	**External**: Aloe, calendula, comfrey, gotu kola, plaintain
BURSITIS AND TENDONITIS (page 142)	Analgesics (acetaminophen, ibuprofen, aspirin, naproxen); corticosteroids (injections)	**Internal**: Cayenne, devil's claw, ginger, kava-kava, licorice **External**: Cayenne, turmeric
CANKER SORES (page 147)	Local anesthetics (Anbesol, Orajel); topical steroids (Aristocort, Fluinide)	**Internal**: Chamomile, ginkgo, goldenseal, gotu kola, licorice
CARDIAC ARRHYTHMIA (page 150)	Lanoxin (Digoxin); propranolol (Inderal); verapamil (Calan, Covera)	**Internal**: Chamomile, hawthorn, kava-kava, reishi, valerian
CARPAL TUNNEL SYNDROME (page 155)	Furosemide (Lasix); hydrochlorothiazide (Dyazide, HydroDiuril); nonsteroidal anti-inflammatories (ibuprofen, naproxen)	**Internal**: Boswellia, ginkgo, turmeric

Condition	Commonly Used Drugs	Herbal Alternatives
Cataracts (page 158)	No drugs can reverse cataract damage once it has occurred; herbs may help prevent such damage	**Internal**: Bilberry, rosemary, turmeric
Cervical Dysplasia (page 162)	No specific drugs can reverse cervical dysplasia or prevent it from progressing into cancer	**Internal**: Astragalus, burdock, milk thistle, red clover, yellow dock
Chronic Fatigue Syndrome (page 167)	Adrenal gland hormones; benzodiazepines (Valium, Xanax); immunoglobulin therapy; nonsteroidal and anti-inflammatory drugs (Motrin, Aleve)	**Internal**: Astragalus, licorice, reishi mushroom, shiitake mushroom, Siberian ginseng
Cold Sores (page 172)	Analgesics (aspirin, acetaminophen, ibuprofen); antiviral drugs (Avirax, Zovirax); lip balms (Carmex Blistex, Lip Medex); topical anesthetics (Viscous Xylocaine, Anbesol)	**Internal**: Echinacea, lemon balm, mullein, St.-John's-wort **External**: Clove, echinacea, lemon balm, mullein, St.-John's-wort
Colds and Flu (page 176)	Analgesics (aspirin, acetaminophen); antihistamines (Comtrex, Contac); antivirals (Symmetrel, Flumadine); oral and nasal decongestants (Sudafed, Dimetapp); saline nasal sprays and drops (Ocean, NaSal Saline Moisturizer)	**Internal**: Astragalus, echinacea, elderberry, ephedra, garlic
Constipation (page 189)	Bulking agents (Maltsupex, Citrucel); enemas (Fleet); laxatives (Diocto-K Plus, Ex-Lax); osmotics (Evalose, Citroma); stool softeners (Correctol, Agoral)	**Internal**: Cascara sagrada, flaxseed, papaya, psyllium seed, senna

Condition	Commonly Used Drugs	Herbal Alternatives
CUTS AND SCRAPES (page 193)	Antibiotic ointments (Baciguent, Neosporin); hydrogen peroxide; povidone-iodine (Betadine); rubbing alcohol; topical analgesics (Bactine)	**External**: Aloe, calendula, cayenne, comfrey
DANDRUFF (page 198)	Ketoconazole shampoos; shampoos containing tar, zinc pyrithion, or selenium; topical corticosteroids	**Internal and external**: Evening primrose oil **External**: Flaxseed oil, tea tree oil
DEPRESSION (page 200)	Monoamine oxidase (MAO) inhibitors: phenelzine sulfate (Nardil), tranylcypromine sulfate (Parnate); sedatives: bupropion (Wellbutrin), nefazodone (Serzone),trazodone (Desyrel), velafaxine (Effexor); selective serotonin reuptake inhibitors (SSRIs): fluoxetine (Prozac), fluvoxamine (Luvox), paroxetine (Paxil), sertraline (Zoloft); trycyclic antidepressants: amitriptyline (Elavil, Limbitrol), doxepin (Adapin, Sinequan), imipramine (Tofranil)	**Internal**: Ginkgo, kava-kava, oats, St.-John's-wort, vervain **External**: Lavender
DIABETES (page 206)	Biguanides (Glucophage); insulin (injection); sulfonylureas (Orinase, Tolinase)	**Internal**: Bilberry, bitter melon, fenugreek, gymnema

Condition	Commonly Used Drugs	Herbal Alternatives
DIARRHEA (page 212)	Antibiotics (E-Mycin, Erybid); attapulgite (Diar-Aid, Diasorb); bismuth subsalicylate (Pepto-Bismol, Helidac); kaolin and pectin (Donnagel-MB, Kaopectate); loperamide (Imodium, Maalox Anti-Diarrheal)	**Internal**: Agrimony, blackberry or raspberry leaf, carob, goldenseal, Oregon graperoot, peppermint
DIVERTIC-ULOSIS (page 217)	Antibiotics (Cipro, Floxin); anti-inflammatories (aspirin, ibuprofen, naproxen); antispasmodics (Levsin, Donnatal)	**Internal**: Aloe vera, cat's claw, peppermint, psyllium, wild yam **External**: Peppermint
EAR INFECTIONS (page 221)	Analgesics (acetaminophen, ibuprofen); antibiotics (oral and ear drops) (Cortisporin, Swim-EAR); antinausea medications (Compazine); nonantibiotic ear drops (Auralgan)	**Internal**: Echinacea, Oregon graperoot, shiitake mushroom
ECZEMA (page 225)	Antihistamines (Benadryl, Claritin); coal-tar preparations (Aquaphor, Fotar); corticosteroids (Kenelog, Cortaid)	**Internal**: Burdock, dandelion, gotu kola **External**: Burdock, echinacea, gotu kola, oats
ENDOMETRI-OSIS (page 231)	Birth control pills: ethinyl estradiol norethindrone acetate (Loestrin); GnRH agonists: nafarelin (Synarel), leuprolide (Lupron); natural progesterone: creams (ProGest, PhytoGest); capsules, vaginal or rectal suppositories; synthetic	**Internal**: Chamomile, cramp bark, dandelion root, motherwort, yarrow

Condition	Commonly Used Drugs	Herbal Alternatives
	progesterone: medroxypro-gesterone acetate–injection (Depo-Provera); medroxy-progesterone—oral (Provera); testosterone derivatives: danazol (Danocrine)	
EYESTRAIN (page 238)	No specific drugs are used for eyestrain	**Internal:** Bilberry, eyebright **External:** Calendula, chamomile, eyebright, witch hazel
FATIGUE (page 243)	There are no specific drugs for everyday fatigue; the remedy most doctors recommend is rest	**Internal:** Astragalus, licorice, reishi, schisandra, Siberian ginseng
FIBROIDS (page 249)	Gonadotropin-releasing hormone (GnRH): leuprolide (Lupron); gonadorelin (Factrel); nafarelin (Synarel)	**Internal:** Burdock, milk thistle, red raspberry, vitex
FIBRO-MYALGIA (page 253)	Anti-inflammatories (naproxen, ibuprofen); injections of local anesthetics and corticosteroids; tricyclic antidepressants (Endep, Elavil)	**Internal:** Devil's claw, ginkgo, grapeseed, St.-John's-wort, willow **External:** Cayenne
FLATULENCE (page 258)	Activated charcoal (Carcocaps, Charcoal Plus); antacids (Mylanta II, Di-Gel); prokinetic agents (Propulsid, Reglan)	**Internal:** Chamomile, fennel, ginger, peppermint

Condition	Commonly Used Drugs	Herbal Alternatives
Fungal Skin Infections (page 261)	Antifungals (topical: Micatin, Lotrimin; oral: Fulvicin, Grifulvin); selenium-sulfide-containing shampoos (Selsun Blue, Head and Shoulders Intensive Treatment)	**Internal**: Garlic **External**: Arnica, garlic, geranium essential oil, grapefruit seed extract, lemongrass, tea tree essential oil
Gallstones (page 264)	Bile salts (Chenix, Actigall)	**Internal**: Artichoke, dandelion, milk thistle, peppermint essential oil, turmeric
Genital Warts (page 269)	No known drugs can eliminate the virus that causes genital warts	**Internal**: Garlic, licorice, St.-John's-wort
Glaucoma (page 271)	Adrenergics: brimonidine, apraclonidin (Iopidine); beta blockers: timolol (Timoptic), betaxolol (Betoptic); carbonic anhydrase inhibitors: acetazolamide (Diamox), dichlorphenamide (Daranide); cholinergics: pilocarpine (Isopto Carpine, Ocusert); prostaglandins: latanoprost (Xalatan)	**Internal**: Bilberry, ginkgo
Gout (page 274)	Nonsteroidal anti-inflammatories (Indocin, Zyloprim, Benemid, Anturane)	**Internal**: Boswellia, celery seed, devil's claw, turmeric, yucca
Gum Disease (page 280)	Antibiotics (Pen-Vee K, Doryx, Flagyl)	**Internal**: Echinacea, goldenseal **External**: Aloe, blood root, calendula

Condition	Commonly Used Drugs	Herbal Alternatives
HANGOVER (page 283)	Analgesics (aspirin, acetaminophen, ibuprofen)	**Internal**: Cinchona, dandelion, ginkgo, willow
HAY FEVER (page 288)	Antihistamines; oral and nasal decongestants (Contac, Dristan); intranasal corticosteroids (Vancenase, Rhinocort); immunotherapy	**Internal**: Ephedra, garlic, licorice, peppermint essential oil, stinging nettle
HEADACHES (page 294)	Beta-blockers (Inderal, Corgard); ergotamine (Ergostat, Gynergen); methysergide (Sansert); over-the-counter and prescription analgesics (aspirin, Midrin, Anacin); triptans (Imitrex)	**Internal**: Cayenne pepper, feverfew, ginger, peppermint
HEART DISEASE (page 301)	Aspirin; beta blockers: propranolol (Inderal); calcium channel blockers: nifedipine (Adalat, Procardia); diltiazem (Cardizem, Dilacor); isorbide dinitrate (Dilatrate-SR, Isordil); isorbide monoitrate (Imdur, Ismo); labetalol (Normodyne, Trandate); metroprolol (Lopressor); nitrates: sublingual nitrogylcerine (tablets or spray); nitro-gylcerine ointment (Nitrobid); verapamil (Calan, Covera)	**Internal**: Bilberry, garlic, ginkgo, hawthorn, motherwort, onion

Condition	Commonly Used Drugs	Herbal Alternatives
HEARTBURN (page 309)	Antacids (Tums, Maalox); histamine-2 receptor antagonists (Tagamet, Zantac); promotility agents (Propulcid, Reglan); proton pump inhibitors (Prevacid, Prilosec)	**Internal**: Aloe, cabbage juice, calendula, licorice root
HEMOR-RHOIDS (page 314)	External: anti-inflammatories and anesthetics (Analpram, Anusol, Cortifoam, Epifoam); over-the-counter preparations (Anusol, Tonolane, Preparation H)	**Internal**: Butcher's broom, dandelion, ginkgo, horse chestnut, yellow dock **External**: Horse chestnut
HERPES (page 318)	Analgesics (acetaminophen, aspirin, ibuprofen); antiviral drugs: acyclovir (Avirax, Zovirax); valacyclovir (Valtrex)	**Internal**: Bupleurum, echinacea, lemon balm, licorice, St.-John's-wort **External**: Bupleurum, lemon balm, licorice, St.-John's-wort
HIGH BLOOD PRESSURE (page 322)	Alpha blockers (Catapress, Tenex); beta blockers (Inderal, Kerlone); calcium channel blockers (Norvasc, Calan); diuretics (Dyazide, Lozol)	**Internal**: Dandelion, forskolin, garlic, hawthorn
HIGH CHOLES-TEROL (page 329)	Bile acid sequestrates (Questran, Colestid); fibric acid derivatives (Lopid, Atromid-S, Tricor); HMG CoA reductase inhibitors (Mevacor, Zocor)	**Internal**: Artichoke, garlic, guggul, psyllium

Condition	Commonly Used Drugs	Herbal Alternatives
HIVES (page 334)	Antihistamines (Zyrtec, Claritin, Benadryl); corticosteroids; epinephrine; hydroxyzine (Anxanil, Apo-Hydroxyzine)	**Internal:** Chamomile, licorice, stinging nettle, yarrow **External:** Aloe, chamomile, yarrow
HYPO-THYROIDISM (page 338)	Thyroid supplements (L-Thyroxine, Armour Thyroid)	**Internal:** Bitters (look for products containing gentian and wormwood), bladderwack, myrhh **External:** Myrhh
INDIGESTION (page 340)	Antacids (Gelusil, Maalox); antimuscarinic agents (Valpin, Darbid); bismuth salicylates (Pepto-Bismol); histamine H2 antagonists (Zantac, Pepcid); prokinetic agents (Populsid, Reglan)	**Internal:** Chamomile, ginger, licorice, marshmallow, peppermint essential oil
INSECT BITES AND STINGS (page 346)	Analgesics (aspirin, acetaminophen, ibuprofen); antihistamines (Benadryl); corticosteroids (Deltasone); epinephrine (inhalation or injection); topical calamine products (Dermarest, Aveeno Anti-itch Cream)	**Internal:** Aloe, calendula, echinacea, plaintain, tea, witch hazel
INSOMNIA (page 351)	Antihistamines (Benadryl Allergy, Nytol Quick Caps); benzodiazepines (Ativan, Halcion, Valium); zolpidem (Ambien)	**Internal:** California poppy, chamomile, kava-kava, passionflower, valerian

Condition	Commonly Used Drugs	Herbal Alternatives
INTERMITTENT CLAUDICATION (page 357)	Antiplatelet agents (aspirin); dipyridamole (Persantin); pentoxyfylline (Trental)	**Internal:** Garlic, ginger, ginkgo, hawthorn, onion
INTESTINAL PARASITES (page 362)	Albendazole (Albenza, Zentel); furazolidone (Furoxone); mebendazole (Vermox, Mebendacin); metronidzaole (Flagyl, Apo-Metronidazole); niclosamide (Niclocide); thiabendazole (Mintezol, Minzolum)	**Internal:** Epazote, garlic, ginger, Oregon graperoot, quassia bark
IRRITABLE BOWEL SYNDROME (page 366)	Antidiarrheal agents (Imodium A-D, Lomotil); antispasmodics (Levsin, Donnatal); laxatives (Ex-Lax, Dulcolax); surfactants (Gas-X, Di-Gel)	**Internal:** Chamomile, peppermint essential oil, psyllium
KIDNEY STONES (page 371)	No specific drugs are used except in rare metabolic conditions	**Internal:** Corn silk, khella, skullcap, valerian, wild yam
LIBIDO PROBLEMS (page 376)	Hormone replacement therapy: oral testosterone (Testex, Metandren), testosterone patch (Testoderm); testosterone with estrogen (Estratest); sildenafil (Viagra)	**Internal:** Damiana, ginseng, ginkgo, oats, saw palmetto, wild yam
LIVER DISEASE (page 383)	With rare exceptions, there are no drugs for most nonhepatitis types of liver disease	**Internal:** Bupleurum, dandelion root, licorice, milk thistle, schisandra
LYME DISEASE (page 388)	Antibiotics (penicillin, tetracycline)	**Internal:** Bupleurum, echinacea, garlic, licorice

Condition	Commonly Used Drugs	Herbal Alternatives
MACULAR DEGENERA-TION (page 393)	Western opthamalogists often suggest antioxidant supplementation with combinations of vitamins	**Internal**: Bilberry, ginkgo
MEMORY LOSS (page 395)	Acetylcholinesterase inhibitors (THA, Aricept); MAO-B inhibitors (Eldepryl, Hydergine)	**Internal**: Ginkgo, Siberian ginseng, water hyssop
MENOPAUSE (page 400)	Hormone replacement therapy (DepGynogen, Premarin, Evista, Estrates)	**Internal**: Black cohosh, dang gui, St.-John's-wort
MENSTRUAL PROBLEMS (page 408)	Analgesics (ibuprofen, acetaminophen); antidepressants (Prozac, Zoloft); benzodiazepines (Xanax, Ativan); nonsedating antianxiety drugs (Buspar); testosterone derivatives (Danazol)	**Internal**: Black cohosh, cramp bark and black haw, feverfew, vitex, yarrow
MORNING SICKNESS (page 416)	Drugs are seldom prescribed for morning sickness because of the potential effect on the fetus; women with severe vomiting are sometimes treated with intravenous fluids	**Internal**:Chamomile, ginger, peppermint
MOTION SICKNESS (page 420)	Over-the-counter and prescription antihistamines (Benedryl, Dramamine, Antivert), promethazine scopolamine (Transderm Scop)	**Internal**: Fennel, ginger, peppermint

Condition	Commonly Used Drugs	Herbal Alternatives
MULTIPLE SCLEROSIS (page 423)	Immune-system suppressants (Cytoxan, Imuran, Avonex); muscle relaxants (Dantrium); steroids (Meticorten)	**Internal:** Black currant, evening primrose, and flaxseed oils; ginkgo, purslane
NAUSEA (page 426)	Dimenhydrinate (Dramamine, Apo-Dimenhydrinate); metoclopramide (Reglan, Emex); phenothiazines (Compazine, Phenergan)	**Internal:** Catnip, chamomile, ginger, lemon balm, peppermint
NERVE PAIN (page 429)	Anticonvulsants (Dilantin, Tegretol); narcotics (Tylenol #3, Percodan); Nonsteroidal anti-inflammatory drugs (aspirin, ibuprofen); tricyclic anti-depressants (Elavil, Pamelor)	**Internal:** Corydalis, Jamaican dogwood, St.-John's-wort **External:** Cayenne
OBSESSIVE-COMPULSIVE DISORDER (page 434)	Selective serotonin reuptake inhibitors (SSRIs; Prozac, Luvox, Paxil); tricyclic antidepressants (Anafranil)	**Internal:** Bergamot essential oil, California poppy, kava-kava, St.-John's-wort, valerian
OSTEO-POROSIS (page 437)	Estrogen replacement therapy: conjugated estrogens (Premarin), dienestrol (Ortho Dienestrol), estradiol (Estrace); selective estrogen-receptor modulators: raloxifene (Evista); combination estrogen plus progesterone (Prempro, Premphase); alendronate (Fosamax); etidronate (Didronel); calcitonin (Calcimar as injection, Miacalcin as a nasal spray)	**Internal:** Horsetail, red clover, stinging nettle

Condition	Commonly Used Drugs	Herbal Alternatives
OVERWEIGHT (page 444)	Amphetamine (Biphetamine), phentermine (Fastin, Ionamin), benzphetamine (Didrex), diethylpropion (Tentuate), mazindol Sanorex); antidepressants: fluoxetine (Prozac), sertraline (Zoloft); sibutramine (Meridia), tetrahydrolipstatin (Xenical); over-the-counter: phenylpropanolamine (Dexatrim, Acutrim)	**Internal**: Garcinia, psyllium, Siberian ginseng, yohimbe
PARKINSON'S DISEASE (page 449)	Amantadine (Aman-Symmetrel); anticholinergics (Artane, Cogentin); dopamine-affecting drugs (Dopar, Parlodel, Permax)	**Internal**: Evening primrose, ginkgo, grapeseed extract
PINKEYE AND STIES (page 453)	Anti-allergy eye drops (Livostin, Alomide); antiviral eye drops (Trifluorothymidine, Herpex); over-the-counter antibacterial eye drops and ointments	**External**: Eyebright, gold thread, golden-seal, Oregon graperoot, tea, yarrow
PNEUMONIA (page 457)	Antibiotics (erythromycin, tetracycline, trimethopeim sulfamethoxazole); cephalosporins (Cefalexin, Clindamycin); antifungal drugs (ketoconazole)	**Internal**: Elecampane, garlic, goldenseal, horehound, mullein, Oregon graperoot
POISON IVY/ OAK/SUMAC (page 465)	Corticosteroids (Cortaid, Sarna HC); topical antihistamines (Benadryl); topical calamine products (Calaldryl, Ivarest)	**Internal**: Aloe, grindelia, jewelweed, plantain, witch hazel

Condition	Commonly Used Drugs	Herbal Alternatives
Prostate Enlargement (page 469)	Alpha adrenergic receptor antagonists (Hytrin, Cardura); finasteride (Proscar)	**Internal:** Pumpkin seed, pygeum, saw palmetto, stinging nettle root
Raynaud's Phenomenon (page 474)	Calcium channel blockers (Procardia, Lotrel, Lexxel)	**Internal:** Bilberry, cayenne pepper, garlic, ginger, ginkgo, hawthorn
Scabies (page 479)	Corticosteroids (Aristocort, Kenacort); insecticides (Lindane); oral ivermectin (Mectizan); permethrin 5 percent cream (Nix, Elimite)	**External:** Clove essential oil, neem essential oil, rosemary, tansy, tea tree essential oil
Shingles (page 482)	Acyclovir (Avirax, Valtrex); analgesics (aspirin, ibuprofen); foscarnet (Foscavir); interferon-alpha; vidarabine (Vira-A)	**Internal:** Licorice **External:** Cayenne, ginger, lemon balm, licorice, St.-John's-wort, turmeric
Sinus Infections (page 488)	Antibiotics; intranasal corticosteroids (Vancenase, Becocnase, Rhinocort); oral and nasal decongestants (Sudafed, Contac, Dristan)	**Internal:** Astragalus, echinacea, ephedra, shiitake mushroom
Smoking Addiction (page 493)	Nicotine and nicotine chewing gums(Habitrol, Nicotrol, Prostep); transdermal (patch)	**Internal:** Coltsfoot, elecampane, lobelia, mullein, schisandra
Sore Throat (page 499)	Analgesics (aspirin, acetaminophen, ibuprofen); antibiotics; narcotic analgesics (Aceta with Codeine, Allay)	**Internal:** Echinacea, eucalyptus, marsh-mallow, shiitake mushroom, slippery elm

Condition	Commonly Used Drugs	Herbal Alternatives
SPORTS INJURIES (page 504)	Analgesics (aspirin, acetaminophen, ibuprofen, naproxen)	**Internal**: Cayenne, ginger, kava-kava, turmeric **External**: Arnica, cayenne, comfrey, turmeric
STRESS (page 509)	Many drugs can alleviate specific symptoms of stress such as headache and anxiety; refer to chapters on these specific conditions	**Internal**: Ashwaganda, Asian ginseng, gotu kola, schisandra, Siberian ginseng
STROKE (page 518)	Aspirin; clot reducers: dipyradamole (Persantine), toclopidine (Ticlid); warfarin (Coumadin)	**Internal**: Garlic, ginger, ginkgo, hawthorn, onion
SUNBURN (page 523)	Analgesics (aspirin, acetaminophen, ibuprofen); topical anesthetics (Bactine, Solarcaine, Foille)	**External**: Aloe, calendula, St.-John's-wort, tea, witch hazel
TOOTHACHE (page 525)	Analgesics (aspirin, acetaminophen, ibuprofen, naproxen)	**Internal**: Chamomile **External**: Clove essential oil, licorice, turmeric
ULCERS (page 528)	Antacids (Maalox, Tums); hydrochloric acid blockers: (Tagamet, Zantac); misoprostol (Cytotec); omeprazole (Prilosec)	**Internal**: Calendula, chamomile, licorice, marshmallow root, meadowsweet, slippery elm

Condition	Commonly Used Drugs	Herbal Alternatives
VAGINAL INFECTIONS (page 534)	Antibiotic creams: clindamycin (Cleocin); antifungals: nystatin (Micostatin, Nilstat); clotrimazole (Gyne-Lotrim); metronidazole (Metrogel); miconazole (Monistat)	**Internal**: Echinacea, garlic, goldenseal, Oregon graperoot, Tea tree
VARICOSE VEINS (page 538)	No known drugs can remove varicose veins	**Internal**: Butcher's broom, gotu kola, hawthorn, horse chestnut
WARTS (page 542)	Cantharidin (Cantharone, Cantherone-Plus); over-the-counter salicylic acid preparations (Compound W, Mediplast, Wart-Off)	**External**: Birch bark, bloodroot, celandine, piñon blanco, white cedar

PART III

EXPLORING
YOUR
TREATMENT
OPTIONS

ACNE

SOME PEOPLE HAVE ACNE as teenagers, kiss it goodbye in their early twenties, and never see it again. Others get through their oily teens without skin problems but for some reason encounter major eruptions late in adulthood. And an unlucky few suffer through teen acne only to face breakouts again as adults.

Multiple factors contribute to acne. One is a change in keratin, a protein produced by skin cells. Excess keratin can clump together to block the oil ducts within hair follicles, producing those telltale bumps you know as pimples. The bacteria that inhabit these tiny hair follicles can also play a role, especially in teen acne.

While teen acne affects boys and girls in equal numbers, adult acne seems more common in women than in men. Some experts attribute this to hormonal changes that occur during the menstrual cycle.

Other things that have long been blamed for acne remain unproved. For example, remember your mother telling you that chocolate would give you zits? This and other diet-related theories have no good evidence behind them.

When used regularly, certain drug treatments can control acne. They take several weeks to work, however, and some treatments cause an initial worsening in acne before the skin begins to clear.

DRUG TREATMENT

Topical Retinoids
Tretinoin (Retin-A, Renova), adapalene (Differin), tazarotene (Tazorac). *Function*: increase generation of new cells and sloughing of old cells to decrease pore blockage. *Side effects*: mild dryness, itching, chapping, and peeling, particularly during first few weeks; may cause acne to worsen initially; may increase skin reactions to sunlight. *Caution*: Do not use during pregnancy or while attempting to become pregnant.

Keratolytics
Salicylic acid (Propa pH, StriDex); salicylic acid and sulfur (Fostex); resorcinol (R.A.), resorcinol and sulfur (Bensulfoid Cream).

Function: soften and loosen keratin, aiding its removal from the skin. *Side effects*: warmth, tingling, peeling, sensitivity to wind or cold, pigment change in treated area.

Antibiotics

Topical types: erythromycin, erythromycin plus benzoyl peroxide, clindamycin (many trade names). *Function:* kill bacteria on the skin. *Side effects:* initial burning or stinging on contact. *Oral types:* tetracyclines (many products). *Function:* kill bacteria in all body systems. *Side effects:* stomach upset, nausea, vomiting, diarrhea, dizziness, lightheadedness; doxycycline can increase photosensitivity.

Oral Contraceptives

Many trade and brand names. *Function*: counteract the effects of male hormones called androgens on the oil glands. *Side effects*: fluid retention, breast tenderness, breakthrough bleeding, nausea, vaginal discharge, brown skin blotches, headaches.

Other Drugs

Benzoyl peroxide (Oxy-10). *Function*: act as an antibacterial agent. *Side effects*: skin dryness and mild irritation with redness and chapping, especially in first weeks of use; do not use with tretinoin or similar products.

Isotretinoin (Accutane). *Function*: reduce oil gland size and activity (usually reserved for stubborn acne.) *Side effects*: lip scaling, dry, itchy, and peeling skin, dry mouth, eye inflammation, skin reactions to sun exposure; less commonly bone and joint pain, tendonitis, elevated blood triglycerides and liver enzymes; can cause serious birth defects.

HERBAL REMEDIES

Tea Tree (*Melaleuca alternifolia*)

The pungent oil from this Australian tree, used externally, acts against the bacteria associated with acne. One study found that a 5 percent tea tree oil preparation worked as well as 5 percent benzoyl peroxide in treating acne, but with fewer side effects. To use tea tree oil for acne, gently cleanse skin and pat dry. Then apply a 5 to

WASH LESS, SMILE MORE

Many people with acne have the mistaken impression that the cause is dirty skin. As a result, they become overzealous face-scrubbers. Aggressive and frequent washing actually aggravates the condition. Besides, washing the skin's surface doesn't rid the follicles of bacteria and excess oils. It's better to wash gently with a mild cleanser. Morning and evening is probably often enough.

15 percent dilution of the oil to problem areas (purchase a diluted product or dilute your own in jojoba oil). Repeat twice daily, morning and evening. *Caution*: May cause a rash, so try a test spot and wait 24 to 48 hours. Do not take internally.

Lavender (*Lavandula angustifolia*)

The essential oil of lavender is antibacterial, anti-inflammatory, and somewhat astringent; it's good to have around the house for general skin irritations and minor burns. To use lavender essential oil, dot it onto individual blemishes with a cotton swab as needed.

Burdock (*Arctium lappa*)

Taken internally, this root promotes sweating and urination. The roots, leaves, and seeds of burdock all can be used, but in commercial preparations, you'll most commonly find the root. Rich in minerals, this plant is used as a food by many cultures. *Typical dosage:* up to 4 cups of tea per day (simmer 1 tablespoon of dried root in 2 cups of water for 15 minutes); or two 400- to 500-milligram capsules three times per day; or 1 to 2 teaspoons of fluid extract three times per day. To use burdock tea as a face wash, make the tea, then cool it and use a clean cloth to apply it to the skin. Rinse with cool water.

Burdock

Dandelion (*Taraxacum officinale*)

Like burdock, dandelion root helps the body dispose of unwanted skin bacteria. It also stimulates digestion and supports the liver— the major organ that helps rid the body of toxins and excess hormones, including the androgens that trigger breakouts. Dandelion leaves are also chock-full of vitamins and minerals, many of which help maintain healthy skin. You can eat the young, fresh leaves raw in salads or steam them. The root, which is usually dried, chopped, and roasted, is moderately anti-inflammatory. *Typical dosage*: 3 to 4 cups of tea per day (simmer 2 teaspoons of dried chopped root in 1 cup of water for 20 minutes or steep 2 teaspoons of dried leaf in 1 cup of hot water for 15 minutes); or two 400- to 500-milligram capsules three times per day; or 1 to 2 teaspoons of fluid extract three times per day.

Calendula (*Calendula officinalis*)

This herb is a traditional remedy for many types of skin problems. Its orange petals are antibacterial and anti-inflammatory, properties that can relieve acne symptoms. To use it, make a tea by steeping 1 teaspoon of dried flowers in 1 cup of hot water for 5 to 10 minutes. Strain, let cool, and apply to the face with a cotton ball or clean cloth.

Vitex (*Vitex agnus-castus*)

If your acne seems hormone-related or is among your premenstrual symptoms, vitex can help. *Typical dosage*: 40 drops liquid

FACE SMOOTHIES

Fruit acids help get rid of excess amounts of the protein keratin and those dead skin cells that may otherwise clog pores. They act like commercial salicylic acid formulas without the side effects. Herbalist Sunny Mavor, coauthor of *Kids, Herbs, and Health,* suggests putting fruits, such as grapes and strawberries or pineapple husks, into a blender. Apply the mixture like a mask; leave on for 10 to 15 minutes, and wash off. Or look for natural face products that contain fruit acids.

ANTIBACTERIAL WASH OR PASTE

These two recipes use the antibacterial properties of two berberine-containing herbs.

To make a wash:

> **2 teaspoons chopped dried Oregon graperoot or goldenseal root**
> **2 cups water**

Simmer all ingredients for 10 to 15 minutes. Strain and cool; use to wash face or soak a clean cloth and use as a compress.

To make a paste:

> **1 teaspoon powdered Oregon graperoot or goldenseal root**
> **A few drops of water**
> **5 drops lavender oil**

Mix all ingredients. Apply to pimples; let dry. Rinse or gently wash off.
NOTE: Oregon graperoot stains fabric.

extract each morning; or 1 capsule dried extract each morning. *Caution*: Do not use during pregnancy.

Oregon Graperoot (*Berberis aquifolium*) and Goldenseal (*Hydrastis canadensis*)

Each of these herbs may help acne in two ways. First, each promotes good digestion and liver function, which help the body get rid of toxins. Second, berberine, which both herbs contain, is a potent antibacterial herb. To use as a wash, see "Antibacterial Wash or Paste." *Typical dosage*: up to six 500- to 600-milligram capsules per day in divided doses; or 10 to 20 drops of tincture three times per day. *Caution*: Do not use either herb internally during pregnancy (external use is safe).

Chamomile (*Matricaria recutita*)

Here's a cheery flowering herb containing the anti-inflammatory essential oil azulene, named for its blue color. To use chamomile, make a skin wash by steeping 1 tablespoon dried flowers in 1 cup of hot water for 10 minutes. Strain and apply with a cotton ball or clean cloth. You can also dab the essential oil onto blemishes, or look for skin-care products that contain chamomile or azulene.

Rose (*Rosa* spp.)

Heavenly smell, soothing, antiseptic action—what's not to love about roses for natural skin care? Look for rosewater made with real rose essential oil. Put it into a spray bottle, close your eyes, and spritz on your face as often as you like.

Grapefruit Seed Extract

This potent antimicrobial agent is useful in any condition that involves fighting bacteria. To use, add 5 drops of grapefruit seed extract to ½ cup of water and use as a face wash; or add 5 drops to ¼ cup of witch hazel mixed with ½ cup of apple cider vinegar and use as a toner when you wash your face.

Aloe (*Aloe vera*)

This soothing, anti-inflammatory, antibacterial gel helps heal wounds of all kinds. Buy only the pure gel and use topically as needed.

Altitude Sickness

For some people, exercising is challenging enough at sea level. But if you're at heights of 8,000 feet or above and are unaccustomed to these altitudes, exercise—or even a moderate stroll—can produce altitude sickness.

Symptoms of altitude sickness may mimic those of flu or a mild hangover. You may feel headache, insomnia, weakness, poor appetite, nausea, and an all-over ill feeling. When you exert yourself,

WARNING SIGNS TO TAKE SERIOUSLY

The following symptoms may indicate altitude-induced accumulation of fluid in the brain (cerebral edema) or lungs (pulmonary edema). Both are very serious, even life-threatening, conditions. If you or a companion shows any of the following symptoms, get immediate medical assistance and arrange to descend immediately.

- ◆ Lack of coordination or stumbling gait
- ◆ Bad headache unrelieved by pain medication
- ◆ Severe nausea and vomiting
- ◆ Impaired judgment, confusion
- ◆ Shortness of breath at rest
- ◆ Coughing or gurgling sounds when breathing
- ◆ Coughing of white or pink foamy sputum

you might be short of breath. If you have a headache—the most common altitude sickness complaint—it'll be throbbing, focused at the front of your head. It'll be worse in the morning and upon lying down, and exercise will aggravate it.

Perhaps worst of all, people with altitude sickness often can't sleep, despite an almost overwhelming fatigue. The hands, feet, and tissues around the eyes sometimes swell. In severe cases, nausea and vomiting may occur.

What causes altitude sickness? At higher altitudes, the amount of available oxygen is less. This drop in oxygen affects the muscles, heart, lungs, and nervous system. Making an altitude transition too quickly increases the likelihood, severity, and duration of symptoms you may experience. Unfortunately, no one can predict your chances of getting altitude sickness. Ironically, being in good physical shape doesn't lower your risk.

Now the good news: For most people, symptoms subside within one to five days as their bodies begin to adjust. And although it's unpleasant, altitude sickness usually isn't serious.

Your best bet for avoiding altitude sickness is to ascend gradually. If you have the time, give your body a chance to adjust by resting for a day at an intermediate elevation (5,000 to 7,000 feet) before continuing to loftier destinations. If symptoms such as headache, nausea, dizziness, or impaired mental processes occur, don't ascend farther until they disappear.

◆ **Drink lots of water.** You lose more fluids at drier, higher altitudes, especially when exercising. While maintaining your fluid intake doesn't prevent altitude sickness, it does help you avoid headache caused by dehydration alone.

◆ **Avoid alcohol.** It increases urination, aggravating dehydration. Also, high alcohol consumption depresses your breathing rate, further lowering blood oxygen.

◆ **Don't take sleeping pills.** Like alcohol, they can slow your breathing. Instead, try a bedtime bath—or at least a foot bath, if you're camping—for a safer sleep aid than pills. Adding about 10 drops of lavender essential oil to the water can help unwind your muscles and your mind.

A few herbs have been researched for preventing or treating altitude sickness. Most herbalists recommend starting to take them one to three days before departure.

Drug Treatment

Pain relievers
Aspirin, acetaminophen, ibuprofen, naproxen. *Function*: ease the headaches that come with altitude sickness (only aspirin has been studied for its ability to prevent such headaches). *Aspirin side effects*: heartburn, indigestion, stomach irritation, and mild nausea or vomiting. *Acetaminophen side effects*: chronic use or higher dosages may damage the liver and kidneys. *Ibuprofen and naproxen side effects*: continuous use may irritate stomach lining; long-term high-dose use may damage the liver and kidneys.

Other Drugs
Acetazolamide (Diamox, Acetazolam). *Function*: prevent altitude sickness when used in advance of climbing, or treat altitude sick-

ness that has already occurred. *Side effects*: increased urination, drowsiness, tingling and numbness of fingers and lips, gastrointestinal upset, blurred vision, flat taste when drinking carbonated drinks.

Dexamethasone (Deronil, Dexasone, Dexone). *Function:* treat altitude sickness. *Side effects:* acne, nausea, vomiting, headache, insomnia, euphoria, dizziness, increased appetite.

HERBAL REMEDIES

Ginkgo (*Ginkgo biloba*)

This herb improves the brain's circulation and its ability to tolerate low oxygen levels, inhibits brain swelling due to trauma or toxins, and inactivates damaging substances called free radicals. Ginkgo's effectiveness in preventing altitude sickness has been borne out by research in humans.

In one study, researchers gave 44 people headed for a Himalayan expedition either 80 milligrams of ginkgo extract or a placebo (fake pill) twice a day for several days before they began the expedition. None of the climbers taking ginkgo experienced headache, nausea, or a feeling of sickness. The group that took ginkgo had fewer respiratory symptoms and fewer problems keeping their hands and feet warm after being exposed to the cold. *Typical dosage*: 3 capsules containing at least 40 to 50 milligrams of standardized extract per day. *Caution*: Allergic reactions are rare but possible. Some people may experience gastrointestinal upset or headaches. Experts have some concerns about combining routine use of aspirin or blood thinners with ginkgo.

Reishi (*Ganoderma lucidum*)

This time-honored Chinese remedy seems to improve blood oxygenation. According to James A. Duke, Ph.D., renowned herbalist and author of *The Green Pharmacy* and *Dr. Duke's Essential Herbs,* a study of Chinese people who climbed above 15,000 feet over three days in Tibet found that reishi greatly reduced altitude sickness.

Reishi

Typical dosage: up to five 420-milligram capsules per day; or 2 teaspoons of tincture three times per day; or up to three 1,000-milligram tablets up to three times per day. One study suggests that travelers to high-altitude destinations take reishi throughout their journey and for several days after.

Ginseng (*Panax ginseng*)

Shown to improve respiratory function and blood oxygenation, ginseng may help people with asthma or bronchitis tolerate altitude. It may also help prevent symptoms of altitude sickness. *Typical dosage*: up to four 500- to 600-milligram capsules per day; or 100 milligrams of standardized products once or twice per day. Take for as long as symptoms persist. *Caution*: Don't take Panax ginseng if you have high blood pressure or are pregnant; do not combine with caffeine, MAO-inhibiting antidepressants, or blood thinners such as warfarin (Coumadin). Many practitioners recommend taking a one-week break after three weeks of use.

Siberian Ginseng (*Eleutherococcus senticosus*)

Studies in China have shown this herb helps prevent altitude sickness. Siberian ginseng is also a well-known tonic herb, one that improves overall health when taken long-term. If you visit the mountains regularly, you can take it for six to eight weeks, followed by a one- to two-week break. If you want it to prevent altitude sickness for a particular trip, some research suggests that you need to begin taking it one to two days before ascending. *Typical dosage*: up to nine 400- to 500-milligram capsules per day; or up to 20 drops of tincture up to three times per day.

Ginger (*Zingiber officinale*)

This spice is a proven nausea remedy. It can come in handy for the nausea associated with altitude sickness or provoked by driving on winding mountain roads. Take it in whatever form seems most appetizing: as a tea, tincture, capsules, raw, or crystallized. Be aware that many commercial ginger ales use flavoring, not real ginger. *Typical dosage*: up to eight 500- to 600-milligram capsules per day; or ½ to 1 teaspoon of the ground root per day; or 10 to 20 drops of tincture in water per day, as needed. *Caution*: Don't take ginger if you have gallbladder disease.

ANGINA

A NGINA, SOMETIMES CALLED angina pectoris, is the pain that oc-curs when your heart isn't getting enough oxygen. You feel a sensation of heaviness or pressure in the middle of your chest. Sometimes the pain radiates to your left arm, throat, or jaw.

Exercise, a large meal, emotional upset, or stress can bring on an attack of angina. But the condition that makes such attacks possible is narrowing of the coronary arteries, which carry oxygen-rich blood to the heart.

What makes these arteries leading to the heart become narrower? Little clumps of cholesterol-based substances called plaques, which accumulate along the artery walls. It's similar to the gunk that builds up in the pipe draining your kitchen sink.

Elevated blood cholesterol is one cause of plaque, but it's not the sole cause. According to current theories, the initial step for plaque formation is an injury to the inner lining of the artery, called the endothelium.

What causes that injury? Scientists don't yet know for certain. But as in the beginning of a murder mystery, many suspects have been implicated. Cigarette smoking is one common cause, as are the normal chemical processes of aging. Vitamin B_6 deficiency is thought to play a role. Other possible factors include immune-system malfunctions; physical injury; viral, bacterial, or chemical assaults; drug use; and poor diet. Also, certain chemical agents can cause blood cells called platelets to clump together, helping plaque to form.

Angina is a serious problem and should never be ignored; it can lead to a heart attack. This is no time to play the stoic. If angina-like symptoms begin to occur with greater frequency or with less provo-cation than usual, they could be a sign of worsening heart disease and impending heart attack. And if you have any undiagnosed chest pain, see your doctor immediately for an evaluation.

Because angina is such a serious disease, you must continue to see your family physician or cardiologist on a regular basis. If you are on medications for angina, work with an experienced herbalist—there are many potentially dangerous ways that drugs for

Three Supplements to Investigate

People whose diets are habitually deficient in certain nutrients tend to be more prone to heart disease. In addition to overhauling your own eating habits, you may want to check with a nutritionist about supplementing your diet with a broad spectrum of vitamins. Meanwhile, supplementing your diet with the following three nutrients can help if you experience angina.

◆ **Bromelain.** Made from certain enzymes in pineapple, bromelain has anti-inflammatory effects, stops platelets from sticking together, and has been shown in studies to break down arterial plaques and ease angina. *Typical dosage:* 250 to 500 milligrams three times per day on an empty stomach. *Caution:* Bromelain may occasionally cause stomach upset—just as eating too much fresh pineapple can.

◆ **L-carnitine.** This amino acid is involved with energy production at the cellular level. It increases the efficiency of oxygen use within the heart muscle; it also lowers cholesterol. In clinical studies, angina patients who took L-carnitine could exercise more, and when they exercised as much as they could, their EKG readings were improved. *Typical dosage:* 750 to 1,500 milligrams per day in divided doses.

◆ **Coenzyme Q$_{10}$.** Like L-carnitine, this vitamin-like substance is involved with energy production in the cells. In one small study, patients with stable angina reduced their episodes of chest pain by more than half, and the amount of time they could spend on a treadmill before experiencing chest pain increased by a full minute. *Typical dosage:* 150 milligrams per day in divided doses.

the heart and herbs can interact. Do not stop taking prescribed medications on your own.

Herbal treatments for angina focus on preventing attacks. Once an episode of angina is occurring, take your nitroglycerin. Herbs can do much for angina—lower blood cholesterol, prevent and heal injuries to the endothelium of arteries, prevent the clumping of blood platelets, shrink plaques, and expand or dilate involved arteries. Herbs can also strengthen the heart in general, especially the herbs that improve energy metabolism within the heart.

DRUG TREATMENT

Nitrates
Under-the-tongue nitroglycerin (tablets or spray), isorbide dinitrate (Dilatrate-SR, Isordil, Sorbitrate), isorbide mononitrate (Imdur, Ismo, Monoket), nitroglycerin ointment (Nitrobid). *Function*: reduce angina pain by relaxing the smooth muscles in the coronary arteries. *Side effects*: headache, slight decrease in blood pressure.

Beta Blockers
Propranolol (Inderal), metroprolol (Lopressor), labetalol (Normodyne, Trandate), others. *Function*: decrease the heart's oxygen consumption by reducing the strength of its contractions, as well as blood pressure and heart rate. *Side effects*: heart failure, too-low heart rate, spasms and narrowing of airway passages, decrease in HDL cholesterol, memory and concentration problems, depression, sexual dysfunction, altered sleep, fatigue.

Calcium Channel Blockers
Nifedipine (Adalat, Procardia), diltiazem (Cardizem, Dilacor, Tiazac), verapamil (Calan, Covera, Isoptin), others. *Function*: inhibit the movement of calcium into cells, dilate coronary vessels and reduce the heart's demand for oxygen. *Side effects*: flushing, low blood pressure, dizziness, swelling, headache, heart failure, heart rhythm irregularities.

Other Drugs
Aspirin. *Function*: decrease risk of heart attack by preventing platelets from sticking together. *Side effects*: heartburn, indigestion, stomach irritation, mild nausea or vomiting.

HERBAL REMEDIES

Garlic (*Allium sativum*) and Onion (*A. cepa*)

These two wonderful foods are good medicine for the heart. Both contain substances that discourage platelets from sticking together and prevent blood clots. They also lower total cholesterol and triglycerides, another type of blood fat, all the while increasing HDL, the "good" cholesterol. Just include one clove of garlic or half a small onion in your daily diet; use them raw or cook them as little as possible to preserve their beneficial compounds.Only garlic comes in supplement form. *Typical dosage*: standardized capsules that deliver a daily dose of at least 10 milligrams of allicin.

Ginkgo (*Ginkgo biloba*)

Much scientific research has confirmed the traditional value of ginkgo in the prevention of angina and the treatment of cardiovascular disease. Ginkgo is an antioxidant and helps neutralize harmful molecules called free radicals. It makes heart cells more efficient and increases blood supply to the extremities. It also has a tonic effect on blood vessels, gradually improving their overall health, and it keeps platelets from sticking together. *Typical dosage*: 40 to 80 milligrams of capsules standardized to 24 percent heterosides, three times per day. *Caution*: Rare cases of gastrointestinal upset, headache, and dizziness have been reported.

Hawthorn (*Crataegus* spp.)

We now know that this traditional European herb used in treating heart disease dilates coronary arteries, thus increasing blood supply to the heart. It improves energy-producing processes in the heart, including oxygenation and energy metabolism, and it decreases lactic acid, the waste product of exertion that causes heart muscle pain. Hawthorn also helps strengthen artery walls. It's antioxidant and anti-inflammatory, and it reduces cholesterol. Products typically use either the flowers and leaves or the berries; both are helpful but the berries are stronger. *Typical dosage:* 1 cup of tea three times per day (simmer 1 teaspoon of dried berries or steep 1 teaspoon of leaves and flowers in 1 cup of hot water for 10 to 15 minutes); or ½ to 1 teaspoon of tincture three times per day; or 100 to 250 milligrams of capsules standardized to 20 percent proanthocyanidins three times per day.

Coleus (*Coleus forskohlii*)

Coleus works primarily by activating an enzyme called cAMP. Among other things, cAMP prevents platelets from sticking together, relaxes arterial muscles, and improves heart function. *Typical dosage*: 50 milligrams of capsules standardized to 18 percent forskolin two or three times per day. *Caution*: Use coleus carefully if your blood pressure is already too low or if you are on medication for your blood pressure. Coleus can also increase the effects of antihistamine drugs.

Coleus

Khella (*Ammi visnaga*, syn. *Daucus visnaga*)

This herb dilates coronary arteries. Several scientific studies have verified its effectiveness in treating angina. It also improves exercise tolerance and normalizes heart rhythms in patients with angina. *Typical dosage*: 250 or 300 milligrams of capsules standardized to 12 percent khellin per day. *Caution*: At higher dosages, nausea, decreased appetite, and dizziness may occur. If this happens, reduce your dose.

Ginger (*Zingiber officinale*)

This aromatic herb may help reduce angina episodes by lowering cholesterol and preventing platelets from sticking together. It works best if eaten fresh and on an empty stomach. *Typical dosage*: up to ¼-inch slice of an average-size root daily; or 250 milligrams per day of freeze-dried fresh root in capsules. *Caution*: Ginger may cause upset stomach, especially at higher doses.

ANXIETY

YOU'RE WALKING ALONE to your car after a late-night meeting. You hear footsteps behind you and a menacing voice says, "Hey you!" Immediately you are flooded with feelings of fear. Your heart pounds, your palms sweat, you feel nauseated. And it doesn't matter that the stranger turns out to be the garage attendant returning the glove that fell from your coat pocket. You still feel the effects of what you thought was a threat.

What you're experiencing is known as the fight-or-flight response, a series of profound physiological changes that occur in reaction to a perceived threat. Your body's nervous system has signaled your adrenal glands to prepare your body to run away or stand your ground. In a split second, a cascade of biological events takes place that affects every organ in your body.

On anxiety-provoking occasions, large amounts of stress hormones, including epinephrine (adrenaline), are secreted into the bloodstream. These hormones cause your heart rate to increase. Your body diverts blood from your skin and internal organs to your muscles and brain. Your blood sugar spikes upward, while your digestive juices decrease dramatically. You breathe faster, and you sweat more. The purpose of all these changes is to enable you to perform the strenuous physical exertions that might be required to fend off an attack or flee whatever is causing your anxiety.

The problem with this elaborate biological response is that it occurs even when the source of anxiety doesn't require physical action, such as when your boss calls you into his office on the spur of the moment, or the IRS informs you that you're being audited. These brief, episodic events provoke a stress response.

That response may be related to specific stimuli (sometimes called phobias), such as flying on an airplane, driving over a bridge, or standing at the edge of a cliff. Or it can be chronic and generalized, not caused by any specific event. Some people seem to be anxious all the time. Their nervous systems and adrenal glands are overactive and respond inappropriately to all kinds of environmental stimuli.

When such anxiety is frequent or chronic, adrenal exhaustion re-

IF YOU'RE TAKING ANTIANXIETY DRUGS, READ THIS

If you are taking antianxiety or antidepressant drugs, do not try to self-medicate with herbs. Some unusual negative side effects, including excessive sedation, have been observed with combinations of herbs and drugs. Also, do not try to withdraw from long-term use of antianxiety drugs on your own. This can be very dangerous. If you are currently using antianxiety drugs, you must work with an experienced physician if you want to switch to natural remedies or combine them with drugs.

sults. You experience fatigue, decreased ability to handle stress, and increased susceptibility to disease of all kinds.

If you experience chronic anxiety and it is recent or unexplained, or if you have new physical symptoms or are taking a new medication, it's important to get a medical evaluation. Occasionally, anxiety can have a physical or biochemical basis.

For phobias and irrational fears, various forms of psychotherapy, such as hypnosis, can be sufficient. Try to choose a therapist with experience in treating phobias.

HOW TO TAKE HERBS FOR ANXIETY

Many plant medicines alleviate occasional anxiety. This chapter lists them from mildest to strongest. It's a good idea to try out these herbs before an anxiety-producing event so that you can gauge your body's response, decide how much of a product you need to take, and identify any side effects.

Sensitivity to this group of herbs is extremely individualized; some people can relax with one cup of chamomile tea, while for others, it takes several doses of a much more potent herb. Although falling asleep while on an airplane is no problem, that's not the reaction you want during an important business presentation.

So start with a small dose, but pay attention to your body's reac-

Other Ways to Ease the Worries

The following strategies may help you keep anxiety at bay.

◆ Avoid stimulants. Various common stimulants increase anxiety by activating the adrenal glands. When used regularly, such stimulants contribute to adrenal exhaustion. These include caffeine as well as caffeine-containing herbs such guarana and kola nut. Ephedra (ma huang) is another stimulant herb that can dramatically increase anxiety.

◆ Improve your diet and nutrition. Deficiencies of certain vitamins and minerals have all been associated with anxiety. These include the B vitamins, vitamins C and E, calcium, magnesium, phosphorus, potassium, selenium, and omega-3 and omega-6 essential fatty acids. The stress of chronic anxiety may increase your need for these nutrients. Consider consulting a nutritionist to check for deficiencies, especially if your diet hasn't been the greatest.

◆ Work it all out. Exercise is one of the best anxiety-management techniques. It can stimulate the brain to produce its own calming chemicals. Because anxiety prepares the body for physical exertion, exercise may help to dissipate all those stress hormones in the most appropriate way. Any physical activity can be effective, but aerobic activity—walking briskly, running, bicycling, or any exercise that gets the heart rate up for a sustained period of time—has additional benefits.

tions. You can repeat dosages of antianxiety herbs as often as every two hours if necessary. If you are taking capsules, follow directions on the bottle, but increase the dose if needed. As long as you are increasing your dosage gradually and you are not overly sedated or experiencing other negative effects, these herbs are all safe. (If you want to take half a capsule of powdered herb or herbal extract, open the capsule, discard half of the contents, and put the two halves of the capsule back together.)

Most antianxiety herbs are compatible and enhance each other's effects, so don't be afraid to try combining these products. But be sure to check out "If You're on Antianxiety Drugs, Read This" on page 85, which explains the dangers of combining herbs with antianxiety drugs.

If your anxiety is frequent or chronic, the herbs you use should be taken every day on a regular schedule. If your anxiety occurs only during a specific activity, such as flying on an airplane or giving a speech, take the herbs a half-hour to one hour before you get on the airplane or step up to the podium.

DRUG TREATMENT

Benzodiazepines
Alprazolam (Xanax), chlordiazepoxide (Librium), clonazepam (Klonipin), diazepam (Valium), others. *Function*: bind to specific receptor sites in the brain, prompting it to produce anxiety-reducing chemicals. *Side effects*: sedation, impaired memory; tolerance and physical dependence with long-term use.

Beta Blockers
Propranolol (Inderal). *Function*: block symptoms of short-term anxiety, such as rapid heart rate and sweating. *Side effects*: oversedation, drop in heart rate, low blood pressure.

Selective Serotonin Reuptake Inhibitors (SSRIs)
Fluoxetine (Prozac), sertraline (Zoloft), paroxetine (Paxil), fluvoxamine (Luvox), others. *Function*: prevent the breakdown of serotonin, a mood-controlling brain chemical. *Side effects*: agitation, anxiety, insomnia, tremor, headache, nausea, sexual dysfunction; less commonly, paradoxical sedation.

Tricyclic Antidepressants
Amitriptyline (Elavil, Limbitrol), imipramine (Tofranil), doxepin (Adapin, Sinequan), others. *Function*: adjust the metabolism of several hormones and brain chemicals. *Side effects*: sedation, dry mouth, constipation, low blood pressure.

Other Drugs

Buspirone (Buspar). *Function*: inhibit the breakdown of serotonin, a mood-controlling brain chemical. *Side effects*: none common.

Herbal Remedies

Oats (*Avena sativa*)

Soothing and nourishing, oats are good for anyone whose nervous system feels frayed or stressed. In selecting the dried herb for tea, pick green- to yellow-colored seeds, not something that looks like chopped straw; the seeds are stronger medicinally. *Typical dosage*: 1 cup of tea up to every two hours (steep 1 to 2 teaspoons of seeds in 1 cup of hot water for 10 minutes); or ⅛ to 3 teaspoons of tincture up to every two hours; or follow manufacturer's directions for capsules.

Chamomile (*Matricaria recutita*)

This old-time remedy for anxiety still works, relaxing and toning the nervous system, relaxing the muscles, and easing the digestive complaints that may accompany anxiety. *Typical dosage*: 1 cup of tea up to every two hours (steep 1 to 2 teaspoons of dried flowers in 1 cup of hot water for 10 minutes); or ⅛ to 3 teaspoons of tincture up to every two hours; or follow manufacturer's directions for capsules.

Linden (*Tilia* spp.)

Gently relaxing with antispasmodic effects that ease muscle tension, linden is also a remedy for high blood pressure (especially when it's made worse by anxiety or stress) and a tonic for the cardiovascular system in general. It makes a pleasant-tasting cup of tea. *Typical dosage*: 1 cup of tea up to every two hours (steep 1 to 2 teaspoons of dried flowers in 1 cup of hot water for 10 minutes); or ⅛ to 3 teaspoons of tincture up to every two hours; or follow manufacturer's directions for capsules.

Linden

Vervain (*Verbena officinalis*)

This herb soothes and calms the nervous system and addresses any depression that might be present. It is also beneficial for the liver, if that organ is stressed or damaged. *Typical dosage*: 1 cup of tea up to every two hours (steep 1 to 2 teaspoons of dried herb in 1 cup of hot water for 10 minutes); or ⅛ to 3 teaspoons tincture up to every two hours; or follow manufacturer's directions for capsules.

Motherwort (*Leonurus cardiaca*)

A tonic for the cardiovascular system in general, this traditional remedy has many beneficial actions. It is particularly useful when anxiety is associated with rapid heart rate. It can be considered a specific aid for anxiety associated with a heart condition called mitral valve prolapse. *Typical dosage*: 1 cup of tea up to every two hours (steep 1 to 2 teaspoons of dried herb in 1 cup of hot water for 10 minutes); or ⅛ to 3 teaspoons of tincture up to every two hours; or follow manufacturer's directions for capsules. *Caution*: Do not use with other cardiac drugs unless under a doctor's supervision; avoid during pregnancy or nursing.

Lavender (*Lavandula angustifolia*)

Lovely, fragrant, relaxing, and uplifting—these words describe lavender, which relieves both anxiety and depression. Because of its wonderful smell, consider using the essential oil applied to the skin, inhaled, or added to a warm bath. To use, add 10 to 12 drops to a bath, or dilute with an equal amount of vegetable oil (almond, olive, or sesame) and use as a massage oil. *Caution*: Don't use essential oils internally.

St.-John's-Wort (*Hypericum perforatum*)

While more commonly used to treat depression, this herb is really a tonic, or overall health booster, for the entire nervous system. Do not use St.-John's-wort as a tea, however; it loses its potency as it dries. *Typical dosage*: ⅛ to 3 teaspoons of tincture up to every two hours; or 300 milligrams (standardized to 0.3 percent hypericin) of capsules three times per day.

Hops (*Humulus lupulus*)

A moderately strong remedy for relaxing the central nervous system, hops is also a good herb to use for insomnia and for tension headaches. Some herbalists recommend avoiding this herb if depression is part of the picture, as hops might worsen those feelings. *Typical dosage*: 1 cup of tea before bedtime (steep one heaping teaspoon of whole dried herb in 1 cup of hot water for 10 to 15 minutes); or ⅛ to 3 teaspoons of tincture up to every two hours.

Skullcap (*Scutellaria lateriflora*)

Skullcap is nourishing and relaxing to the entire nervous system. It is useful for anxiety of all kinds, particularly for the anxiety and irritability associated with hormonal swings, such as in premenstrual syndrome and in menopause. *Typical dosage*: 1 cup of tea up to every two hours (steep 1 to 2 teaspoons of dried herb in 1 cup of hot water for 10 minutes); or ⅛ to 3 teaspoons of tincture up to every two hours; or follow manufacturer's directions for capsules.

Kava-Kava (*Piper methysticum*)

Significant scientific research on this important antianxiety herb from the South Pacific Islands has identified its active constituents, called kavalactones. They appear to work by modifying, but not binding to, benzodiazepine and certain receptors in the brain. These are the same receptors that allow drugs such as Valium to work. Kavalactones mainly act in the limbic system, a part of the brain that influences all other parts of the nervous system and is considered the principal seat of emotions.

Unlike most pharmaceuticals used to treat anxiety, kava does not cause addiction or tolerance over time. One study among menopausal women showed that kava not only decreased their anxiety but also reduced hot flashes. Kava can also help alleviate pain. Moreover, despite its relaxing effects, it does not decrease intellectual functioning. It might even improve intellectual ability, such as memory, according to a study that compared kava with a placebo (fake pill) and with the antianxiety drug Oxazepam. Volunteers who took kava

Kava-kava

did better than the placebo group in several measures of memory; the Oxazepam group did worse.

This means kava is a good choice to treat short-term situational anxiety. *Typical dosage*: up to six 400- to 500-milligram capsules per day; or ⅛ to 3 teaspoons of tincture up to every two hours. *Caution*: Do not use during pregnancy or nursing. Do not combine with alcohol.

Valerian (*Valeriana officinalis*)

Here is a good, strong antianxiety herb. Its active ingredients, valepotriates, bind to benzodiazepine receptor sites in the brain—a mechanism similar to the action of drugs such as Valium. The herb, however, seems to be more beneficial to the nervous system, and it does not cause dependence or tolerance.

Several studies show that valerian also improves the quality of sleep. It is an excellent muscle relaxant for both skeletal and smooth muscles (those in the digestive tract, the blood vessels, and the uterus, for example). *Typical dosage*: 300 to 400 milligrams standardized to 0.5 percent essential oil in capsules per day (one hour before bedtime if using as a sleep aid); or ⅛ to 3 teaspoons of tincture up to every two hours. *Caution*: For a small percentage of the population, valerian increases anxiety and causes an unpleasant restlessness. If this happens, discontinue use.

Passionflower (*Passiflora incarnata*)

Generally used for treating insomnia, passionflower is a strong calming herb and is occasionally useful for severe daytime anxiety. It is also a good antispasmodic. *Typical dosage*: 1 cup of tea up to every two hours (steep 1 to 2 teaspoons of herb in 1 cup of hot water for 10 minutes); or ⅛ to 3 teaspoons of tincture up to every two hours; or follow manufacturer's directions for capsules. *Caution*: Do not use with MAO-inhibiting antidepressants unless under the supervision of a doctor.

Siberian Ginseng (*Eleutherococcus senticosus*)

This herb restores overstressed adrenal glands, working wonders for people who are chronically stressed. It's one of the primary tonic herbs, meaning that it works its magic slowly over time, so you'll need to take it for several months to see results. The quality of commercial products varies widely; purchase from a reputable manufacturer. *Typical dosage*: up to nine 400- to 500-milligram capsules per day; or 20 drops of tincture up to three times per day.

Ginseng (*Panax ginseng*)

This type of ginseng, also known as Chinese ginseng, comes in many forms and strengths, so it can be tricky to use if you are not experienced with herbs. However, like Siberian ginseng, it's an effective herb for those who suffer from chronic or long-term anxiety. If you do choose to self-medicate with *Panax ginseng,* use the dried root, or white Asian ginseng, which is the mildest form, rather than the steamed root, known as red ginseng. *Typical dosage*: up to four 500- to 600-milligram capsules per day; or 100 milligrams of standardized products one or two times per day. *Caution*: Ginseng may worsen anxiety in some people, so be sure to use it only under the supervision of an experienced herbalist.

Licorice (*Glycyrrhiza glabra*)

Among its many medicinal benefits, licorice is considered an adrenal tonic; in particular, it increases production of the very chemicals that aid in the body's recovery from chronic anxiety. *Typical dosage*: 1 to 3 cups of tea per day (simmer 1 to 2 teaspoons of dried root in 1 cup of water for 10 minutes); or ⅛ to ½ teaspoon of tincture one to three times per day. *Caution*: Some people find licorice too stimulating; avoid it if you have high blood pressure or heart or liver disease, are pregnant, or are taking diuretics or digitalis-based heart medications.

ARTHRITIS

D O YOU HAVE TROUBLE getting out of bed in the morning—even when you're not sleepy? If you have morning stiffness that lasts 30 minutes or longer, creakiness climbing stairs, or difficulty gripping the lid of a jar to open it, you may have arthritis. You're not alone: This disease affects about 40 million Americans of all ages.

Arthritis is the inflammation of a joint, which makes movement difficult and causes redness, swelling, and sometimes warmth. It can occur in any joint, but it most commonly begins in the fingers, knees, and hips.

There are more than a hundred different types of arthritis, the most common being osteoarthritis and rheumatoid arthritis. Arthritis can also be a symptom of other treatable diseases including infections, Lyme disease, lupus, and Reiter's disease (also called reactive arthritis).

Most Americans show some signs of osteoarthritis by the time they are 40 years old; their symptoms typically worsen with age. Osteoarthritis means that the actual structural components in the joints are wearing out. It sometimes follows a previous injury and is more common among people who have participated in competitive contact sports.

To understand how arthritis produces pain, you need to take a look inside a joint, the place where two or more bones meet. Bones do not actually touch—they are separated by a small space referred to as the synovial space. This space is filled with fluid to allow movement. The fluid is contained in a capsule by a synovial membrane. Finally, the ends of each bone are covered with smooth cartilage, which allows movement with less friction.

In rheumatoid arthritis, the synovial membrane is inflamed. This inflammation creates additional tissue that causes distortion of the joints, which you can see from the outside. Unlike other types of arthritis, the rheumatoid form is an autoimmune disorder. This means that the inflammation in the joints is caused by the body's own immune system, which is not functioning properly. Rheumatoid arthritis usually produces symptoms in a few joints, most commonly the wrists. The inflammation that it causes can also affect the heart, lungs, and brain. Sometimes an attack of rheumatoid arthritis is set off by stress, either emotional or physical.

In those who have osteoarthritis, the joints themselves—especially those in the fingers—sometimes swell and become deformed. Osteoarthritis has less inflammation associated with it than rheumatoid arthritis. One of its distinguishing characteristics is that the affected joint is cool and hard to the touch rather than warm and spongy as in rheumatoid arthritis. Destruction of the cartilage that surrounds the ends of the bones is common in os-

Supplements to Help Relieve Arthritis

The following nutrients can help keep your joints limber and pain-free.

◆ **B vitamins.** One small study showed that arthritis patients improved when they took 6.4 milligrams of folic acid per day and 20 micrograms of vitamin B_{12} per day. Niacin (vitamin B_3) may also provide some relief.

◆ **Vitamins C and D.** This duo has been shown to help osteoarthritis. Vitamin C is essential to the body for making collagen, an important component of joints. Two hundred milligrams of C per day is probably enough; try 500 IU of vitamin D.

◆ **Vitamin E.** This vitamin may help relieve some pain of arthritis. *Typical dosage:* 400 to 600 IU daily.

◆ **Boron.** The Rheumatoid Disease Foundation recommends 3 milligrams of boron per day. Doctors don't know how it works, but where people ingest 1 milligram or less of boron per day, the rate of arthritis is higher.

◆ **Calcium.** This element is an important component of bone. It has been shown to decrease the amount of bone loss that occurs from long-term steroid use. *Typical dosage:* 1,000 milligrams per day.

◆ **Glucosamine sulfate.** This compound makes up the main component of cartilage in joints. It has received much attention, and many people claim that it works wonders. Although it also has its skeptics, many well-designed, short-term studies have shown that glucosamine can decrease arthritis patients' symptoms. Glucosamine is not a pain reliever, however, and it takes four to eight weeks before you feel results. *Typical dosage:* 500 to 1,500 milligrams daily. *Caution:* Glucosamine can cause mild digestive problems and should not be used by people with heart disease or diabetes.

teoarthritis. Small bone spurs then grow from the surface of the bone into the joint. These spurs decrease the mobility of the joint.

Osteoarthritis also tends to run in families. If you have a family history of this disorder, keeping your weight at an optimal level has been shown to decrease your risk of developing it in knee joints.

Ankylosing spondylitis is yet another type of arthritis. It typically affects the spinal column, causing pain and stiffness in the back.

Arthritis can also be associated with inflammatory bowel disease. This type of arthritis can usually be controlled by focusing on controlling the intestinal inflammation.

There is no known cure for arthritis. Doctors prescribe drugs to reduce pain and inflammation in the joints and to prevent further joint damage and deformities. For osteoarthritis, acetaminophen may help, while anti-inflammatory drugs are typically used for rheumatoid arthritis. You'll notice that some pain drugs also reduce inflammation, but acetaminophen isn't one of them.

DRUG TREATMENT

Analgesics

Acetaminophen, acetaminophen with codeine, aspirin. *Function:* decrease pain; codeine helps decrease more severe pain. Aspirin reduces both pain and inflammation. *Acetaminophen side effects:* dizziness, excitement, disorientation, liver damage. *Acetaminophen with codeine side effects:* constipation, dizziness, drowsiness, nausea, weakness, tiredness, vomiting, dependency. *Aspirin side effects:* abdominal cramping and pain, deafness, stomach bleeding, ulcers, nausea and vomiting, ringing in the ears, increased tendency to bleed.

Nonsteroidal Anti-Inflammatories

Indomethicin (Indocin), ibuprofen (Motrin, Advil, Nuprin), mefenamic acid (Ponstel), naproxen (Naprosyn, Naprelan), piroxicam (Feldene). *Function:* block production of prostaglandins, body chemicals that favor inflammation. *Side effects:* abdominal pain and indigestion, dizziness, stomach ulcers and bleeding, nausea, nightmares.

Cox-2 (cyclooxygenase type II) Inhibitors

Celecoxib (Celebrex), refecoxib (Vioxx). *Function:* relieve pain by blocking inflammatory prostaglandins. *Side effects:* abdominal pain, indigestion, dizziness, stomach ulcers and bleeding, nausea, nightmares.

Nonacetylated Salicylates

Magnesium trisalicylate (CMT, Tricosal, Trilisate), choline salicylate (Arthropan), magnesium salicylate (Magan, Doan's Pills, Mobidin), salsalate (Disalcid, Mono-Gesic, Salflex), sodium salicylate (Uracel 5). *Function:* relieve inflammation and pain without stomach upset. *Side effects:* bloating, confusion, deafness, diarrhea, dizziness, heartburn, stomach irritation, rash, ringing in the ears.

Corticosteroids

Cortisone (Cortone Acetate), dexamethasone (Decadron, Hexadrol), hydrocortisone (Cortef), methylprednisolone (Medrol), prednisolone (Prelone), prednisone (Deltasone, Orasone), triamcinolone (Aristocort). *Function:* reduce inflammation. *Side effects:* with long-term use or high dosage, may cause cataracts, high blood pressure, weight gain, thinning of the skin, weakened bones, increased appetite, elevated blood sugar, indigestion, insomnia, mood changes, restlessness, worsened arthritis, increased susceptibility to infection.

Other Drugs

Methotrexate (Rheumatrex). *Function:* suppress the immune system to slow the progression of rheumatoid arthritis. *Side effects:* cough, diarrhea, hair loss, loss of appetite, bleeding, bruising.

Chrysotherapy, gold salts (Auranofin). *Function:* alter the immune system to slow the progression of rheumatoid arthritis. *Side effects:* stomach cramps, bloating, loss of appetite, diarrhea, indigestion, nausea, vomiting, mouth sores, skin rash, sun sensitivity, headaches, lowered white blood cell count, decreased red blood cell numbers, and increased tendency to bleed.

Cyclosporine (Sandimmune, Neoral). *Function:* suppress the immune system to slow the progression of rheumatoid arthritis. *Side effects:* sore gums, high blood pressure, increased hair growth, kidney and liver problems, loss of appetite, tremors.

EASE THE PAIN THESE EASY WAYS

Lifestyle changes can make a difference in controlling arthritis symptoms. Here's what experts recommend.

◆ **Take the waters.** Most practitioners suggest a program of regular exercise, but water exercise is especially good, since it doesn't put additional pressure on the joints. This exercise must be coupled with periods of rest.

◆ **Do a dietary check-in.** Many doctors recommend increasing the amount of whole, unprocessed foods you eat. Some people with arthritis find that a vegetarian diet can reduce the symptoms. You might also find it helpful to cut back on coffee, alcohol, chocolate, and dairy products, since these foods tend to foster inflammation. Food sensitivities or allergies may also play a role in arthritis, and many people find some relief by eliminating certain foods. The most common foods that can affect arthritis are members of the nightshade family, such as eggplants, tomatoes, peppers, and potatoes.

◆ **Watch your weight.** Yes, you've heard it before. But being overweight in relation to the size of your frame and the thickness of your bones puts undue stress on the joints of the lower extremities.

Cyclophosphamide (Cytoxan). *Function:* suppress the immune system to slow progression of rheumatoid arthritis. *Side effects:* blood in the urine, burning on urination, confusion, cough, dizziness, fever and chills, infertility, loss of appetite, nausea and vomiting, bleeding and bruising, weakness and tiredness, missed menstrual periods, infection.

Hydroxychloroquine sulfate (Plaquenil). *Function:* ease the effects of rheumatoid arthritis, though how it works is not well understood. *Side effects:* loss of vision, nerve and muscle weakness.

Penicillamine (Cuprimine, Depen). *Function:* alter the immune system to slow progression of rheumatoid arthritis. *Side effects:*

mouth sores, impaired sense of taste, fever, rash, bleeding, infection, aplastic anemia, kidney damage.

Herbal Remedies

Cayenne and Other Peppers (*Capsicum* spp.)
Peppers contain a strong analgesic and anti-inflammatory agent known as capsaicin. This compound blocks a chemical in the body that acts as a pain signal. You can find capsaicin in many commercial creams and ointments for arthritis pain. *Typical dosage*: a cream containing 0.25 percent to 0.75 percent capsaicin applied daily. *Caution*: Some people experience a slight burning of the skin with capsaicin use. If you do, try a cream with a lower percentage of capsaicin.

Evening Primrose (*Oenothera biennis*)
The seed from this plant contains the essential fatty acid gamma-linolenic acid (GLA), which has an effect on inflamma-

KEEPING JOINTS FROM CREAKING

Remember the Tin Man in *The Wizard of Oz*? His joints were so rusted he could barely squeak out the words, "Oil can. Oil can. . . ." Consuming the following oils won't work on painful joints as quickly as the Tin Man's solution—but they are good substitutes for costly evening primrose oil because of their high levels of either gamma-linolenic acid (GLA) or of the chemicals your body uses to make GLA.

◆ Borage seed oil
◆ Black currant seed oil
◆ Fish oils
◆ Flaxseed oil
◆ Nut oils
◆ Safflower oil

tion. For this reason, the seed oil may significantly help arthritis pain, especially in cases of rheumatoid arthritis. One study showed that patients taking 12 capsules per day of evening prim-rose oil or 540 milligrams of GLA were able to reduce the amount of nonsteroidal anti-inflammatory drugs they were tak-ing. (Evening primrose oil is expensive, but other good sources of GLA are available; see "Keeping Joints from Creaking.") *Typical dosage:* up to 12 capsules per day; or ½ teaspoon of oil per day.

Flaxseed (*Linum usitatissimum*)

The linoleic acid found in flaxseed oil may also be beneficial for arthritis because it alters how the body breaks down prostaglandins, chemicals involved in inflammation. *Typical dosage:* 2 tablespoons of oil per day in food (use on top of cereal or as a salad dressing).

Stinging Nettle (*Urtica dioica*)

This plant is used by some in a process called urtication, accord-ing to James A. Duke, Ph.D., author of *The Green Pharmacy*. What this involves is swatting the aching joint with the whole plant so the nettles scratch the skin. Such a procedure probably works both by distracting the patient—or victim, depending on how you look at it—and by injecting anti-inflammatory chemicals from the plant. There's a much less painful way to take nettles: steaming or drying the leaves removes their sting. Nettles are high in boron, a mineral recommended for arthritis. *Typical dosage:* up to six 435-milligram capsules per day; or 1 cup of tea per day, divided into two or three doses (steep 1 teaspoon of dried herb in 1 cup of hot water for 10 minutes).

Ginger (*Zingiber officinale*)

This root has traditionally been used in India to treat arthritis. Com-ponents of ginger such as gingerol can inhibit the production of prostaglandins possibly more effectively than the arthritis drug in-domethicin. *Typical dosage:* up to eight 500- to 600-milligram cap-sules per day; or ½ to 1 teaspoon fresh ground root per day; or 10 to 20 drops of tincture in water three times per day. *Caution:* Doses of ginger higher than these should not be used by people with diabetes, heart problems, or bleeding problems.

Devil's Claw (*Harpagophytum procumbens*)

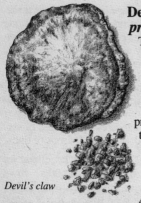

Devil's claw

This herb from Africa has traditionally been used for most types of arthritis. The tubers contain a group of chemicals called iridoids that have anti-inflammatory activity. One clinical study showed patients with arthritis improved when taking one 500-milligram tablet of devil's claw three times per day. Other studies conclude, however, that devil's claw provides no relief for arthritis. It may be best to find out for yourself. *Typical dosage:* up to six 400- or 500-milligram capsules per day; or 30 drops of tincture three times per day. *Caution:* Do not take if you have gastric or duodenal ulcers.

Green Tea (*Camellia sinensis*)

Most of the Eastern world has been drinking green tea for centuries, but only recently has it become the darling of medical research. Scientists now know that green tea—from the same plant as black tea, but processed in a different way—contains compounds called polyphenols that may help the symptoms of rheumatoid arthritis. A study from Case Western Reserve University in Cleveland showed that mice given polyphenols isolated from green tea were protected from developing a disease similar to rheumatoid arthritis. Although this experiment was conducted on mice, similar results might be found in humans. Black tea may also be beneficial. *Typical dosage:* several cups of green tea per day is safe (follow manufacturer's instructions for tea bags). Because green tea extracts vary widely in concentration, follow manufacturers' recommendations on dosage of extracts.

Feverfew (*Tanacetum parthenium*)

Typically thought of as a relief for headache, feverfew has also been used for arthritis. Although no conclusive human studies have been done, in some laboratory studies extracts of feverfew were able to stop certain processes involved in rheumatoid arthritis. *Typical dosage:* up to three 300- or 400-milligram capsules per day;

or two average-sized fresh leaves per day; or 15 to 30 drops of tincture per day. *Caution*: Do not take during pregnancy.

Turmeric (*Curcuma longa*)

A common Indian spice, turmeric has also been used as a treatment for arthritis. Its active ingredient, curcumin, inhibits the production of prostaglandins. This anti-inflammatory property has been confirmed in animal studies. Turmeric can be taken in food, or applied topically to the joint as a poultice to relieve pain. *Typical dosage:* 250 to 500 milligrams of standardized capsules up to three times daily; or up to 1 teaspoon per day in food; or 10 to 30 drops of tincture up to three times per day.

Yucca (*Yucca brevifolia*)

Many Native American tribes use yucca as a food, especially the fruits of this cactus-like plant. It has traditionally been used as an arthritis remedy and studies have confirmed its effectiveness. Human studies have shown that an extract of yucca reduces the swelling, pain, and stiffness of arthritis, though the studies were controversial. Yucca can be used either internally or externally on the joint. *Typical dosage:* up to four 490-milligram capsules per day.

Willow (*Salix alba* and other *Salix* spp.)

Willow is probably the oldest herb known to treat pain and inflammation. The inner bark of this plant contains salicin, which is changed to salicylic acid in the body. The compound in aspirin, acetylsalicylic acid, is derived from salicylic acid. *Typical dosage:* up to six 400-milligram capsules per day.

Boswellia (*Boswellia serrata*)

This gum resin is an Ayurvedic remedy for arthritis. Studies in India have documented its usefulness and products containing boswellia are marketed there. Boswellia is sometimes mixed with turmeric and another Ayurvedic remedy, ashwaganda. *Typical dosage:* up to three 400-milligram capsules per day.

Pineapple (*Ananas comosus*)

When fresh, not canned, this fruit contains bromelain, a compound with anti-inflammatory properties that many people find useful for arthritic conditions. *Typical dosage:* three to four 40-milligram capsules per day; or simply enjoy eating more pineapple in your regular diet.

ASTHMA

THINK OF ASTHMA AS A FORM of respiratory high drama. Just as an actress might wring as much emotion as possible from a simple prop, so the lungs of a person with asthma seize and wheeze over something as innocuous as a pillow covered with cat hair. The difference? The actress has control over her scene; the person with asthma doesn't.

What's going on? People without asthma breathe easily despite a swamp of pollens, molds, animal dander, and cigarette smoke. For a person with asthma, inhaling certain irritants triggers a cascade of events. The smooth muscle encircling the airways constricts, diminishing their diameters. The mucous membranes swell and produce excessive mucus, further narrowing the air passages.

Unfortunately, asthma has become more common in recent years. About 14 million Americans—one-third of them children—have asthma.

Doctors prescribe asthma medications according to the disorder's severity and how frequently attacks happen. Although many asthma drugs cause side effects, they have also saved lives. If you have asthma, you should work in close partnership with your doctor to try herbal remedies; never stop taking any asthma medication or change your dosage without your doctor's approval. Some of the herbs traditionally used for asthma can interact with asthma drugs in negative ways. That said, there are herbs that have been shown through either years of traditional use or medical studies to help people with asthma regain their respiratory health.

DRUG TREATMENT

Beta-Agonists, Bronchodilators

Albuterol (Proventil), pirbuterol (Maxair), metaproterenol (Alupent), salmeterol (Serevent), terbutaline (Brethaire), bitolterol (Tornalate). *Function:* relax the smooth muscle encircling the airways to widen their diameter, also known as bronchodilation. *Side effects:* hand tremor, increased heart rate and blood pressure, dizziness, nervousness.

Inhaled Corticosteroids
Triamcinolone (Azmacort), flunisolide (AeroBid), beclomethasone (Vanceril, Beclovent), budesonide (Pulmicort), fluticasone
(Flovent). *Function:* reduce or prevent inflammation. *Side effects:*
at higher dosages, hoarseness, cough, and oral thrush.

Anticholinergics
Ipratroprium bromide (Atrovent). *Function:* open the airways by
blocking nerves that would otherwise constrict the airways. *Side
effects:* dry mouth, cough.

Adrenergics
Theophylline (Accurbron, Aerolate, Bronkodyl, Pulmophylline,
Slo-Bid, Slophyllin, Theobid, Theo-Dur). *Function:* bronchodilation. *Side effects:* irritability, restlessness, nausea, vomiting, rapid
heartbeat, headache, insomnia.

Oral Corticosteroids
Prednisone (Deltasone), methylprednisolone (Medrol). *Function:* reduce or prevent inflammation. *Side effects:* increased appetite, fluid
retention; with long-term use, muscle weakness, easy bruising, high
blood pressure, depressed immune function, osteoporosis, cataracts.

Leukotriene Antagonists
Zafirlukast (Accolate), montelukast (Singulair), zileuton (Xyflo).
Function: inhibit the formation or action of inflammatory chemi-
cals called leukotrienes. *Side effects:* headache and nausea.

OTHER DRUGS

Cromolyn sodium (Intal, Fivent, others). *Function:* inhibit the release of inflammation-causing chemicals from cells called mast
cells; must be taken every day to be effective. *Side effects:* slight
throat irritation, dry cough.

HERBAL REMEDIES

Ginkgo (*Ginkgo biloba*)
This herb has long been used by the Chinese to treat asthma. The
leaves contain ginkgolides, which inhibit platelet-activating factor,

a chemical involved in asthma and allergies. Small studies on humans show that taking ginkgolides orally reduces narrowing of the airways in response to inhaled allergens and it partially protects against exercise-induced asthma. *Typical dosage:* 40 milligrams of standardized extract three times per day, for six to eight weeks. *Caution:* Rare cases of skin allergies or gastrointestinal upset have occurred. Consult your doctor before using ginkgo if you use aspirin daily or take a blood-thinning drug such as warfarin.

Coffee (*Coffea arabica*) and Tea (*Camellia sinensis*)

Both of these beverages contain caffeine, a chemical cousin to the asthma drug theophylline. Researchers have found that a caffeine dose of 7 milligrams per 2.2 pounds of body weight significantly improves the lung function of people with asthma and prevents exercise-induced asthma attacks. Coffee has between 135 and 150 milligrams of caffeine per 8-ounce cup; tea has about 60 milligrams plus beneficial antioxidants. That means a 150-pound man would have to drink 3 to 3½ cups of coffee to break an asthma attack. Because consuming a lot of caffeine isn't good for your health, taking coffee or tea to prevent asthma is hardly practical. Still, if you start wheezing and have no other asthma drugs or herbs handy, a cup of java might be worth a try.

Garlic (*Allium sativum*) and Onion (*A. cepa*)

These allium family members have long been used to treat bronchitis and asthma. Lab tests show that onion extracts can block the production of certain chemicals involved in inflammation, thereby inhibiting allergen-induced asthmatic responses. The ingredients responsible for this action include mustard oils and quercetin. You can find quercetin, an anti-inflammatory and antioxidant substance, sold as a dietary supplement; follow the package directions for dosage. You can also include lots of onions in your diet. And don't forget onion's cousin, garlic. It also possesses anti-inflammatory, immune-stimulating, and antimicrobial properties. *Typical dosage:* up to three 500- to 600-milligram capsules per day; look for products that contain at least 5,000 micrograms of allicin in a daily dose. Or simply eat one or more raw cloves per day.

Licorice (*Glycyrrhiza glabra*)

This herb acts as an expectorant, demulcent, anti-inflammatory, immune stimulator, and antiviral—all properties of potential

HERBAL STEAMS: GOOD FOR ASTHMA?

Steam inhalation is an age-old remedy for loosening the respiratory mucus associated with colds and coughs. Adding aromatic herbs such as eucalyptus, peppermint, thyme, and rosemary as infusions or essential oils boosts the therapeutic effect. Theoretically, it would seem that an herbal steam is a good idea.

Well, maybe. Some essential oils, notably spruce needle and pine needle oil, can worsen bronchial spasms. And for some people with asthma, just inhaling plain steam can trigger coughing. Proceed with caution if you want to try steam therapy for your asthma. Try plain steam first. If that doesn't provoke an attack, try simmering ½ cup of herbs in 4 cups of water for 10 minutes and breathing the steam. If you tolerate the herbs well, then try substituting 3 drops of essential oil for the herbs.

In all cases, carefully pour water in a heat resistant bowl and place it on a sturdy table. Put a towel over your head and hold your face at least 12 inches away from the steam. If any of these steams sets off a bout of coughing or wheezing, stop.

benefit for people with asthma. Licorice slows the breakdown of the body's corticosteroids such as cortisol, thus prolonging the anti-inflammatory effects of this hormone. *Typical dosage:* up to six 400- to 500-milligram capsules per day; or 20 to 30 drops of tincture up to three times per day. (Note: If you have asthma, you'll want to use whole-root products rather than deglycyrrhizinated, or DGL, licorice, which does not contain the active ingredient glycyrrhizin.) *Caution:* Do not take licorice for more than six weeks unless under the supervision of a health practitioner. People who take corticosteroids should not take licorice without consulting their doctor. Do not take licorice at all if you have high blood pressure, diabetes, disease of the thyroid, kidney, liver, or heart; if you're using diuretics; or if you are pregnant or nursing.

Other Ways to Ease Asthma

Besides herbs, other therapies may help reduce your asthma symptoms.

◆ **Acupuncture.** Researchers have found that acupuncture often leads to significant improvement of asthma and other chronic lung conditions and often results in reduced need for medication. Side effects are minimal.

◆ **Yoga.** A number of studies have found that yoga training improves overall well-being, promotes greater relaxation, increases exercise tolerance, and lessens the need for asthma medications.

◆ **Diet changes.** Studies have shown that putting adults on a vegan diet—a diet that eliminates all animal products, including dairy and eggs—significantly improves asthma. Researchers believe this diet may work because it increases antioxidants and other helpful botanical chemicals and reduces pro-inflammatory chemicals that are abundant in animal foods. Even if you're not interested in becoming a strict vegetarian, your asthma may improve when you decrease the amount of meat, eggs, and dairy in your diet and increase the amount of fruits, vegetables, and grains.

Ephedra (*Ephedra sinica*)

This herb has a 5,000-year history of use in Chinese medicine as an asthma treatment. It contains ephedrine, which is similar in structure to your body's own adrenaline. It decreases congestion and opens the airways. But because ephedra stimulates the cardiovascular and nervous systems, it can also produce restlessness, anxiety, tremor, insomnia, headache, and elevated blood pressure and heart rate. Ephedra is best used under the supervision of a trained herbal practitioner. *Typical dosage:* 15 to 30 drops of tincture in water up to four times per day; or follow manufacturer's or practitioner's directions. *Caution:* Do not use if you have high blood pressure, heart disease, glaucoma, anorexia, hyperthroidism, or diabetes, nor by those taking theophylline or MAO-inhibiting antidepressants. If you're taking other asthma drugs, check with your doctor before taking ephedra. Do not combine with caffeine use; do not use while pregnant.

Coleus (*Coleus forskohlii*)

This plant is used in Ayurvedic remedies in India. It contains forskolin, a substance that relaxes the smooth muscle of airways, opening them for easier breathing. In an Austrian study, forskolin inhaled as a dry powder helped open the airways in asthma patients. So far, no studies have investigated the impact on asthma patients of whole coleus or forskolin taken in capsules. Despite this lack of research, forskolin is used in inhalers in Europe. In the United States, it's available as a standardized extract in capsules. For dosage, follow manufacturer's or practitioner's instructions.

Ephedra

Reishi (*Ganoderma lucidum*)

This medicinal mushroom boasts several healthful effects, including an ability to reduce allergies. Reishi inhibits some of the chemical mediators of inflammation, including histamine. In China, it is used to treat asthma and other allergic diseases. Reishi can also benefit people with asthma because it acts as an immune tonic. Increased resistance to infections might derail colds and the flu, which often provoke asthma symptoms. *Typical dosage:* up to five 420-milligram capsules per day; or up to three 1,000 milligram tablets per day.

Turmeric (*Curcuma longa*)

This herb is one of the main spices in curry. It contains curcumin, which has anti-inflammatory, antiviral, antioxidant, and antitumor activity. Further research is needed to prove that this spicy component helps once it's in the human body, but in the meantime, it won't hurt to include turmeric on your spice shelf. *Typical dosage:* 250 to 300 milligrams in standardized capsules, up to three times per day; up to 1 teaspoon of ground spice in food per day; or 10 to 30 drops of tincture up to three times per day. *Caution:* Do not use if you have gallstones or any obstruction of the bile ducts.

Rosemary (*Rosmarinus officinalis*)

This common culinary herb has been used traditionally to ease asthma. One laboratory study conducted in Jordan shows that rosemary's volatile oils can block the airway constriction induced by histamine, the chemical culprit of both asthma and other allergy symptoms. To a warm bath, add 5 to 10 drops of rosemary essential oil or a quart of rosemary tea (steep ¼ cup of the needles in 4 cups of hot water for 10 minutes). You can also use the tea for steam inhalation, or just drink up to 3 cups per day.

Astragalus (*Astragalus membranaceus*)

This herb can be taken as a tonic—part of your long-term daily regimen—to strengthen the immune system's natural defenses. *Typical dosage:* eight or nine 400- to 500-milligram capsules daily; or 15 to 30 drops of tincture, twice daily.

Mullein (*Verbascum thapsus*)

Antispasmodic and anti-inflammatory, mullein also fights some of the respiratory viruses that tend to plague people with asthma. *Typical dosage:* up to 6 cups per day of tea (steep 2 teaspoons of dried leaves and flowers in 1 cup of hot water for 10 to 15 minutes); or 25 to 40 drops of tincture every three hours.

Bladder Infections

Uh-oh, that urgent feeling. You think you have to urinate—but when you get to the toilet, you produce just a few dribbles. Even that little bit stings. The area above your pubic bone aches. So does your lower back. Such symptoms are particularly familiar to women, nearly half of whom suffer one or more episodes of urinary tract infections at some point in their lives. Sexual intercourse raises the risk. So does using a diaphragm and spermicidal jelly; so does delaying urination after sex.

If you think you have a urinary tract infection, do see your doctor. Untreated, such infections can travel to the kidneys, where they cause more severe illness and possibly permanent damage. Pregnant women with urinary tract infections are more likely to deliver premature and low-birth-weight infants.

DRUG TREATMENT

Antibiotics

Trimethoprim-sulfamethoxazole (Bactrim, Septra), ciprofloxacin (Cipro), levofloxacin (Levaquin), cefixime (Suprax). *Side effects:* diarrhea, nausea, vomiting, stomach pain, headache, vaginal yeast infection, allergic reactions; others that vary with the specific antibiotic used.

HERBAL REMEDIES

Cranberry (*Vaccinium macrocarpon*)

These tart red berries can help prevent urinary tract infections and may also help cure them. For some time, it's been a controversial question whether just drinking cranberry juice can acidify the urine. It can, but you have to drink a little over five cups to achieve this effect. But cranberries do prevent *Escherichia coli* bacteria—the ones that most frequently cause urinary tract infections—from adhering to the urethra and bladder. And if bacteria can't stick, they get washed out by urination and can't infect tissue. The same anti-stick chemical is also present in blueberries. Don't substitute berries for your antibiotics when you have an infection, but if you have recurring infections, try drinking 1¼ cups of unsweetened cranberry juice per day. *Typical dosage for the concentrated juice extract*: one 300- to 400-milligram capsule morning and evening.

Uva Ursi (*Arctostaphylos uva-ursi*)

Also called bearberry or kinnikinnik, this low-growing shrub has long been used to prevent and treat urinary tract infections. Its leaves contain arbutin, which acts against *E. coli* and increases urination. In a study of women prone to bladder infections, uva ursi prevented infection. Germany's Commission E, the counterpart to our Food and Drug Administration, has approved it for inflammatory disorders of the urinary tract. *Typical dosage:* up to nine 400- to 500-milligram capsules per day, or 30 to 60 drops of tincture diluted in a cup of water three times per day, or ½ cup of strong tea three times per day (soak ⅓ ounce of dried leaves in 4 cups of cold

water for 24 hours; remove leaves and simmer liquid down to 2
cups). *Caution:* Not recommended for use beyond seven days unless under medical supervision. Do not use while pregnant, nor if
you have kidney disorders or inflammatory conditions of the gastrointestinal tract. Overdose can produce stomachache, nausea,
vomiting, and ringing in the ears.

Goldenrod (*Solidago virgaurea*)
This herb is popular in Europe for treating bladder infections and the
Commission E endorses it. Varro Tyler, Ph.D., distinguished professor emeritus of pharmacognosy at Purdue University and author of
Herbs of Choice, judges goldenrod one of the safest and most effective herbs for increasing urine flow and inhibiting bacteria. It also
decreases the inflammation and painful spasms that can accompany
bladder infection. *Typical dosage:* 2 to 3 cups of tea per day (steep
1 teaspoon of dried herb in 1 cup of hot water for 10 minutes).

Oregon Graperoot (*Berberis aquifolium*)
Like goldenseal (*Hydrastis canadensis*), barberry (*Berberis vulgaris*), and gold thread (*Coptis* species), Oregon graperoot also
has a place in traditional treatment of bladder infections. Studies
show that berberine may kill many types of bacteria, including *E.*

PREVENTING RECURRENT BLADDER INFECTIONS

If you tend to get bladder infections over and over, here
are some things you can do to keep them away.

◆ Drink lots of fluids, at least eight glasses per day. One
  beverage you might want to include is cranberry juice.

◆ Urinate often, at least every three hours during the day. If
  you drink liberally, this should come naturally. The goal is
  to frequently flush the bladder and urethra (the tube that
  drains the bladder), thereby washing out any bacteria.

◆ If you use a diaphragm and spermicidal jelly, consider
  switching to another form of birth control. Discuss these
  options with your doctor.

coli, and prevent bacteria from adhering to the bladder lining. *Typical dosage:* 1 teaspoon of tincture three times per day. *Caution:* Do not use during pregnancy.

Echinacea (*Echinacea purpurea, E. angustifolia, E. pallida*)

Antibacterial and anti-inflammatory echinacea also revs up the immune system, which can be helpful to people with recurrent bladder infections. *Typical dosage:* up to nine 300- to 400-milligram capsules per day; or up to 60 drops of tincture three times per day. *Caution:* If you're allergic to other members of the aster family, such as ragweed, you may be allergic to echinacea. Start with small doses and build up slowly.

Dandelion (*Taraxacum officinale*)

Herbs that increase urine flow, although they don't kill bacteria, help rid the urinary tract of microbes simply by washing them out. Dandelion is among the foremost of these; it's popular among herbalists because it also contains potassium. *Typical dosage:* 1 cup of tea morning and evening (steep 1 to 2 teaspoons of dried root in 1 cup of hot water for 10 to 15 minutes); or 30 to 60 drops of tincture three times per day.

Horsetail (*Equisetum arvense*)

Also known as shavegrass, this herb is common in European medicine for blood in the urine and urinary stones. It's a mild diuretic that works its wonders without depleting electrolytes, so you don't get that "washed out" feeling. *Typical dosage:* up to six 400- to 500-milligram capsules per day; or 15 to 30 drops of tincture three times per day; or up to 6 cups of tea per day (steep 2 teaspoons of dried herb in 1 cup of hot water for 10 to 15 minutes).

Marshmallow (*Althaea officinalis*)

A far cry from the confections you've probably toasted over a campfire, this marsh-growing plant has a root whose compounds can coat the urinary tract and prevent further inflammation, thus easing pain. *Typical dosage:* up to six 400- to 500-milligram capsules per day; 1 cup of tea per day in three divided doses (steep 1 to 2 teaspoons of dried root in 1 cup of hot water for 10 to 15 minutes); or 20 to 40 drops of tincture up to five times per day.

Making Use of the Good Bacteria

Whether or not you want to picture this, our skin and mucous membranes are normally colonized by millions of bacteria. These "good" bacteria perform many functions, including an ability to prevent "bad" microorganisms from taking hold. In the case of urinary tract infections, they seem to prevent *Escherichia coli* from sticking to the urethra (a first step in establishing an infection). Lactobacilli, the kind of bacteria present in live-culture yogurt and kefir and in acidophilus supplements can help prevent bladder infections. Preliminary research suggests that taking such bacteria with antibiotics hastens elimination of *E. coli*. And it can help prevent the chances of getting a vaginal yeast infection—a common adverse effect of antibiotic treatment.

Corn Silk (*Zea mays*)

Another herb that soothes the urinary tract, corn silk is easy to obtain in summer; when it's not sweet corn season you can take it in capsules or tincture. *Typical dosage:* 2 to 3 cups of tea per day (steep 1 teaspoon of dried herb or 2 teaspoons of fresh herb in 1 cup of hot water for 15 minutes); or up to six 300-milligram capsules per day; or 20 to 60 drops of tincture up to three times per day, taken with a glass of water.

Corn silk

Cramp Bark (*Viburnum opulus*) and Black Haw Bark (*V. prunifolium*)

You may have heard of both of these barks as treatments for menstrual cramps; they're both antispasmodic, meaning they will help with cramps in the bladder or lower back. *Typical dosage:* 1 cup of tea up to three times per day (steep 1 scant teaspoon of dried herb in 1 cup of hot water for 15 minutes). *Caution:* Do not use either herb if you have a history of kidney disease or kidney stones.

BLISTERS

Y OU WORE THE WRONG SHOES to go hiking. You spent an entire Saturday hoeing the garden. You brushed your exposed ankle against the hot exhaust pipe of a motorcycle. The result: a painful, fluid-filled pocket known as a blister.

Blisters result from physical trauma to the skin—whether it's repeated rubbing or a minor burn. Your body creates a little "cushion" of fluid to protect the damaged skin—a fairly effective protective strategy. The collected fluid and the raw, red underlying skin contain specialized cells that the body has rushed to the area to limit the injury and begin the process of healing. For this reason, it's usually best to leave a blister intact so that the inflamed underlying skin can heal.

For the average blister, vulnerary herbs (herbs that promote healing) can help speed generation of new skin. Other herbs can help cool and heal inflammation and fight bacteria. All the herbs discussed below are readily available in the form of ointments,

BASIC BLISTER CARE

Clean the area by soaking it briefly in warm water, or apply a small amount of hydrogen peroxide solution. Pat dry. Do not drain an intact blister unless it is very large or is interfering with movement at a joint.

If you need to drain the blister, pierce it with a sterilized needle, allow the fluid to drain and pat dry. Do not remove the protective covering of skin until it begins to dry and peel on its own; you can then remove it with your fingers or a pair of clean scissors. Apply a small amount of herbal salve or cream to a bandage or soft piece of gauze and gently cover the blister. Avoid further stress to the area for several days. Repeat the cleaning and application of the herb cream and dressings two or three times per day until the blister is healed.

creams, salves, and oils and are found in health food stores. You don't need all of them; just find a topical application that includes one or more of them.

Lavender and tea tree can each be purchased as a highly concentrated and fragrant essential oil. To use essential oils on a blister, dilute them by adding five times as much of a neutral vegetable oil, such as olive, almond, sesame, vitamin E, or avocado oil. To make an infused oil with any of the herbs described below, pack a small, clean jar with the herb, then cover the herbs with vegetable oil. Put a tight lid on the jar. Allow it to steep in a sunny spot for two weeks, shaking it every other day. After two weeks, strain the herbs out of the oil and put it into a clean bottle. Store it in a cool place.

Drug Treatment

Conventional over-the-counter treatment for blisters is usually recommended only if a blister has torn, exposing the skin underneath. Antibacterial creams and ointments can be applied, along with adhesive bandages that keep the wound clean.

Herbal Remedies

Comfrey (*Symphytum officinale*)
This wonderful, traditional herbal wound healer appears to work, in part, because it is rich in allantoin, a chemical that stimulates cell proliferation, thus speeding the growth of healthy new skin. Salves containing comfrey can be spread on blisters as needed.

Calendula (*Calendula officinalis*)
The yellow or orange flowers of this common garden herb are wound-healing, anti-inflammatory, and antiseptic. You'll see calendula as an ingredient in many first-aid creams. It makes a wonderful, skin-healing infused oil. Use commercial products as directed on the package or as needed.

Chamomile (*Matricaria recutita*)
In addition to having wound healing properties, chamomile is also anti-inflammatory and antiseptic. If you have chamomile tea on hand, you can simply dampen a tea bag in warm water and hold it against the blister as often as you need to.

Lavender (*Lavandula angustifolia*)

Lavender speeds healing and is mildly antiseptic. As an added benefit, just the smell of lavender has traditionally been used to lift mood. Use commercial products as directed; dilute lavender essential oil as directed above and use as often as needed.

St.-John's-Wort (*Hypericum perforatum*)

When applied topically in an infused (not essential) oil, St.-John's-wort is wound-healing, anti-inflammatory, and antiseptic. Simply dab it on the blister with a clean swab or cotton ball several times per day.

BLISTER BALM

This herbal ointment is also appropriate for minor cuts, abrasions, burns, and fungal infections.

- ½ ounce dried calendula blossoms
- ½ ounce dried comfrey root
- 2 cups almond, olive, or other vegetable oil
- ½ cup finely chopped beeswax
- 10 drops lavender essential oil
- 10 drops tea tree essential oil

Combine the herbs and vegetable oil in a crock pot. Turn the crock pot to its lowest setting, cover, and allow to heat gently two to four hours, checking and stirring frequently to prevent burning. When the oil is yellow in color and has an "herby" smell, it's done. Strain through a coffee filter or piece of clean cloth into a large measuring cup. This oil is now an infused herbal oil.

To each cup of infused oil (you'll lose some in the straining process), add ¼ cup of the beeswax. Heat the oil and beeswax together over very low heat until the beeswax is completely melted. Do not allow to boil or burn. Test the consistency by placing one tablespoon of the mixture in the freezer for a minute or two until cool. The balm should be the consistency of an easily spreadable paste. If it seems too thin, add a little more beeswax; if too thick, add a little oil. Remove from the heat. Quickly add the essential oils. Pour into clean glass containers and cover tightly. Cool to room temperature.

Body Odor

Hollywood legend has it that great actor Rex Harrison had bad breath and that famed forties pin-up Betty Grable battled body odor. So don't feel singled out if, in your natural state, you smell a bit more natural than you (and your friends) would prefer. When it's not a hygiene problem and you didn't step in anything during your lunchtime stroll, something else can be to blame.

Body odor comes from the skin, which produces two different types of sweat from two different types of sweat glands: eccrine and apocrine. These glands do their thing in response not only to heat, but also to stress, anger, nervousness, and sexual excitement. Bacteria that thrive on secretions from the apocrine sweat glands can grow and multiply, producing an aroma that comes from the bacteria breaking down the fluids in sweat.

Body odor can also be caused by skin infections. The most common of these is athlete's foot (see Fungal Skin Infections on page 261). But body odor can also be a result of serious diseases of the liver and kidney, conditions that you want to diagnose as soon as possible for the best treatment. If yours persists, see your doctor for help.

Drug Treatment

There are no drugs that specifically treat body odor, but perhaps deodorants and antiperspirants should be labeled as drugs because they can contain compounds such as aluminum chloride hexahydrate, benzalkonium chloride, boric acid, and hexachlorophene. Any of these agents can cause skin irritation and be absorbed through the skin into the body, so be sure to read labels carefully if you're searching for a new deodorant or antiperspirant. And if you're switching to a stronger product, do a patch test first on a small area of skin.

Herbal Remedies

Sage (*Salvia officinalis*)
Compounds found in sage can dry up perspiration, while the oils contained in sage are antiseptic and antibiotic. Using sage on the

skin can help lessen a body odor problem caused by perspiration or by infectious agents. One way to use the herb is as a body powder (see the recipe below). Another way is to wash the body in a tea made from sage. Sage tea helps reduce excessive sweating (steep 2 teaspoons of dried herb in 1 cup of hot water for 5 minutes). *Caution:* If used internally, take small amounts as needed rather than taking routinely. Prolonged use can result in dizziness, hot flashes, and seizures. Do not use internally if you are pregnant or nursing.

Rosemary (*Rosmarinus officinalis*)

This aromatic culinary herb contains agents that are antiseptic and antibiotic. Its piney scent is also refreshing. Use the ground, dried herb as a body powder to treat odor caused by perspiration and bacteria or by fungus on the skin. You can also make a tea from rosemary to use as a body wash (steep 1 teaspoon of dried leaf in 1 cup of hot water for 10 to 15 minutes). *Caution:* If irritation occurs, discontinue use.

Fennel (*Foeniculum vulgare*)

As early as the tenth century A.D., the mystic Hildegard of Bingen recommended fennel seed as a treatment for body odor. At Indian restaurants you might see fennel seeds instead of after-dinner mints. Fennel not only improves digestion but also can reduce bad breath and body odor that originates in the intestines. *Typical*

SWEET-SMELLING BODY POWDER

You can use this powder under the arms or wherever odor originates.

- ½ **cup cornstarch**
- ½ **cup baking soda**
- 1 **tablespoon ground sage**
- 1 **tablespoon ground rosemary**

Mix ingredients together.

'Twas Something You Didn't Eat. . .

Zinc deficiency may contribute to body odor. If this might be the case for you, check out the following foods, which are rich in zinc, to add your diet.

◆ Spinach
◆ Whole grains
◆ Legumes
◆ Rice
◆ Nuts

dosage: Eat whole seeds after a meal as desired; or drink 1 cup of tea per day (simmer 2 to 3 teaspoons of crushed seeds in 1 cup of water for 10 to 15 minutes).

Breast Cysts

B ENIGN BUT PAINFUL LUMPS characterize the most common form of noncancerous breast disease: chronic cystic mastitis, also known as fibrocystic breast disease. This condition affects one in five women, typically those in their thirties and forties. It often subsides after menopause.

Because breast tissue is very sensitive to hormonal changes, it can enlarge and thicken by as much as half, then shrink again by the same amount, at various times during the menstrual cycle. Normally, fluid from the breast tissue is collected and transported out of the breasts by means of the lymphatic system. If there is more fluid than the lymphatic system can handle, small spaces in breast tissue may fill with this fluid and form cysts. These pockets of fluid can appear alone or in clusters. Although cysts are not in themselves considered dangerous, they can make it harder to detect a possible cancerous lesion or lump. If you suspect that you have a cyst, you should have it checked by your doctor—both for your health and for your peace of mind.

Medical treatment for breast cysts sometimes involves inserting a needle into one of the cysts to withdraw a sample of fluid for evaluation. Often, draining the cyst can prevent its return in the future. Other treatment options are hormone drugs and surgical removal of the cyst.

DRUG TREATMENT

Hormone-Based Drugs

Danazol (Danocrine). *Function:* shrink breast lumps by decreasing levels of follicle-stimulating hormone and luteinizing hormone, thereby reducing estrogen production. *Side effects:* weight gain, acne, increased body and facial hair, voice changes, menstrual disturbances, and reversible liver dysfunction.

Oral contraceptives (Norinyl, Ortho-Novum, many others). *Function:* reduce both size and occurrence of cysts by minimizing hormone fluctuations and reducing overall levels of estrogen. *Side effects:* nausea, weight gain, bloating, increased risk of blood clots.

HERBAL REMEDIES

Evening Primrose (*Oenothera biennis*)

Oil from this plant's seed contains essential fatty acids that have natural antiprostaglandin properties, which may help to reduce breast lumps. Prostaglandins are a group of chemicals that the body produces; some of them favor inflammation and are believed to contribute to breast cysts. Studies have found that women reporting breast tenderness responded well to evening primrose oil therapy. *Typical dosage:* 1,500 milligrams in capsules two times per day.

Evening primrose

Vitex (*Vitex agnus-castus*)

Also known as chaste berry, vitex boosts progesterone production, helping to correct estrogen-progesterone imbalances that can be at fault in breast cysts. *Typical dosage:* 200 milligrams standardized to 5 percent agnuside content per day; or up to three nonstandardized 650-milligram capsules per day; or 15 to 40 drops of tincture per day; or 1 cup of tea per day (steep a scant teaspoon of dried, ground berries in a cup of hot water for 10 to 15 minutes). *Caution:* Do not use during pregnancy or while taking hormone replacement therapy.

A Diet for Breast Health

Women who develop breast cysts may find that retooling their diets can ease a lot of the pain and swelling associated with the cysts. Concentrate on low-fat, high-fiber foods, with lots of raw foods, seeds, nuts, and grains. Use olive oil in place of saturated fats. Fresh bananas, apples, grapes, grapefruit, fresh vegetables, and yogurt (check the label to see if a product contains live cultures) are all good foods to include.

Soy-based foods such as tofu are highly recommended because they contain isoflavones. These compounds help neutralize excess estrogen so your body can filter it out. Cruciferous vegetables such as cabbage, broccoli, and Brussels sprouts contain another class of chemicals called indoles. They also work to protect breast tissue from excess estrogen. Finally, the culinary immune-boosters garlic, onions, and shiitake mushrooms may help keep your whole system operating healthfully.

Avoid alcohol; also refrain from drinking coffee, tea, and other caffeine-containing foods and beverages. Cut down on dairy products and animal meats, along with the hydrogenated fats found in margarine and the saturated ones that pack fried foods. Salt, sugar, and white flour are also enemies—so leave out processed cookies, crackers, and cakes.

Butcher's Broom (*Ruscus aculeatus*)

This bushy perennial contains chemicals that are related to diosgenin, the hormonelike component of wild yam. It may help to inhibit the inflammatory processes in the breasts that lead to the formation of cysts. *Typical dosage:* 100 milligrams of product standardized to 10 percent saponins, one to three times per day; for nonstandardized products, take 400 milligrams or two to six capsules per day. Do not use if you have high blood pressure.

You can take several supplements to help speed the shrinking of breast cysts.

◆ **Vitamin E.** This skin-boosting vitamin also protects breast tissue because of its antioxidant ability and it helps keep hormones in balance. Clinical studies have found that breast tenderness and cysts dramatically improved with vitamin E therapy. *Typical dosage:* 800 to 1,200 IU daily of d-alpha tocopherol.

◆ **Vitamin A.** The vision vitamin also helps to keep breast ducts functioning properly and scavenges for damaging molecules called free radicals in breast tissue. Studies have shown its ability to reduce breast pain. *Typical dosage:* 15,000 IU daily. *Caution:* If you are pregnant, do not exceed 10,000 IU daily.

◆ **Isoflavones.** These are the same compounds found in tofu and soy-based foods. They have the ability to protect breast tissue from the formation of tumors. *Typical dosage:* 20 to 40 milligrams daily (including 6 to 12 milligrams of genistein, one of the key isoflavones).

◆ **Indoles.** These are the cyst- and tumor-fighting phytochemicals in cabbage-family vegetables. Now available in capsule form, they are new enough that practitioners haven't formed a consensus on dosage. Take them as recommended by your practitioner or by the manufacturer.

Gotu Kola (*Centella asiatica*)

This herb is an important tonic or general health-booster in Ayurvedic medicine. *Typical dosage:* 250 milligrams of product standardized to 10 percent triterpenes, two or three times per day; or up to eight 400- to 500-milligram capsules of nonstandardized product per day; or 20 to 40 drops of tincture up to twice per day; or 1 cup of tea per day (steep 1 teaspoon of dried herb in 1 cup of hot water for 10 to 15 minutes).

Black Cohosh (*Cimicifuga racemosa*)

This herb seems to reduce the fluctuation of estrogen and its influence on the breast. Black cohosh is also credited with regulating hormones. *Typical dosage:* 500 milligrams of product standardized to 0.2 percent triterpenes, one to three times per day. *Caution*: Do not take while pregnant.

Saw Palmetto (*Serenoa repens*)

This herb has a significant anti-inflammatory effect that helps reduce inflammation of the breast. It also can help regulate estrogen influence on the breast. *Typical dosage:* 160 milligrams in capsules standardized to 85 to 95 percent fatty acid content, two times per day.

BREAST PAIN

FOR SOME WOMEN, BREAST PAIN or tenderness is so great that even a blouse brushing against the skin causes intense pain. This condition, also called mastalgia, is often misdiagnosed as fibrocystic breast disease, which is usually accompanied by one or more lumps in the breast.

But the American Cancer Society emphasizes that mastalgia is not a disease. It is caused by normal changes in breast tissue related to monthly fluctuations in levels of estrogen and progesterone, which cause the glands and ducts in the breast to enlarge.

MANY WAYS TO GET YOUR GLA

Evening primrose oil is a perfectly fine way to supplement your diet with gamma linolenic acid (GLA), but it can be costly. (It's also trendy, so your health food store might be out of it when you need it.) Other seed oils containing GLA are black currant (*Ribes nigrum*) and borage (*Borago officinalis*).

Because linoleic acid, a common compound in some foods, can be converted to gamma-linolenic acid by the body, including such foods in your diet is another option. High sources of linoleic acid include safflower, soy, and flaxseed oils. Put a dressing made with one of these on a big salad filled with fiber and nutrients and you've done your body a world of good.

As a result, the breasts become swollen, painful, tender, and lumpy. For many women, these symptoms occur as part of the premenstrual syndrome and usually disappear during or after menstruation.

Breast pain can be present at other times when ovarian hormone levels change, such as during puberty, pregnancy, approaching menopause, and estrogen replacement therapy. It can occur after pregnancy because of milk engorgement, but breastfeeding usually relieves this discomfort. During nursing, however, painful infections or abscesses can form in the breast tissue. Pain can also be a side effect of certain drugs, such as diuretics used for high blood pressure, and heart drugs. On rare occasions, pain can be a sign of breast cancer, so it's prudent to consult a doctor about breast pain.

DRUG TREATMENT

Analgesics
Aspirin, acetaminophen, ibuprofen. *Function:* relieve pain. *Aspirin side effects:* stomach upset. *Acetaminophen side effects:* dizziness,

excitement, disorientation, liver damage. *Ibuprofen side effects:* gastrointestinal irritation and bleeding, rash.

Hormone-Based Drugs

Oral contraceptives (many types and trade names). *Function:* decrease the levels of hormones secreted by the ovaries, thereby easing breast pain. *Side effects:* nausea, headache, vaginal bleeding, weight gain, vaginal infections, blood clots, changes in metabolism, increased blood pressure, skin pigment changes. *Note:* The side effects of oral contraceptives vary greatly depending upon the amount of estrogen and progesterone in the preparation.

Synthetic Steroids

Danazol (Danocrine). *Function:* suppress the function of the ovaries and mimic progesterone somewhat; typically used only in cases of severe breast pain. *Side effects:* weight gain, decreased

FOUR QUICK PAIN-EASERS

These strategies may not work for every woman, but they're all non-invasive, relatively inexpensive, and natural.

◆ **Give yourself some support.** Invest in good support bras, or make sure that the ones you have fit properly. You might be surprised at the difference this makes, especially for larger-breasted women.

◆ **Try a heat treatment.** Many herbalists recommend warm castor oil packs or just plain heat packs, which seem to help move fluid out of the breasts.

◆ **Trim the fat.** Although not all doctors agree on this, some research indicates that high levels of dietary fat can contribute to breast pain.

◆ **Cut the caffeine.** Again, doctors disagree, but eliminating or reducing your caffeine intake is definitely worth a try, especially if you describe yourself as a java junkie. Don't forget to count sodas and iced teas in your caffeine totals, especially if you're sensitive to this stimulant.

breast size, acne, increased male characteristics such as hair growth and deepening of the voice, headache, hot flashes, changes in libido, liver damage.

HERBAL REMEDIES

Evening Primrose (*Oenothera biennis*)

The seeds of the evening primrose furnish an oil that contains gamma-linolenic acid (GLA). In the body, this oil increases the level of a particular type of prostaglandin that helps fight inflammation. Some studies have shown that GLA significantly helps women with breast pain; others have shown that it doesn't. It seems that the oil may be useful for mild discomfort but not severe pain. *Typical dosage:* capsules totaling 3,000 to 4,000 milligrams per day; or ½ teaspoon of the oil per day; take either for three months to see results.

Vitex (*Vitex agnus-castus*)

The fruit of this herb, also known as chaste berry, has hormonelike effects on the body and normalizes progesterone activity. It can make many symptoms of premenstrual syndrome—including breast pain—go away. Again, as with evening primrose or other GLA products, vitex may need to be taken for three months before significant effects are seen. *Typical dosage:* 200 milligrams of a standardized extract containing 0.5 percent agnuside, one to three times per day. *Caution:* Do not take during pregnancy, or if you are on hormone replacement therapy. If you are taking other hormonelike drugs, consult your doctor before using vitex.

Breastfeeding Problems

B REAST MILK IS THE BEST nourishment you can give a baby, for whom it has been custom-made. It contains so many nutrients that all have not been identified yet. The American Academy of Pediatrics recommends that infants be breastfed exclusively for six months and that breastfeeding continue for at least the first year. But any amount that you breastfeed provides some benefit to your child. And breastfeeding is a nurturing and rewarding experience for most mothers that will long be remembered with joy.

But for some mothers, breastfeeding brings frustration and feelings of inadequacy, usually because their milk supply is not enough for their baby. The initial days of breastfeeding are often time-consuming and tiring. That can make matters worse, because stress and fatigue contribute to a lowered milk supply. It can take a month before a new mother feels comfortable nursing her baby.

Lactation, or the production of milk, depends upon several hormones produced by the mother's body. During pregnancy, high levels of estrogen and progesterone prevent milk from being made. After birth, estrogen and progesterone decrease and prolactin levels increase. Prolactin is responsible for stimulating milk production in the breast.

But prolactin does not work alone. Oxytocin, which a mother's body releases in response to the baby's suckling, has two roles. It helps maintain the levels of prolactin necessary for milk production and it stimulates the release of milk from the breast—sometimes called ejection.

Mothers have used herbs to foster better production of breast milk for centuries. Many of these herbs can't be taken during pregnancy, however, because they may stimulate uterine contractions. Once your baby is born, herbs not only can help boost the supply of your breast milk while you're nursing, but once you're finished they also can help your body reduce the supply and eventually eliminate it. Some can help ease nipple soreness or other minor complaints associated with nursing.

In addition, many hospitals now have a lactation consultant. This person is usually a nurse trained in breastfeeding who can help a new mother get started. Licensed nurse/midwives also are often knowledgeable in natural health care for nursing mothers. Finally, the La Leche League is a long-established organization that assists new mothers with breastfeeding.

DRUG TREATMENT

At one time doctors prescribed hormones to help dry up the initial milk supply and relieve breast engorgement for mothers who did not intend to breastfeed. This is no longer done, because the side effects of such hormone treatment can be severe. No drug options exist for the reverse situation: inadequate milk supply. Because any drugs taken by the mother while breastfeeding are also passed along to the baby, doctors generally err on the side of caution with even the mildest of over-the-counter drugs.

HERBAL REMEDIES

Fenugreek (*Trigonella foenum-graecum*)
These seeds are an ancient treatment for increasing milk production. They have oxytocin-like effects on the body, stimulating milk production and contracting the uterus. Start with a low dose and slowly increase it if necessary. *Typical dosage:* up to six 600- or 700-milligram capsules per day; or up to ½ teaspoon of seeds per day. *Caution:* Do not use fenugreek while pregnant.

Fennel (*Foeniculum vulgare*)
Another age-old treatment for increasing milk flow, fennel works in a way similar to the body's hormones. You can eat fennel seeds in food or drink them as a tea. A side benefit to fennel is that it typically eases any mild post-pregnancy digestive problems. *Typical dosage:* up to three 400- or 500-milligram capsules per day; or one cup of tea per day (simmer 2 to 3 teaspoons of crushed seeds in 1 cup of hot water for 10 to 15 minutes). *Caution:* Do not use fennel during pregnancy.

Fenugreek

Tips for Successful Nursing

Here are some guidelines to increase your success at breastfeeding:

♦ Begin as soon as possible after birth.

♦ Nurse whenever your baby appears to want to, up to a dozen times every 24 hours.

♦ Set up a comfortable nursing station—a good chair, a footstool, a pillow, and a nearby supply of water.

♦ Do not give the baby any supplements such as water, juice, or formula unless your pediatrician specifically recommends them.

♦ Avoid pacifiers; they confuse your baby's suckling response.

♦ Air-dry your nipples after nursing to prevent cracking and infection.

♦ Eat right and get enough rest.

♦ If you are wearing breast pads in your nursing bra, change them after each feeding to avoid infection.

Aniseed (*Pimpenilla anisum*)

This seed contains a volatile oil component known as anethole, which can promote prolactin secretion and thus milk production. Like fennel, aniseed promotes digestion. *Typical dosage:* 1 cup of tea per day (simmer 2 to 3 teaspoons of crushed seeds in 1 cup of hot water for 10 to 15 minutes). *Caution:* Do not use aniseed during pregnancy.

Aloe (*Aloe vera*)

It may not increase your milk supply, but pure aloe vera gel soothes the skin and can be applied to nipples after you nurse to avoid cracking and dryness. Use topically as necessary.

BRONCHITIS

Many maladies aren't obvious to an observer. You may have a headache, but unless you grasp your forehead and shriek in agony, no one knows. Perhaps you have athlete's foot, but as long as you keep your shoes on, who can tell? But develop a cough and just watch—you're an instant outcast.

Bronchitis is different from run-of-the-mill coughs. In bronchitis, the bronchi—the main, branching passageways of the lungs—are inflamed. Bronchitis comes in two main varieties: acute (sudden) and chronic (continuing). Acute bronchitis is usually a complication of a viral infection such as a cold or the flu. The bronchitis cough typically starts off dry and hacking. Then it becomes rattling and produces gray or yellow mucus, possibly with wheezing or mild shortness of breath. For half of those with acute bronchitis, the cough lingers three weeks or longer. In most cases, it eventually goes away without any conventional treatment.

In chronic bronchitis, persistent inflammation results in a mucus-producing cough that lasts at least three months. Coughing is worse in the morning. Symptoms often intensify over time, with breathlessness and wheezing. The best treatments for chronic bronchitis are quitting smoking and avoiding air pollutants. No herbal or conventional treatments can substitute for these two crucial steps.

DRUG TREATMENT

Cough Suppressants

Dextromethorphan (Benylin DM, Comtrex, many others); codeine (Actifed with Codeine Cough, Brontex, many others); either of the above may be combined with decongestants or expectorants. *Function:* act directly on the cough center in the brain. *Dextromethorphan side effects:* few when taken as directed but many people experience side effects from the decongestants in combination products. *Codeine side effects:* increased effects of central nervous system depressants such as alcohol, tranquilizers, and many antidepressants; dizziness, drowsiness, headache, nausea, vomiting, stomachache, constipation, over-excitement; can be habit-forming.

Expectorants
Guaifenesin (Dimetane Expectorant, Robitussin, many others). *Function:* loosen respiratory secretions so they are more readily expelled in coughing.

Inhaled Bronchodilators
Albuterol (Proventil, Ventolin), fenoterol (Berotec), salmeterol (Serevent), terbutaline (Brethaire, Brethine, Bricanyl). *Function:* relax smooth muscle encircling airways to widen their diameter, thus easing breathing. *Side effects:* none common.

HERBAL REMEDIES

Licorice (*Glycyrrhiza glabra*)
This root is a one-stop herb shop for bronchitis. It soothes mucous membranes and is expectorant, anti-inflammatory, and directly antiviral. It also stimulates cells to produce interferon, the body's own antiviral compound. *Typical dosage:* six 400- to 500-milligram capsules per day; or 20 to 30 drops of tincture up to three times per day; or 3 to 4 cups of tea per day (simmer ¼ cup of root in 2 cups of water for 10 to 15 minutes). *Caution:* Do not take for longer than six weeks. Do not use if you are pregnant or nursing or if you have severe liver, kidney, or heart disease or high blood pressure. Do not use with diuretics that cause potassium loss.

Mullein (*Verbascum thapsus*)
If your cough is wet, mullein helps you expel mucus; if your cough is dry, it helps ease that rasping pain. *Typical dosage:* 25 to 40 drops of tincture every three hours; or up to 6 cups of tea per day (steep 2 teaspoons of dried leaves and flowers in 1 cup of hot water for 10 to 15 minutes).

Marshmallow (*Althaea officinalis*)
An excellent mucous-membrane soother, marshmallow is a good choice for dry coughs. It also has a mild stimulating effect on the immune system. *Typical dosage:* up to six 400- or 500-milligram cap-

DON'T TREAT THIS CONDITION AT HOME

Bronchitis is a matter for prompt medical attention if the following symptoms occur.

◆ You feel breathless or have difficulty breathing

◆ You have severe chest pain

◆ You develop a fever over 102°F

◆ You cough up blood

◆ Your symptoms persist longer than four weeks

◆ Your symptoms worsen

sules per day; or 20 to 40 drops of tincture up to five times per day; or 3 to 4 cups of tea per day (simmer 1 teaspoon of dried root in 1 cup of water for 10 minutes). Or use marshmallow blended with other tea herbs (some people find its taste off-putting when used alone).

English Plantain (*Plantago lanceolata*)

This herb has a strong reputation as a gentle cough suppressant, demulcent, and antibacterial agent. The German Commission E, that country's counterpart to the American Food and Drug Administration, endorses it as safe and effective for bronchial conditions. *Typical dosage:* up to 6,000 milligrams in capsules per day; or up to 4 cups of tea per day (steep 2 teaspoons of dried leaf in 1 cup of boiling water for 10 to 15 minutes).

Garlic (*Allium sativum*)

This expectorant fights many bacteria and some of the viruses that cause flus and colds. Its aromatic oils are excreted through the lungs (which is why eating the bulb produces garlic breath). In the process, those oils act directly to kill microorganisms and to help you cough up mucus. *Typical dosage:* up to three 500- to 600-milligram capsules per day (look for products that deliver 4,000 micrograms of allicin daily); or 1 to 3 fresh cloves per day (mince and eat raw, or crush and add to cooked foods just before serving).

TWO EASY LUNG-EASERS

Here are two old-fashioned strategies for loosening bronchitis.

◆ Drink a lot of liquids, especially water, teas, broths. This helps thin respiratory secretions and makes them easier to cough up. Warm liquids also help relax the airways.

◆ Steam inhalation also thins respiratory mucus and promotes expectoration (a fancy word for getting rid of that gunk in your chest). You can use a commercial steamer, steam room, or the old-fashioned pot of boiling water. For the latter, simply boil water, pour it carefully in a heat-resistant bowl, and place it on a sturdy table. Cover your head with a towel and hold your face at least 12 inches from the steam so that it feels warm but not unpleasantly hot. Herbal steams can be doubly helpful. Many herbs contain volatile oils that rise with the steam and have antiseptic, expectorant, and airway-relaxing properties. Good choices include eucalyptus, thyme, peppermint, and rosemary; use about a total of ¼ cup of herbs for every 4 cups of water. You can also add 3 to 5 drops of the essential oil of these herbs.

Wild Cherry (*Prunus serotina*)

The bark of this tree inhibits the cough reflex. Although herbal cough suppressants tend to have a more subtle action than dextromethorphan and codeine, you should nevertheless use these natural alternatives only for dry, hacking coughs. You'll find wild cherry bark most often blended with other herbs in teas and syrups; follow the manufacturer's recommendations on dosage. *Caution:* While cherry bark is safe when used for short-term ailments at recommended dosages, it is not recommended for long-term use.

Wild cherry

Thyme (*Thymus vulgaris*)

Expectorant, antispasmodic, and antibacterial, thyme is endorsed by Commission E for treating bronchitis. It turns up in cough syrups and other blended liquid extracts. In addition to drinking thyme tea, you can make a thyme steam to inhale (see "Two Easy Lung-Easers" on page 132). *Typical dosage:* up to 4 cups of tea per day (steep 1 teaspoon of dried leaves in 1 cup of just-boiled water for 10 minutes).

Horehound (*Marrubium vulgare*)

You'll see horehound in both lozenge and syrup products on the shelves of health food stores; these products soothe sore throats and promote expectoration. *Typical dosage:* up to 3 cups per day of tea (steep 2 teaspoons of dried leaves in 1 cup of hot water for 10 minutes); or take lozenges or syrup as manufacturer recommends.

Peppermint (*Mentha × piperita*)

The menthol in peppermint relaxes the airways and fights bacteria and viruses. To do an herbal steam with peppermint, add 3 to 5 drops of the essential oil to 4 cups of just-boiled water. *Typical dosage:* 1 cup of tea as needed (steep 2 teaspoons of dried leaves in 1 cup of hot water for 5 to 10 minutes); or 10 to 20 drops of tincture three or four times per day.

Hyssop (*Hyssopus officinalis*)

This bee-attracting herb is antiviral and expectorant; you can find it in syrups and liquid extracts. *Typical dosage:* 10 to 40 drops of tincture up to four times per day; or 1 cup of tea as needed (steep 1 teaspoon of dried herb in 1 cup of hot water for 10 to 15 minutes).

Lobelia (*Lobelia inflata*)

Both the leaves and the seeds of this potent expectorant and antispasmodic are used. *Typical dosage:* 20 to 30 drops of tincture three times per day. But note that the other common name for this plant is puke weed—and for good reason: even small doses can cause nausea or vomiting. For this reason, it may be best to purchase a blended product containing this herb and follow the manufacturer's instructions, or consult a qualified practitioner for instructions on using it. *Caution:* Do not use if you are pregnant or have heart conditions.

Echinacea (*Echinacea angustifolia, E. purpurea, E. pallida*)

This herb stimulates white blood cell activity, increases the body's production of antiviral substances such as interferon, and helps immune cells engulf and destroy invading microbes. It combats some of the viruses that commonly cause bronchitis. *Typical dosage:* up to nine 300- to 400-milligram capsules per day (taken in several doses); or up to 60 drops of tincture three times per day. Most herbalists agree that you should take echinacea for no more than two weeks, then discontinue it for one week. *Caution:* Not recommended for people with multiple sclerosis, HIV infection, or other autoimmune disease. Rarely, people with allergies to other members of the daisy family may also be allergic to echinacea.

BRUISES

B RUISES COME IN ALL SHAPES and sizes and exhibit a spectrum of shifting colors—midnight blue, the purplish red of raw liver, and olive green mottled with sickly yellow. Injury to the soft tissues of skin and muscle causes most bruises. Surgery, major or minor, can cause extensive bruising. Sometimes the injury that causes the bruise is serious; sometimes the trauma, especially as we get older, is so mild we don't even register the bump until there's a change in skin color. But if you habitually bruise without injury, see your doctor. This can be a sign of illness such as a platelet disorder, leukemia, or nutrient deficiency. If a snake bite produced your bruise, or you feel ill and break out in a rash of tiny bruises, get medical help immediately.

DRUG TREATMENT

Analgesics

Acetaminophen, aspirin, ibuprofen. *Acetaminophen and aspirin side effects:* heartburn, mild nausea or vomiting. *Ibuprofen side effects:* dizziness, stomachache, nausea, headache, diarrhea.

BRUISE CURES FROM YOUR FREEZER

Simple, old-fashioned, and effective, a cold application right after an injury can help reduce swelling. Cold temperatures encourage blood vessels to narrow, thus stanching their flow and minimizing swelling. Cover your skin with a thin cloth, then apply a bag of frozen vegetables (peas and corn conform nicely), a plastic bag of ice cubes, or a commercial cold pack. Elevate the injured part and keep it cold for 10 to 15 minutes. Repeat three to four times per day the first day of the injury.

HERBAL REMEDIES

Arnica (*Arnica montana*)

Pain-relieving, antiseptic, and anti-inflammatory, arnica is most commonly used topically for traumatic injuries and is said to speed the disappearance of bruises. In fact, Germany's Commission E, that country's equivalent to the United States' Food and Drug Administration, has approved arnica's external use for injuries. Many gels, creams, ointments, and salves contain arnica. You can also make your own compress with arnica flowers you purchase in bulk. Just steep 2 teaspoons of dried flowers in 1 cup of hot water for 10 minutes, strain and cool; or add 1 dropperful of tincture to 1 cup of water. Wet a clean cloth with the solution and apply to the injured area for about half an hour three times per day, preferably beginning as soon as the injury occurs. With manufactured products, follow package directions. *Caution:* Do not apply products containing arnica to broken skin or open wounds.

Arnica

Calendula (*Calendula officinalis*)

Anti-inflammatory, astringent, antiseptic, and cooling: Pretty calendula has all of these properties, plus it inhibits bleeding. A tra-

FOR SENIORS WHO BRUISE EASILY

Have you ever seen a scattering of bruises on your forearms or shins and wondered how they got there? Older people sometimes develop capillary fragility. Capillaries are the smallest of blood vessels and the ones that tend to leak blood into tissues. Vitamin C and bioflavonoids, the nutrients that often accompany vitamin C in foods, help keep blood vessels strong and less likely to leak. You can either take a vitamin C supplement (at least 500 milligrams per day) or eat foods rich in vitamin C and bioflavonoids: peppers, guavas, parsley, dark green leafy vegetables, broccoli, cabbage, citrus fruits, and strawberries.

ditional remedy for wounds of all sorts, it can also be applied externally to bruises in the form of a compress, gel, cream, or salve. Steep the dried flowers in the same way as for arnica to make a compress. Apply to the injured area three times per day.

Comfrey (*Symphytum officinale*)
This herb contains allantoin, a substance that helps "knit" cells back together. It's also anti-inflammatory. The Commission E endorses its external use in treating bruises, sprains, and strains. You can make a poultice to apply to an injury, wrapping wet comfrey leaves in a clean cloth. Or make a tea of the roots or leaves (steep ¼ cup of dried roots or leaves in 2 cups of hot water for 15 minutes), cool, strain, and moisten a cloth with this solution. Apply for about an hour at a time. Repeat four times per day or as needed. Comfrey is contained in many commercial first-aid salves; apply these as the manufacturer recommends.

Tea (*Camellia sinensis*)
Both green and black tea contain tannins, astringent compounds that help shrink swollen tissue and narrow blood vessels. Here's a simple remedy: Grab a tea bag (plain old black or green tea), moisten it with water, and slap it on your bruise. Herbalist Sunny

Mavor, coauthor of *Kids, Herbs, and Health,* says she always keeps tea bags in her first-aid kit. She finds them a handy remedy for black eyes, among other mishaps.

St.-John's-Wort (*Hypericum perforatum*)
This bright yellow flower is anti-inflammatory and can be used topically to reduce pain and speed healing. Germany's Commission E endorses its external use for bruises. The flowering tops tinge the infused oil a lovely red. To use such an oil, simply apply it as necessary. *Caution:* May cause skin reactions to sun exposure, so cover your oil-anointed bruise if you're going out in the sun.

Cayenne (*Capsicum annuum, C. frutescens*)
These peppers contain a pain-reducing substance called capsaicin that also speeds wound healing. If your bruise aches, try massaging it with a commercial cream or ointment that contains cayenne. Again, apply according to manufacturer's directions. *Caution:* Wash your hands immediately after applying cayenne products—it's just too easy to apply the ointment and then rub an eye, with predictable stinging results.

Bilberry (*Vaccinium myrtillus*)
These fruits have a great reputation for strengthening and protecting capillaries and improving circulation, making them a good choice for bruises. *Typical dosage:* 240 to 480 milligrams of capsules standardized to 25 percent anthocyanoside per day, divided into two doses.

MEDICINAL GARNISH

Two common kitchen items can help heal bruises.

◆ Parsley. Its leaves can be crushed and applied repeatedly to a bruise. This remedy may help speed the disappearance of black-and-blue marks.

◆ Potato. Spud slices, raw and cool, are an old home remedy for bruises, including black eyes.

A SWEET SOURCE OF HEALING

Bromelain, the protein-digesting enzyme from pineapple, may be worth a try if you've suffered a serious injury accompanied by bruising. One study found that it reduced swelling, pain, and tenderness in patients who had suffered blunt trauma.

The potency of bromelain is measured in milk clotting units or MCUs; a typical dose might be one to four 2,400-MCU capsules two or three times per day between meals. Bromelain should be taken as soon as possible after the injury and continued for several days afterward. *Caution:* If you have gastric or duodenal ulcers or gastritis, you should not take bromelain.

Ginkgo (*Ginkgo biloba*)
While most famous for increasing blood flow to the brain, ginkgo also increases blood flow to the extremities. *Typical dosage:* 120 to 240 milligrams extract standardized to 24 percent ginkgo flavone glycosides and 6 percent terpene lactones per day, divided into two or three doses. *Caution:* Don't combine ginkgo with blood thinners.

BURNS

B URNS ARE A FACT OF LIFE—and will likely continue to be one until the sun explodes or until the human species learns to cook without heat. Burns can be as common as a kitchen scald or as rare as being struck by lightning; what they have in common is that proper first aid is important in all types of burns.

Skin damage in burns is measured by degrees. A first-degree burn involves only the surface skin, producing mild redness and pain. In second-degree burns, injury extends to deeper skin layers to produce darker redness along with swelling, pain, and blisters. A third-degree burn destroys all layers of skin, wiping out nervous sensation and, therefore, pain, although the surrounding tissue hurts. The burned skin appears white or charred.

If you receive a first-degree burn or a small second-degree burn (covering an area no larger than the palm of your hand), immediately immerse the injured area in cold water or apply a cold compress. Don't apply ice directly to the burned skin, but you can put ice cubes in the water. Continue for 10 minutes or until the pain stops.

If you receive a chemical burn, remove any chemical-splashed clothing and rinse the skin with cool water for 20 to 30 minutes. Do not apply ointments, oils, or butter. Keep the burn clean by gently washing it twice a day with water and mild soap. Call your doctor if signs of infection develop—redness, swelling, yellow drainage, or a foul smell.

Finally, if you have second-degree burns over an area larger than the palm of your hand, or on your face, hands, feet, or genitals—or any third-degree burn—have someone take you immediately to the doctor. If you can't drive, call 911 or your local emergency number. While awaiting help, cut away overlying clothing, unless it has adhered to the burn. Loosely cover the wound with sterile (nonadhesive) dressings or clean cloths such as linen or muslin. Do not apply anything else, not even water. To prevent swelling, elevate burned extremities. *These burns are a medical matter; do not self-treat them with the remedies in this book unless your doctor directs you to do so.*

DRUG TREATMENT

Analgesics

Aspirin, acetaminophen, ibuprofen, naproxen. *Function:* relieve pain. *Aspirin side effects:* heartburn, indigestion, stomach irritation, mild nausea or vomiting. *Acetaminophen side effects:* long-term use and higher dosages commonly produce liver damage that results in jaundice, malaise, nausea, and vomiting; may damage the kidneys. *Ibuprofen and naproxen side effects:* dizziness, nausea, stomachache, headache.

Grandma's Sunburn Cure

Oatmeal (*Avena sativa*) is soothing to irritated skin. You can use it in one of four ways.

◆ Cook 3 tablespoons of dry oatmeal in ½ cup of water, let cool, wrap in a gauzy cloth, and apply to the burn.

◆ Wrap ½ cup of dry oatmeal in cheesecloth and let steep in 3 cups water 15 minutes. Apply the cool liquid to the burn.

◆ Wrap 1 cup of dry oatmeal in a cloth or pour into a clean athletic sock. Tie a knot at the top. Put it in a tub of tepid water to soak for 10 minutes, then add yourself.

◆ Purchase a commercial oatmeal product that dissolves in water and add to your bath.

Topical Anesthetics

Lidocaine plus the antiseptic benzalkonium chloride (Bactine), benzocaine (Solarcaine, Americaine, Unguentine), benzocaine and menthol (Dermoplast), benzocaine and chloroxylenol (Foille), benzocaine and aloe (Lanacane). *Side effects:* infrequent allergic reactions, with hives, skin rash, tenderness, swelling of tissues of mouth and throat; may increase sun sensitivity.

Herbal Remedies

Aloe (*Aloe vera*)

The gel from inside this plant's leaves reduces inflammation, soothes burn pain, fights bacteria, and speeds healing. That's why many cooks keep an aloe plant in the kitchen window where it's handy for minor burns and scalds. You can also use a commercial preparation of pure aloe vera gel as often as needed.

Calendula (*Calendula officinalis*)

Anti-inflammatory, astringent, antiseptic, cooling, and wound-healing, calendula turns up in many over-the-counter burn products. You can also make a tea from the dried flower petals (steep 2 teaspoons of dried herb in 1 cup of hot water for 10 minutes; strain and let cool) and apply with a clean cloth as often as needed.

Comfrey (*Symphytum officinale*)
Both the leaves and root of this plant contain allantoin, which speeds healing of burned skin. Once again, look for commercial products or make a tea or poultice. To make a tea, steep 1 teaspoon of dried herb in 1 cup of hot water for 10 minutes; strain and let cool. To make a poultice, mash about a cup of fresh leaves, or soak a cup of dried ones in enough water to cover them. Wrap the mash in a thin cloth and apply to the burn as needed.

Lavender (*Lavandula angustifolia*)
The essential oil of this flower relieves pain and enhances the healing of burns. Unlike most other essential oils, it's fine to apply undiluted directly to the skin. If you fear that you may be allergic (or just don't like lavender's scent), dilute it with an equal quantity of vegetable oil such as olive, almond, or sesame oil. Apply as often as needed.

Gotu Kola (*Centella asiatica*)
A compound in gotu kola stimulates collagen synthesis to help repair skin. It helps heal wounds of all kinds and reduces scarring from burns. The easiest way to use it may be to open capsules of powdered gotu kola until you have about a teaspoon. Mix the powder with an equal quantity of aloe gel. Apply as often as needed.

Lavender

Plantain (*Plantago major, P. lanceolata*)
These common weeds contain antimicrobial and anti-inflammatory substances and the tissue-knitting substance allantoin. Crush a fresh plantain leaf and apply the juice directly to a minor burn as often as needed.

St.-John's-Wort (*Hypericum perforatum*)
A tea made from these yellow flowers is anti-inflammatory, and pain-reducing, and speeds healing of wounds and minor burns. Steep 2 teaspoons of dried herb in 1 cup of hot water for 10 minutes. Cool, strain, and use the tea to wet a clean cloth. Apply to

minor burns as needed. *Caution:* May increase skin reactions to sun exposure.

Tea (*Camellia sinensis*)
Both green and black teas are rich in antioxidants and cooling to sunburns. The sun's ultraviolet rays produce free radicals in the skin. Tea's antioxidants can mop up these free radicals to help prevent damage to tissues. Just apply a wet, cool tea bag to a burn.

• Witch Hazel (*Hamamelis virginiana*)
The extract of the bark of this tree—the same witch hazel you see cheaply available in stores—is astringent, decreases inflammation, and soothes sunburns.

BURSITIS AND TENDONITIS

MANY PEOPLE OVERDO. When you spend Saturday repainting the bedroom after sitting in a desk chair all week, how do you treat the sore shoulder that follows? Must be sore muscles, you shrug (or try to), deciding to work out the stiffness by relaxing on the golf course. The pain increases with each swing, but hey, it's only nine more holes. A few days later, you can barely raise the phone to your ear. What's going on?

Any time you put excessive or unaccustomed demands on your body, you risk stirring up inflammation. Repetitive motions are particularly likely to inflame two joint structures: the tendons and the bursae. A tendon attaches muscle to bone. A bursa is a fluid-filled sac that cushions and reduces friction in joints.

Inflammation of these structures is called tendonitis and bursitis, respectively. Tendonitis is likely to affect the wrist, shoulder, elbow, and knee; bursitis, the shoulder, elbow, hip, and knee. Both can occur at once.

WHEN TO CALL YOUR DOCTOR

If you experience any of the following symptoms, check in with your doctor or other health care practitioner. You may have an injury that needs more than home care.

◆ Significant pain and swelling

◆ Loss of significant range of motion in that joint

◆ No improvement in the injury after two or three days of rest and ice

DRUG TREATMENT

Analgesics

Aspirin, acetaminophen, ibuprofen, naproxen, ketoprofen. *Function:* ease tendonitis or bursitis pain. *Aspirin side effects:* heartburn, indigestion, stomach irritation, and mild nausea or vomiting. *Acetaminophen side effects:* chronic use or higher dosages may damage the liver or kidneys. *Ibuprofen, naproxen, and ketoprofen side effects:* continuous use may irritate stomach lining; long-term high-dose use may damage the liver or kidneys.

HERBAL REMEDIES

Turmeric (*Curcuma longa*)

Long prized as an anti-inflammatory and antioxidant agent, turmeric is now the subject of studies examining the effect of its active ingredient, curcumin. In laboratory experiments, curcumin proved as effective in reducing inflammation as the potent anti-inflammatory drugs hydrocortisone and phenylbutazone, but without the side effects. In Ayurvedic medicine, turmeric is used both topically and internally for sprains and other muscle injuries. *Typical dosage:* 400 to 600 milligrams in capsules three times per day. (Some products formulate curcumin with bromelain to improve absorption from the intestines, or with flaxseed oil to boost anti-inflammatory effects.) *Caution:* High doses of curcumin may irri-

tate the lining of the stomach and intestines. Do not take if you
have ulcers, gallstones, or bile duct obstruction. Not recommended
during pregnancy.

Ginger (*Zingiber officinale*)

With its anti-inflammatory, antioxidant, and pain-relieving properties, ginger works in not-so-mysterious ways. Scientists now know
that it inhibits the production of inflammatory chemicals called
prostaglandins and leukotrienes. A compound in ginger called 6-
shogaol can mildly reduce pain, probably by blocking the nerves'
transmission of pain signals. *Typical dosage:* up to eight 500-
milligram capsules per day; or 10 to 20 drops of tincture three
times per day; or ½ to 1 teaspoon of the ground root per day; or ⅓
ounce of fresh ginger (about a quarter-inch slice) per day. *Caution:*
Do not use if you have gallbladder disease.

Cayenne (*Capsicum annuum*)

Topical use of capsaicin, the compound that gives hot peppers their
kick, has been the focus of a lot of pain research. When first applied to the skin, capsaicin initially activates pain nerves, then

THE COMMONSENSE SORENESS CURE

If you suspect you've inflamed a tendon or bursa, protect
it from further motion. Put your arm in a sling if your shoulder or elbow hurts. Get off your feet if it's your knee or hip.
After a few days of babying the injury, begin to put the affected joint through its full range of motion—gently. Otherwise, you risk getting what's called a frozen joint. Frozen
shoulder syndrome is particularly common and requires
physical therapy to break up the adhesions that begin to
bind the joint.

While lying on the couch, apply a commercial cold pack,
a bag of crushed ice, or a bag of frozen peas or corn—over
a damp cloth to protect your skin. Leave the ice in place for
15 to 20 minutes and repeat three or four times a day for
the first few days.

THE HEALING POWER OF PROTEASES

Proteases are protein-digesting enzymes. They can help resolve inflammation by breaking down some of the inflammatory debris and improving circulation. Studies have shown benefits of proteases following blunt trauma and minor athletic injuries.

Two common proteases are found in fruits: Papaya contains papain and pineapple contains bromelain. These can also be taken, between meals, in supplemental form.

Edmund R. Burke, Ph.D., director of the Exercise Science Program at the University of Colorado at Colorado Springs and author of *Optimal Muscle Recovery,* recommends selecting an enteric-coated protease product to help resist breakdown by stomach acid. Also, he prefers using proteases in a combination that includes bromelain, papain, trypsin, and chymotrypsin. Enzyme combinations vary product to product, so follow manufacturer's directions on dosage.

renders them unresponsive, thereby relieving pain. It will also increase blood flow and make the injured area feel warm. This effect may not do much, however, for the deeper pain of tendonitis and bursitis. You'll have to be the judge of whether these commercial creams work on your pain; apply them as the manufacturer directs. Cayenne has benefits as an antioxidant when taken internally. Furthermore, it contains high concentrations of salicylic acid, the chemical relative of acetylsalicylic acid (aspirin). *Typical dosage:* up to three 400- to 500-milligram capsules per day; or 5 to 10 drops of tincture in water. *Caution:* Be sure to wash your hands with soap after applying cayenne or capsaicin creams to avoid spreading the heat to eyes, nose, or other sensitive tissues.

Willow (*Salix alba* and other *Salix* spp.)

This tree and other salicylate-containing plants—meadowsweet (*Filipendula ulmaria*), wintergreen (*Gaultheria procumbens*), and black birch bark (*Betula lenta*)—are very mild pain relievers. In fact, they're so mild that some experts think they can't possibly have a pain-relieving effect. Others swear by them. *Typical dosage:* three 500-milligram capsules per day; or 5 to 10 drops of tincture in water three times per day. *Caution:* Excessive doses may irritate the gastrointestinal tract. Do not use wintergreen or black birch oil internally.

Licorice (*Glycyrrhiza glabra*)

This sweet-tasting root inhibits inflammation in several ways. It acts much like your body's own natural corticosteroids. It decreases generation of damaging molecules called free radicals at the site of inflammation. And it inhibits an enzyme that's involved in the inflammatory process. *Typical dosage:* one 500-milligram capsule three times per day; or 20 to 30 drops of tincture three times per day; or 3 cups of tea per day (boil ½ teaspoon of herb in 1 cup of water for 15 minutes). Because licorice has an intensely sweet taste, you might want to blend it with other herbs when you make tea. *Caution:* Do not take licorice for more than six weeks. Do not take it if you are on diuretics, if you're pregnant, or if you have high blood pressure, diabetes, thyroid, kidney, liver, or heart disease.

Boswellia (*Boswellia serrata*)

This gum resin extract has anti-inflammatory and analgesic properties. Whether it specifically relieves pain and inflammation has not been studied, but the way it acts on a biochemical level to inhibit inflammation suggests that it would. *Typical dosage:* follow the manufacturer's instructions.

Devil's Claw (*Harpagophytum procumbens*)

Scientific studies have confirmed that devil's claw reduces pain and inflammation. According to Francis Brinker, N.D., author of *Formulas for Healthy Living,* the root of this African plant has become popular in Europe for pain relief. *Typical dosage:* up to six 500-milligram capsules per day; or 30 drops of the tincture three times per day. *Caution:* Do not take if you have gastric or duodenal ulcers.

Peppermint (*Mentha × piperita*)

Mint contains menthol, an aromatic oil. It acts as a counterirritant—a substance that causes an irritation that blocks another form of irritation. In this case, the cooling sensation of mint oil interferes with the sensation of pain. Many commercial and herbal liniments contain menthol; use them as the manufacturer directs. Or combine 10 to 15 drops of peppermint essential oil with 1 ounce of vegetable oil and apply as needed to the sore area. *Caution:* Some people develop an allergic skin rash when they contact peppermint essential oil or pure menthol. Try a test patch before slathering on a menthol-containing ointment.

CANKER SORES

MOUTH ULCERS, COMMONLY CALLED canker sores, can be excruciatingly uncomfortable. Experts disagree on what causes them, but the culprits that turn up frequently in studies include food allergies, immune dysfunction, viral infections, and nutritional deficiencies. In particular, being short on iron, vitamin B_{12}, or folic acid may bring on canker sores. So if these recurrent little sores are giving you trouble all out of proportion to their size, consider checking with your doctor or a qualified herbalist or nutritionist to determine whether you are running low on one of these nutrients.

DRUG TREATMENT

Topical Steroids
Triamcinolone acetonide (Aristocort), fluocinolone (Fluinide). *Function:* decrease inflammation and pain. *Side effects:* thinning of skin, redness, allergic reaction.

Local Anesthetics
Benzocaine (Anbesol, Orajel). *Function:* temporarily decrease pain. *Side effects:* allergic reactions; long-term use can affect the central nervous system.

Herbal Remedies

Gotu Kola (*Centella asiatica*)

Canker sores stem from a breakdown in tissue structure. Gotu kola is widely used to heal wounds and promote connective tissue growth. *Typical dosage:* 1 cup of tea daily (steep 1 teaspoon of dried herb in 1 cup of hot water for 10 minutes). You can also use this tea cold as a soothing rinse.

Echinacea (*Echinacea angustifolia, E. purpurea, E. pallida*)

Echinacea tinctures produce a numbing sensation that may offer relief from a canker sore's throbbing ache. If your sore is large, deep, or excruciatingly painful, however, be aware that the alcohol in tinctures may sting. If that's the case, or if you just want to avoid alcohol, try using a glycerin extract, also called a glycerite. *Typical dosage:* 20 to 40 drops in a few ounces of water up to four times per day. Swish around in the mouth to make sure that the numbing components make contact with the sore. *Caution:* Those allergic to ragweed may be allergic to echinacea. Do not use if you have autoimmune disorders.

Licorice (*Glycyrrhiza glabra*)

This potent anti-inflammatory herb helps tissues heal. Licorice is also antiviral, so if your canker sores have a viral connection, this is a good herb to use. *Typical dosage:* open a capsule and put a pinch of powder right on the sore, or suck on a lozenge made from deglycyrrhizinated licorice.

Chamomile (*Matricaria recutita*)

One study showed that a chamomile mouthwash was effective in treating mouth ulcers caused by chemotherapy, probably because the herb fights inflammation and helps wounds heal. It's also a gentle sedative, so if you think that stress may be depleting your immune system and that's why you're getting canker sores, this is a good herb to choose. *Typical dosage:* up to 4 cups of tea per day (steep 1 to 2 teaspoons of dried flowers in 1 cup of hot water for 10 minutes), taken internally or cooled and used as a mouthwash; or 10 to 40 drops of tincture up to three times per day (the tincture can also be taken internally or used as a mouthwash).

CANKER SORE SWAB

You can use this gel as often as hourly throughout the day, until your canker sore heals.

- 1 teaspoon echinacea tincture
- 1 teaspoon goldenseal tincture
- 1 teaspoon calendula tincture
- 1 teaspoon grapefruit seed extract
- 1 tablespoon aloe vera gel

Mix all ingredients in a small jar with a tight seal. To use, place a pea-size amount of the gel on a clean piece of gauze; hold in the mouth against the sore.

Goldenseal (*Hydrastis canadensis*)

Goldenseal is antiseptic and anti-inflammatory, so it can help fight the infection of a mouth ulcer and ease the swelling and throbbing that makes having one so painful. It also helps inhibit the further growth of bacteria. *Typical dosage:* 20 to 50 drops of tincture, dissolved in a little water and swished in the mouth. *Caution:* Do not use if you're pregnant or nursing.

Ginkgo (*Ginkgo biloba*)

This herb is starting to receive serious attention for its ability to promote healing when applied topically. Ginkgo leaf extract is rich in antioxidants and is anti-inflammatory. For canker sores, you don't need the more expensive extract; just make a strong tea using the leaf. *Typical dosage:* Steep ½ teaspoon of dried leaf in 1 cup of hot water for 15 minutes and apply to the sore with a clean cotton ball as needed.

Cardiac Arrhythmias

T HE HEART IS AN AMAZING ORGAN. It is designed to beat within a basic rhythm, which ensures that it accomplishes its task of moving blood through the body with maximum efficiency.

But when something disturbs that normal rhythm, an arrhythmia occurs. A number of things could cause this irregular beating: a failure of electrical impulses within the heart; scarring from previous heart attacks; a drug reaction; a disruption in body chemicals such as calcium, magnesium, or potassium; or a malfunction of the thyroid gland.

Many people experience "skipped heartbeats," or what feels like heartbeat fluttering, when they become sleep-deprived, experience periods of emotional stress, or overexert themselves physically. In these cases, rest and relaxation can help restore normal rhythm.

Arrhythmias might make you feel anxious, but most are not life-threatening. Whether or not an arrhythmia is serious depends on what is causing it. If structural deformities or heart disease is present, the arrhythmias are symptoms of a greater problem.

If you experience arrhythmias, see your doctor to rule out structural abnormalities or the presence of disease. One non-drug option for people with arrhythmias may be an outpatient surgical procedure to destroy certain muscle fibers responsible for the disturbed beat. In the case of life-threatening arrhythmias, doctors may recommend the implantation of a pacemaker.

Drug Treatment

Calcium Channel Blockers

Verapamil (Calan, Covera, Isoptin, Verelan). *Function:* interfere with exchange of calcium into cells to reduce the electrical ex-

THERAPY AT THE TABLE

You've heard it before and you'll likely hear it again: Diet is a crucial factor in any ailment involving the heart. Cardiac arrhythmia has been linked to food allergies. By all means, consult an allergist, but because these sensitivities are subtle and often elude conventional allergy tests, you may need to work with an experienced practitioner—a clinical nutritionist or naturopathic doctor—to identify them. Meanwhile, here are some foods you can emphasize and some you can cut back on or eliminate.

The "Do" List

Chicken
Cold-water fish
Fresh fruits
Garlic
Olive oil
Onions
Raw almonds
Raw vegetables
Turkey
Water—6 to 8 glasses
   per day

The "Don't" List

Alcohol
Caffeine
Fried foods
Herbal stimulants such
   as ephedra and
   guarana
High-fat dairy products
Margarine
Peanuts
Red meat
Soft drinks
Sugar

citability of certain heart tissues. *Side effects:* low blood pressure, swelling of hands and feet, constipation, dizziness, headache.

Beta Receptor Agonists

Inderal (Propranolol). *Function:* control arrhythmias by affecting chemical processes in the nervous system. *Side effects:* low blood pressure, shortness of breath, low heart rate, depression, fatigue.

SUPPLEMENTS TO HELP KEEP THE BEAT

The following nutrients may help ease arrhythmias:

♦ **Calcium chelate plus magnesium.** Calcium is essential for maintaining a regular heartbeat and it helps all the body's muscles repair after exercise. Magnesium should always accompany calcium for maximum effectiveness of both minerals. Low levels of these two nutrients can occur in people with arrhythmias. *Typical dosage:* 500 to 1,500 milligrams of calcium combined with 400 to 800 milligrams of magnesium per day.

♦ **Coenzyme Q$_{10}$.** This nutrient is an overall heart tonic. *Typical dosage:* up to 400 milligrams per day.

♦ **L-carnitine.** This nutrient reduces levels of triglycerides, a type of blood fat, while boosting the delivery of oxygen to the heart muscle during times of stress. *Typical dosage:* 1,000 milligrams per day in divided doses.

♦ **Selenium.** This nutrient acts as a powerful antioxidant in heart tissue, especially when paired with vitamin E (see below). *Typical dosage:* 200 micrograms per day.

♦ **Vitamin E.** This partner of selenium helps prevent heart tissue damage and naturally thins the blood. *Typical dosage:* 200 to 800 IU per day.

♦ **Potassium.** This mineral helps ensure proper ratios of body chemicals called electrolytes, which are often deficient in people experiencing arrhythmia. *Typical dosage:* aim for about 3,500 milligrams of potassium per day. *Caution:* Have your blood level for this mineral checked by a doctor before deciding on your dosage, because too much potassium is dangerous. A wide range of conditions and medications must not be combined with potassium supplements.

♦ **Fish oil.** Combine this easily obtainable supplement with vitamin E (or increase your consumption of coldwater fish) and you've got a potent heart tonic. *Typical dosage:* 100 to 400 milligrams per day.

Other Drugs

Lanoxin (Digoxin). *Function:* decrease excitability of nerve and muscle fibers in the heart. *Side effects:* nausea, vomiting, diarrhea, yellow-tinted vision, mental confusion.

HERBAL REMEDIES

Kava-Kava (*Piper methysticum*)

This South Pacific root can ease the anxiety that is a major cause of cardiac arrhythmias. And while kava-kava does produce relaxation, it doesn't have the side effects that pharmaceutical sedatives often do. *Typical dosage:* up to six 400- or 500-milligram capsules per day (look for supplements with 55 percent kavalactones); or 15 to 30 drops of tincture up to three times per day. *Caution:* Do not take when pregnant, nursing, depressed, or operating machinery or vehicles.

Valerian (*Valeriana officinalis*)

Many people with arrhythmias suffer also from insomnia, due either to their anxiety about the disorder or other worries. Valerian is another safe but potent herb for anxiety associated with arrhythmias. Precisely because it's so potent, it's the one to choose as a sleep aid. *Typical dosage:* 50 to 100 milligrams of standardized extract containing 0.8 percent valeric acid two or three times per day; or 20 to 60 drops of tincture per day. *Caution:* Continued use of valerian can cause headaches, which can be avoided by taking a break of two or three days every two weeks.

Chamomile (*Matricaria recutita*)

Time-honored, gently relaxing chamomile is often consumed in pill or tea form to soothe anxiety. *Typical dosage:* 50 to 75 milligrams of product standardized to 1 percent apigenin content two or three times per day; or 10 to 40 drops of tincture three times per day; or 3 or 4 cups of tea per day (steep ½ to 1 teaspoon of dried flowers in 1 cup of hot water for 10 to 15 minutes).

Hawthorn (*Crataegus* spp.)

A superior cardiovascular herb, hawthorn helps lower blood pressure and strengthens the heart muscle. In clinical trials, it has proven its ability to treat heart failure and minor arrhythmias. *Typ-*

ALL STRESSED UP AND NOWHERE TO VENT

During times of stress, your adrenaline starts pumping and directly affects your heartbeat. Relaxation therapies such as meditation, biofeedback, massage, and gentle exercises can help control conditions such as arrhythmia. Your health professional can refer you to relaxation classes given at your local hospital. Community recreation centers are also a good place to seek such classes.

ical dosage: up to 750 milligrams per day of extract standardized to 1.8 percent vitexin-2'rhamnoside or 10 percent procyanidins; or up to nine nonstandardized 500- or 600-milligram capsules per day; or 10 to 30 drops of tincture up to three times per day; or 3 cups of tea per day (steep 1 teaspoon of dried berries in 1 cup of hot water for 10 to 15 minutes). *Caution:* Hawthorn increases the effects of some heart medications; if you are taking any, consult your doctor before adding hawthorn to your regimen.

Reishi (*Ganoderma lucidum*)

This medicinal mushroom has long been used in China as a general heart tonic, as well as for a host of other conditions. If your arrhythmias are caused by stress, reishi is a good choice to add to your routine because it acts on the many body systems that can be affected by stress. *Typical dosage:* up to five 420-milligram capsules per day; or up to three 1,000-milligram tablets up to three times per day.

CARPAL TUNNEL SYNDROME

Back in the days before computers, carpal tunnel syndrome seemed to happen only to dairy farmers and needleworkers. Now that so many of us are "mousing and keyboarding"—without even stopping our typing long enough to hit a carriage return—this disorder of a nerve in the wrist affects thousands of people.

Carpal tunnel syndrome involves the compression of the median nerve, which passes between the bones and the ligaments of the wrist through what is called the carpal tunnel. When this nerve is repeatedly compressed, it can react by swelling. Typical symptoms include a tingling feeling in affected fingers, weakness, pain upon gripping, shooting pains that go into the fingers or up into the forearm, a sensation of tingling when the wrist is tapped, or increased pain at night, especially if the wrists are bent. The thumb and any of the next three fingers might be affected. The disorder can occur in one or both hands.

Hairstylists, carpenters, food service workers, and anyone else who uses repetitive hand motions in their work may also be at risk. Pregnancy may also play a role because of the fluid retention that moms-to-be experience. Sometimes the tendons of middle-aged women thicken, narrowing the tunnel and causing pressure on the nerve.

If carpal tunnel is severe enough, doctors may use a steroid injection to alleviate inflammation, although this approach doesn't cure the condition. Sometimes the only course of treatment is surgery to free the affected nerve.

DRUG TREATMENT

Anti-inflammatories

Ibuprofen, naproxen. *Function:* reduce inflammation and swelling by blocking the production of compounds called prostaglandins.

Supplements for Suppleness

If you're at risk for developing carpal tunnel syndrome, you may want to check your intake of the following nutrients:

◆ **Vitamin B$_6$.** Clinical data strongly suggest that a vitamin B$_6$ deficiency may contribute to carpal tunnel syndrome. While 25 milligrams of vitamin B$_6$ is considered adequate, some treatments for carpal tunnel syndrome involve taking 200 milligrams for two or three weeks, then half that dose for another one or two weeks. Results are not usually seen for a month—sometimes six weeks. *Caution:* Discuss your dosage with your doctor, because high doses of vitamin B$_6$ can be toxic. This vitamin also works best in combination with others, so a doctor's advice is doubly crucial.

◆ **Vitamin C with bioflavonoids.** This broad-spectrum nutrient is vital to tissue repair and healing and it can contribute to reducing inflammation. Vitamin C also plays a significant role in connective tissue regeneration. *Typical dosage:* 1,000 milligrams with each of three meals.

◆ **Bromelain.** Anyone who requires surgery for carpal tunnel syndrome should take bromelain for its ability to lessen swelling and inflammation. If you choose not to undergo surgery, bromelain helps prevent further tissue inflammation. *Typical dosage:* 500 milligrams one to three times daily.

◆ **Grapeseed extract.** Also known as pycnogenol, this compound contains powerful compounds that inhibit swelling and inflammation. Added bonus: It's good for your heart. *Typical dosage:* 500 milligrams two or three times per day.

Side effects: gastrointestinal problems such as stomach ulcers and bleeding, constipation, heartburn, dizziness, kidney and liver damage.

Diuretics

Hydrochlorothiazide (Dyazide, HydroDiuril), furosemide (Lasix). *Function:* force the kidneys to excrete fluids at a higher rate, relieving swelling that sometimes plays a role in carpal tunnel. *Side effects:* an imbalance in body chemistry that can affect bowel and heart function; low blood pressure; elevated blood levels of sugar, uric acid, and fats.

CARING FOR HARDWORKING WRISTS

In addition to taking herbs internally, there's a great deal you can do to prevent carpal tunnel syndrome or to treat a mild case before it worsens. You can apply herbs topically, or you can try wearing a wrist splint through the night or while working. Take frequent breaks, stretching your wrist and neck muscles when you do. Many doctors advise consulting a physical therapist for an individually tailored exercise program that takes into account the severity of your condition. One exercise suggested by the American Physical Therapy Association involves resting your forearm on a table or desk. With the other hand, grab the resting hand's fingertips. Pull back gently for 3 to 5 seconds. Repeat for the other hand.

Other ways to take the burden off your wrists:

♦ **Hydrotherapy.** Alternating between cold and hot packs may bring some pain relief, although the effect is usually only temporary.

♦ **Acupuncture or acupressure.** Either technique may help stimulate circulation and relieve pain. Consult a qualified practitioner trained in these disciplines.

Herbal Remedies

Turmeric (*Curcuma longa*)
This common kitchen spice contains a substance that can lower prostaglandin levels and reduce inflammation. *Typical dosage:* one 300-milligram capsule (standardized to 95 percent curcumin, the active ingredient) one to three times per day; or 10 to 30 drops of tincture up to three times per day; or up to 1 teaspoon of powdered spice per day in food.

Boswellia (*Boswellia serrata*)
This tree resin can block the production of leukotrienes and prostaglandins, two body chemicals that favor inflammation. It has a long tradition of use in Ayurvedic medicine for various types of joint, nerve, and muscle pain. *Typical dosage:* 300 to 350 milligrams in capsules two or three times per day (look for products that contain 65 percent boswellic acid).

Ginkgo (*Ginkgo biloba*)
Concentrated extracts of compounds from this tree's leaves increase blood flow and reduce swelling. Ginkgo also protects nerves and helps them heal. *Typical dosage:* 60 milligrams of extract in capsules or tablets standardized to 24 percent flavone glycosides, two or three times per day.

Cataracts

If you've ever driven through heavy fog or tried to see through a frost-covered windshield, you can imagine what cataracts are like—except that your vision doesn't clear when you reach your destination. Some people accept cataracts as part of aging, but blurred and diminished eyesight is not inevitable.

Cataracts are most often caused by overexposure to the sun, but other factors can contribute to them: cigarette smoking, heredity, injury, diabetes, and some medications, such as corticosteroid nasal sprays. Sugar plays a role in the formation of cataracts, but it might do so only for people with diabetes.

Cataracts aren't painful. They usually develop slowly, starting with blurred vision, spots, and the impression that a film is covering the eyes. People with cataracts also tend to see a lot of halos around lights and glare from lamps and the sun; they sometimes have double vision. Eventually, cataracts can lead to blindness. Fortunately, they can be caught early—if you get your eyes checked regularly.

GETTING YOUR DAILY ANTIOXIDANTS

Planning your diet around antioxidant content is a good thing to do even if your high-risk years for cataracts are far away. And you don't even have to memorize a list. Just aim for color: greens (leafy and cruciferous veggies), oranges (the fruit named for the color as well as sweet potatoes); yellows (squashes and bananas); reds (apples, cabbages, and beets); and purples (eggplants, peppers, asparagus, and beans). Some of the herbs in the lists below can also be eaten as leafy greens.

Herbs High in Vitamin A
◆ Dandelion leaves
◆ Purslane leaves
◆ Turmeric

Herbs High in Vitamin C
◆ Parsley
◆ Rose hips
◆ Turmeric

Herbs and Foods High in Vitamin E
◆ Nuts and seeds
◆ Turmeric
◆ Whole grains

DRUG TREATMENT

There is no drug treatment for cataracts and no known way—herbal or pharmaceutical—to reverse lens damage once it has occurred. Surgery to replace the damaged lens is the only treatment available. This surgery is one of the most common operations performed today. For 90 percent of people who have this surgery, vision is greatly improved, which allows most of them to continue driving.

Cataract surgery takes only about 30 minutes. It is performed either as an outpatient procedure or with a hospital stay of one to several days. On rare occasions, the surgery leads to complications such as infection, bleeding, pressure in the eye, pain, swelling, or detachment of the retina.

This procedure consumes the largest proportion of the Medicare budget, costing $3.2 billion annually in the United States. Many unnecessary cataract surgeries are performed, so make sure yours is needed. Sometimes a new prescription for corrective lenses is what's needed instead.

HERBAL REMEDIES

Bilberry (*Vaccinium myrtillus*)

These berries have a long tradition of use in improving vision and protecting the eyes from disease. The fruits of this tree contain high amounts of anthocyanosides and antioxidants, nutrients that can prevent clouding of the eyes. *Typical dosage:* two to three standardized capsules per day. (Bilberries are closely related to blueberries, cranberries, and huckleberries, which also contain anthocyanosides. It's a great excuse to eat these berries daily.)

Rosemary (*Rosmarinus officinalis*)

This common culinary herb contains a variety of powerful antioxidants. It's worth trying, though no formal studies have shown rosemary's effectiveness in

Rosemary

PROTECTING YOUR VISION

Cataracts are one of those disorders that require surgery
to correct. The lens of your eye is what allows you to focus
an image on the back of your eyeball; when the lens is
damaged, the image is flawed. Clouding of the lens results from oxidative damage that causes the proteins of
the lens to clump.

Several studies have suggested that antioxidants, particularly vitamins A, C, and E, may reduce cataract risk. But
because these studies are not conclusive, check with your
doctor if you want to use these vitamins for this purpose.

Wearing hats and the right kind of sunglasses can also
help, because they block the sun's ultraviolet rays. And if
you smoke, quit; cigarettes contribute to a number of oxidative processes in the body.

preventing cataracts. *Typical dosage:* James A. Duke, Ph.D., author of
The Green Pharmacy, recommends one cup of tea made from rosemary, catnip, and lemon balm each day (steep 1 teaspoon of a blend
of equal parts of the dried herbs in 1 cup of hot water for 10 to 15 minutes).

Turmeric (*Curcuma longa*)

This spice is packed with antioxidants, especially the big three that
have already been shown to prevent cataracts: vitamins A, C, and
E. Curcumin, the main component of this seasoning, has also been
shown to prevent cataracts in animals. *Typical dosage:* up to 1 teaspoon per day in food; or 250 to 500 milligrams of standardized
capsules up to three times per day; or 10 to 30 drops of tincture up
to three times per day.

Cervical Dysplasia

T HE WORDS *CERVICAL DYSPLASIA* mean that the cells lining the cervix, the slender entrance to the uterus, are abnormal. But because the condition can be a precursor to cervical cancer, they're among the most unwelcome words a woman can hear at her gynecologist's office.

The truth is, most women diagnosed with cervical dysplasia do *not* develop cancer. They recover fully. About one-third of mild cases spontaneously regress. Of the other cases, the Pap test's early warning offers a chance to prevent the condition from progressing. It usually takes 10 or more years for cancer to develop from mild dysplasia, according to the National Cancer Institute. The more advanced the abnormality is, the more likely the cells will become cancerous. Once a Pap test reveals the dysplasia, what happens next depends on how advanced it is, but even mild dysplasia requires careful monitoring.

You'll see below that herbs that support and repair the liver are an important category in fighting cancer and threatened cancer. Why? Abnormal cell growth is often a response to a continual irritant, such as cigarette smoke, the body's own waste products, waste products of disease-causing bacteria and other organisms, and environmental toxins such as pesticides. The liver produces enzymes that help the body break down and get rid of toxic waste. A decrease in liver function has been linked to an increased chance of developing cervical dysplasia and cancer. The liver is equally important in breaking down and regulating hormones such as estrogen. Certain herbs and foods may help the liver do its job better.

Drug Treatment

Currently, no pharmaceuticals can reverse cervical dysplasia or prevent its progression to cancer. Moderate and advanced cases are sometimes treated with various surgical techniques. Research is under way on the preventive powers of antioxidants such as vitamins A, C, and E, and of a group of chemicals called retinoids. Nonsteroidal anti-inflammatory drugs such as ibuprofen are also being studied. One new oral drug being researched, difluoromenthylor-

PREVENTION STRATEGIES

Women can decrease their risk for developing cervical dysplasia by practicing safe sex and avoiding cigarette smoking. One study found that women with cervical dysplasia are six times more likely than other women to be infected with the human papillomavirus, the same virus that causes genital warts. Dysplasia is also promoted by herpes simplex type II, the virus that causes genital herpes. Dysplasia is two to three times more likely to occur in women who smoke cigarettes. When smokers get it, it's often more severe.

Many women with dysplasia have a deficiency of folic acid, a part of the vitamin B complex. Folic acid also tends to be low among women who take oral contraceptives or drink heavily. Excessive estrogen, whether synthetic or produced by the body, can also increase the chances of cervical dysplasia and cervical cancer. And DES daughters—women exposed prenatally to the synthetic estrogen diethylstilbestrol—are at special risk of cervical dysplasia and vaginal cancer.

Whether you have additional risk factors or not, all women should have regular Pap tests, because one of the keys to treating and preventing cervical cancer is early detection of abnormal cells.

nithine (DFMO), shows some promise. It seems to inhibit the action of a key enzyme that promotes development of cancerous cells.

HERBAL REMEDIES

Burdock (*Arctium lappa, A. minus*)
This traditional detoxifying herb has demonstrated antitumor effects in animal studies; in other research it has acted as an antimutagen. Traditional Western herbalists and practitioners of Traditional Chinese Medicine consider the dried root of this plant a blood purifier. Some research shows that it stimulates the flow of bile, one of the key digestive substances the liver produces. *Typical dosage:* up to six 400- to 500-milligram capsules per day; or three cups of tea per day (steep 1 teaspoon of dried root in 1 cup of hot

SUPPLEMENTS FOR CERVICAL DYSPLASIA

Often, women with cervical dysplasia are deficient in several nutrients. If you are at risk, check whether you're getting enough of the following daily nutrients, or consult your doctor about fashioning a supplement regimen.

◆ Vitamin A (5,000 to 10,000 IU)

◆ Riboflavin (1.6 to 10 milligrams)

◆ Vitamin C (1,000 to 2,000 milligrams)

◆ Folic acid (400 to 600 micrograms)

◆ Vitamin E (400 to 800 IU)

Yellow dock

water for 10 to 15 minutes); or 10 to 25 drops of tincture three times daily.

Yellow Dock (*Rumex crispus*)

Although no research exists to validate its use, yellow dock has traditionally been used to treat enlarged lymph nodes, skin conditions, and respiratory infections. It is a folk remedy of high repute for cancer. *Typical dosage:* up to four 500-milligram capsules per day; or 20 to 40 drops of tincture, up to two times per day. *Caution:* Avoid during pregnancy. If you have kidney stones, consult a health care practitioner before using.

Milk Thistle (*Silybum marianum*)

This herb is not only one of the oldest remedies for any kind of condition involving liver stress, it's also one of the best researched. More than 300 studies have verified the effectiveness of its main compound, silymarin. It also deactivates harmful free radicals and prevents them from attacking the liver. *Typical dosage:* 140 milligrams of standardized silymarin capsules, three times per day; after 6 weeks reduce to 90 milligrams, three times per day; or 10 to 25 drops of tincture up to three times per day.

Turmeric (*Curcuma longa*)

This spice's active ingredient, curcumin, has been shown to reduce the incidence of cell mutation in smokers. *Typical dosage:* 250 to 500 milligrams of standardized curcumin capsules up to 3 times per day; or 10 to 30 drops of tincture up to 3 times per day; or up to 1 teaspoon per day of the ground spice in food.

Ginger (*Zingiber officinale*)

This spice is thought of in Traditional Chinese Medicine as a warming herb that helps remove stagnation. It also helps strengthen digestion and settle the stomach. *Typical dosage:* up to eight 500- to 600-milligram capsules per day; or several ⅛-inch slices of the fresh root taken in cooked foods; or 1 cup of tea per day (simmer 3 to 4 fresh root slices in 1 cup of water for 10 to 15 minutes). *Caution:* Do not exceed recommended dosage; do not take if you have gallbladder disease.

Red clover (*Trifolium pratense*)

Although its action to prevent or cure cancer has not been studied, red clover is a rich source of phytoestrogens—plant chemicals similar to human estrogens. Phytoestrogens may be responsible for the absence of cancer in those who eat a plant-based diet, because these plant-based estrogens lock on to certain cells, preventing the "real" estrogens from overstimulating the body. Red clover flowers are easily obtainable and safe and they make a reasonably tasty tea. *Typical dosage:* up to five 500-milligram capsules per day; or

YOU SAY TOMATO

Lycopene, a carotenoid found in both fresh and cooked tomatoes, seems to protect against dysplasia. Of course, in any condition that challenges the immune system, the more chemical toxins you avoid the better, so consider looking for organic tomatoes or growing your own. If you want to take lycopene as a supplement, take 1 to 5 milligrams daily.

2 or 3 cups of tea per day (steep 1 tablespoon of dried flowering tops in 1 cup of hot water for 10 to 15 minutes); or 15 to 30 drops of tincture up to four times per day.

Echinacea (*Echinacea purpurea, E. angustifolia, E. pallida*)

You'll see this immune booster in many commercial formulas, mainly for colds and flu. To get best results from echinacea, take it for two weeks, then take a one-week break. *Typical dosage:* up to nine 300- to 400-milligram capsules per day; or 60 drops of tincture up to three times per day. *Caution:* Anyone allergic to other members of the aster family such as ragweed may be allergic to echinacea. Do not use with immune disorders such as lupus or HIV.

Astragalus (*Astragalus membranaceus*)

This root has been used as a general tonic by the Chinese for 2,000 years. Studies show it has helped cancer patients' immune systems regain normal function. Astragalus sticks, widely available in Chinese pharmacies or health food stores, can be added to soups during cooking and then removed before serving, though you won't be sure how much you're getting this way. You may see astragalus in formulas blended with ligustrum berries (*Ligustrum lucidum*), another Chinese remedy. *Typical dosage:* eight or nine 400- to 500-milligram capsules daily; or 3 to 4 dropperfuls of tincture, three times per day.

Reishi (*Ganoderma lucidum*) and Shiitake (*Lentinula edodes*)

These edible fungi contain immune-boosting compounds. You can simmer a few dried mushrooms to make a broth, add a few fresh mushrooms per day to soups, or take tablets or liquid extracts. *Typical dosage of reishi*: up to five 500-milligram capsules per day; or up to three 1,000-milligram tablets up to three times per day. *Typical dosage of shiitake:* 500 milligrams standardized extract capsules or tablets 2 times per day.

Vitex (*Vitex agnus-castus*)

Also known as chaste berry or chaste tree, vitex is considered the herb of choice for treating PMS and other hormone-based conditions affecting women. While it hasn't yet been studied for cervical dysplasia, it may be useful in any condition involving the female reproductive tract. *Typical dosage:* up to three 650-milligram capsules per day; or

CERVICAL DYSPLASIA TEA

This tea can be stored in the refrigerator for up to three days; drink 2 to 3 cups per day before meals.

2	**teaspoons vitex berries**
1	**teaspoon burdock root**
1	**teaspoon red clover**
1	**teaspoon astragalus root**
½	**teaspoon stevia leaf (optional)**
½–1	**teaspoon peppermint, spearmint, or winter-green (optional)**
5	**cups water**

Bring herbs and water to a boil. Simmer gently for 5 minutes. Cover pot and let steep 20 more minutes. Strain out herbs.

1 cup of tea per day (steep 1 scant teaspoon of dried, ground berries in 1 cup of hot water for 10 to 15 minutes); or 15 to 40 drops of tincture per day. *Caution:* Do not take vitex if you are also taking hormone-replacement drugs. Do not use it if you are pregnant.

CHRONIC FATIGUE SYNDROME

IF YOU HABITUALLY READ UNTIL 1:00 A.M. and wake up at six feeling tired, that's not what doctors mean when they talk about chronic fatigue syndrome. That kind of tired is normal. Chronic fatigue syndrome (CFS) refers to a relentless, debilitating exhaustion that makes walking out to the mailbox feel like a Himalayan trek. Each year, some six million Americans see their doctors with symp-

Living with CFS

If you're going to conquer chronic fatigue, lifestyle adjustments are probably the most important treatment.

◆ **Rest, rest, rest.** You're going to have to make major modifications in your schedule, especially during flare-ups. This requires flexibility and understanding on the part of employer, spouse, and children—and yourself.

◆ **Reduce stress.** Researchers note that stress reduces immune function, resulting in many of the changes that occur in chronic fatigue syndrome. One theory is that stress-induced immune impairment could increase vulnerability for a viral infection or for reactivation of latent viruses such as herpes.

◆ **Exercise lightly.** Although too much physical activity can trigger a relapse, too little can weaken skeletal and heart muscles, further aggravating fatigue. Pacing is critical. Studies have found that moderate amounts of aerobic exercise can significantly improve fatigue, muscle strength, and overall fitness. Ask your doctor how much exercise is appropriate for you.

◆ **Eat wisely.** Avoid nutrient-depleting junk foods and go for a varied, whole-foods diet that includes ample protein and complex carbohydrates. Frequent, small meals every three hours or so can help maintain energy levels.

◆ **Avoid stimulants.** Flogging your system with stimulants only drains energy reserves, so it makes sense to stay away from caffeine, though it's easier said than done. Try subbing carob-coated nuts for chocolate bars, herb teas for black tea, and decaf or herbal coffee substitutes for the jolt of java.

◆ **Go smoke-free.** Cigarette smoke, including the secondhand form, increases susceptibility to respiratory tract infections, reduces how much oxygen gets to your cells, and generally wreaks immune-system havoc. It's a challenge you don't need.

toms of CFS. Because no one knows its exact cause, a cure remains elusive. Research and doctors' experience both suggest that some herbs and nutritional supplements can help ease the symptoms.

This illness begins as a flu-like cold that won't completely go away, followed by fatigue that rest won't relieve and tiredness that has nothing to do with overexertion. Other symptoms include sore throat, tender lymph nodes in the neck or armpit, muscle pain, joint pain, headaches, impaired memory and concentration, depression, anxiety, and insomnia. Symptoms tend to wax and wane; just when you think you're getting better and attempt to get your life back, you relapse.

If you suspect you have CFS, it's important to see a doctor for a diagnosis. Some easily treatable diseases can mimic CFS symptoms or underlie a full-blown case of CFS.

Drug Treatment

Currently, no "magic bullet" exists; no single drug has proven significantly and consistently helpful. Nonsteroidal anti-inflammatory drugs such as ibuprofen and naproxen can help relieve aching muscles and joints.

Some doctors prescribe benzodiazepine drugs such as Valium, Xanax, Serax, and Restoril when anxiety and insomnia predominate, or antidepressants when sadness is among the symptoms.

Herbal Remedies

Siberian Ginseng (*Eleutherococcus senticosus*)
This well-known tonic supports adrenal function and bolsters resistance to stress. A German study found that taking this herb (10 milligrams of fluid extract) three times daily for four weeks raised the number of immune cells in healthy volunteers. The two cell types that increased—T lymphocytes and natural killer cells—are often low in CFS sufferers. *Typical dosage:* Up to nine 400- to 500-milligram capsules per day; or 20 drops of tincture up to three times per day.

Echinacea (*Echinacea angustifolia, E. purpurea, E. pallida*)
This popular herb has been shown to enhance immune function in people with chronic fatigue syndrome. *Typical dosage:* up to nine

300- to 400-milligram capsules per day; or 60 drops three times per day. Take either for two weeks, followed by a one-week break. *Caution:* If you're allergic to other members of the daisy family, you may be allergic to echinacea.

Astragalus (*Astragalus membranaceus*)

A revered overall tonic in Traditional Chinese Medicine, astragalus rebuilds the immune system and is antibacterial and antiviral. It also improves stamina and is safe for long-term use. All of these qualities make it an ideal choice for chronic fatigue. *Typical dosage:* eight or nine 400- to 500-milligram capsules per day; or 15 to 30 drops of tincture two times per day.

Astragalus

Reishi (*Ganoderma lucidum*)

Another traditional Chinese remedy, reishi has been used as a folk medicine for thousands of years. Today, studies have confirmed that reishi protects the liver and fights allergies, inflammation, and viruses. It's also an antioxidant. Want more? Reishi helps calm anxiety and ease insomnia, and it's safe to use long-term. *Typical dosage:* up to five 420-milligram capsules per day; or up to three 1,000-milligram tablets up to three times per day.

Licorice (*Glycyrrhiza glabra*)

This root delays the body's removal of cortisol, an adrenal hormone that tends to be low in those with chronic fatigue syndrome. The chemical glycyrrhizin produces licorice's effect on cortisol and is responsible for its antiviral properties. This means that taking deglycyrrhizinated (DGL) licorice won't help CFS. Donald Brown, N.D., author of *Herbal Prescriptions for Better Health,* starts his CFS patients on 2,000 to 3,000 milligrams of licorice root twice daily for four to eight weeks. *Caution:* Do not take for longer than six weeks without a doctor's supervision. Do not take if you have high blood pressure, diabetes, or a disease of the thyroid, kidney, liver, or heart, or if you take diuretics. Do not use if you're pregnant.

Lomatium (*Lomatium dissectum*)

This herb has a long history of use by Native Americans. Some research suggests that it is active against many types of viruses and bacteria. Because lomatium root tinctures have been associated with a temporary, full-body rash, practitioners often use an isolate—an extract into either alcohol or glycerin that is specially processed to eliminate the rash-causing resins. *Typical dosage:* Researchers haven't come to a consensus on a dosage for lomatium, so follow the manufacturer's recommendation.

Lemon Balm (*Melissa officinalis*)

This traditional tea herb fights several viruses, including the herpes simplex virus, which has been suspected of contributing to chronic fatigue syndrome. *Typical dosage:* up to nine 300- to 400-milligram capsules per day; or 1 cup of tea per day (steep 2 to 4 teaspoons of dried herb in 1 cup of hot water for 10 to 15 minutes).

St.-John's-Wort (*Hypericum perforatum*)

Many herbalists find that this herb, usually called upon to treat depression, improves appetite and energy levels and calms anxiety. And it's antiviral. *Typical dosage:* 300 milligrams of product standardized to 0.3 percent hypericin three times per day; or 1 cup of tea per day (steep ½ to 1 teaspoon of dried herb in 1 cup of hot water for 10 to 15 minutes); or 15 to 40 drops of tincture up to three times per day.

Valerian (*Valeriana officinalis*)

If sleeplessness due to anxiety is one of your symptoms, valerian can be an important herb in your chronic fatigue regimen (for more alternatives, see Insomnia, page 351). It induces sleep as reliably as strong pharmaceutical sedatives, but without causing a morning hangover, interacting with alcohol, or leading to addiction. *Typical dosage:* 1 cup of tea (simmer 2 teaspoons of dried, minced root in 2 cups of water for 10 to 15 minutes; combine with other herbs or juice if the taste or smell is off-putting); or one 150- to 300-milligram capsule standardized to 0.8 percent valeric acid; or 300 to 400 milligrams in nonstandardized capsules; or ½ to 1 teaspoon of tincture in water. Take 30 minutes before bedtime. *Caution:* Valerian is not addictive, but if you're convinced you can't sleep without it, you could develop a psychological dependence. In rare instances, valerian stimulates instead of sedating. If this occurs, discontinue use.

Cold Sores

Y OU'VE BEEN UNDER A LITTLE STRESS. The boss is on your case, your car needs major repairs, and your in-laws are coming to visit in less than a week. Sitting at your desk one afternoon, you become aware of a tingling in your upper lip. The sensation is familiar—it heralds a cold sore.

Soon, the mirror will show the telltale cluster of small, painful blisters. And you'll be tempted to shroud your face in scarves until the sore goes away—usually within 10 to 14 days. If you get cold sores, chances are you already know that it's stress that triggers them, but the herpes simplex virus that causes them.

Drug Treatment

Oral Antiviral Drugs

Acyclovir (Avirax, Zovirax), valacyclovir (Valtrex). *Function:* inhibit (but not eliminate) the herpes simplex virus to shorten the duration of a cold sore outbreak; also inhibit the virus's ability to infect others. *Side effects:* loss of appetite, nausea and vomiting, constipation or diarrhea, excessive sweating, dizziness, malaise, headache, confusion; may lead to viral resistance.

Analgesics

Acetaminophen, aspirin, ibuprofen. *Function:* relieve pain and (except acetaminophen) inflammation of cold sores. *Aspirin side effects:* heartburn, mild nausea, vomiting. *Ibuprofen side effects:* dizziness, stomachache, nausea, headache, diarrhea.

Topical Drugs

Lidocaine (Viscous Xylocaine), benzocaine (Anbesol, Oragel, Topicaine). *Function:* numb the lesion. *Side effects:* possible allergic reactions.

Lip balms (Carmex, Blistex Lip Medex, Campho-phenique). *Function:* keep lesion moist, reduce pain. *Side effects:* rare to none.

EASY WAYS TO STOP THE SORES

Here are some additional tips for preventing cold sores or shortening their duration.

◆ **Protect yourself from the sun.** Sun exposure is a known trigger of cold sores. An hour before going outside, apply sunscreen to your face and lips and reapply it frequently. (The exception is products that contain titanium dioxide or zinc oxide; such sunblocks do not need to be applied in advance.) Large-brimmed hats can help but are not a substitute for sunscreen. And if you're taking St.-John's-wort internally, be doubly careful, as this herb can increase your skin's reactions to sun exposure.

◆ **Java junkies, rejoice.** The caffeine in coffee and tea inhibits the herpes simplex virus. In a study, a topical caffeine gel (Cafon) reduced the development of cold sore lesions. If you feel a lesion coming on, one of the fastest first-aid tools just might be a wet tea bag or some used coffee grounds. Tea also contains astringents that help dry herpes lesions.

HERBAL REMEDIES

Lemon Balm (*Melissa officinalis*)
This herb inhibits the spread of a variety of viruses, including the herpes simplex virus. A German study of people with cold sores and people with genital herpes found that a cream containing 1 percent lemon balm extract, applied five times per day, eased symptoms and reduced the size of the outbreak, apparently by preventing healthy cells from becoming infected with the virus. Within four days, 60 percent of the patients reported that their cold sores were healed. By the eighth day, 96 percent were lesion-free. Commercial lemon balm creams are available; if you have access to fresh lemon balm, you can make a compress or poultice from its leaves. *Typical dosage:* 3 to 4 cups of tea per day (steep 1 to 2 tea-

spoons of dried leaves in 1 cup of hot water for 10 minutes); or up to nine 300- to 400-milligram capsules per day; or essential oil of lemon balm applied directly to lesions three to five times per day. *Caution:* Do not take the essential oil internally.

Licorice (*Glycyrrhiza glabra*)

In studies, licorice inactivates the herpes simplex virus. It also has a potent anti-inflammatory effect. When an outbreak first occurs, you can apply commercial products that contain licorice extract and pain-relieving menthol from peppermint, or apply a licorice compress or poultice several times per day. *Typical dosage:* 3 cups of tea per day (steep 2 teaspoons of dried, chopped root in 1 cup of hot water for 15 minutes); or up to six 400- to 500-milligram capsules per day; or 20 to 30 drops of tincture up to three times per day. *Caution:* Do not use licorice internally for longer than six weeks. Do not take it at all if you have heart disease, high blood pressure, or liver disease, if you're on diuretics or digitalis, or if you're pregnant.

Mullein (*Verbascum thapsus*)

Laboratory studies have shown that this plant helps fight herpes viruses. It also soothes irritated skin. *Typical dosage:* 6 to 8 cups of tea per day (steep 2 teaspoons of dried flowers and leaves in 1 cup of hot water for 10 minutes); or 25 to 40 drops of tincture every three hours while awake. To make a compress, dampen a clean cloth with the cooled tea and apply it to the cold sore as needed.

Mullein

St.-John's-Wort (*Hypericum perforatum*)

Hypericin, one of the compounds in St.-John's-wort, also fights the herpes viruses. The herb has long been used to heal wounds. *Typical dosage:* 300 milligrams in capsules three times per day; or 15 to 40 drops of tincture three times per day; or 3 cups of tea per day (steep 1 teaspoon of dried plant in one cup of hot water for 10 minutes). You can also apply a compress made with the tea to the cold sores three times per day. *Caution:* May cause increased skin reactions to sun exposure. Do not take internally if you are on an antidepressant drug.

VITAMINS FOR INSIDE AND OUT

The following supplements may help fend off or heal cold sores.

◆ Vitamin C, zinc, and quercetin all fight the herpes simplex virus. In one study, frequent application of a solution containing vitamin C helped heal cold-sore lesions and reduce symptoms. Topical application of a zinc sulfate gel to cold sores also works. Quercetin, a plant pigment found in onions, garlic, and other foods, fights herpes. And bee propolis, which contains quercetin, worked better against herpes simplex type 1 than quercetin alone in a study. You can look for these ingredients either separately or together in manufactured topical products.

◆ The amino acid lysine combats the herpes virus. Because the virus requires arginine, another amino acid, to replicate itself, a diet high in lysine and low in arginine might, in theory, help prevent herpes. Knowing what we do about high-fat diets and their side effects, however, it's hard to recommend that people eat more meat and dairy products, which are high in lysine, and fewer legumes, whole grains, and nuts, all of which contain arginine.

But could lysine supplementation help prevent cold-sore recurrences? Maybe. Some, but not all studies, show it to be effective. In one, 1,000 milligrams of L-lysine three times per day for six months was effective in reducing recurrences. So if you're prone to cold-sore outbreaks, you may want to discuss lysine supplements with your doctor.

Echinacea (*Echinacea angustifolia, E. purpurea, E. pallida*)

Another herb that inhibits herpes viruses, echinacea extracts also produce a numbing sensation that may offer relief from cold-sore pain. Try using echinacea tea in poultices and compresses. If an all-over ill feeling accompanies your cold sores, or a common cold triggered the lesions, take echinacea internally. *Typical dosage:* up to nine 300- to 400-milligram capsules per day; or 60 drops of tincture three times per day.

Clove (*Syzygium aromaticum*)

In a laboratory study, clove was used in combination with acyclovir. The drug-plus-herb combination performed better than either treatment given alone. So even if you're taking antiviral drugs, you might try applying essential oil of clove to your cold sore. *Caution:* Don't take this oil internally.

Garlic (*Allium sativum*)

Pungent and potent, garlic fights many viruses, including herpes simplex viruses. During cold-sore outbreaks, you may want to include plenty of garlic in your diet. To preserve the antimicrobial activity, cut, crush, or press the cloves, then mix them into cooked foods at the last minute. *Typical dosage:* one to three fresh cloves per day.

Colds and Flu

Some people seem to head into the cold and flu season as though forging into a blizzard—head down, shoulders hunched, hands jammed deep into pockets. Even if they don't physically adopt this defensive posture, their mental attitude assumes a gloomy crouch. You'd think they could already hear the wind howl—a wind that seems to blow thousands of respiratory viruses their way.

While it's true that the cold and flu season rides in on winter's coattails, it's really not the weather that causes all the misery. It's the time spent indoors, sharing air space with sick people. The viruses that cause colds and flu are highly contagious and there's no denying that they play havoc with our health. Colds and flu are a leading cause of doctor's office visits and missed days from work. Adults get an average of four colds a year. They get more if they smoke or spend a lot of time around small children.

IS IT A COLD, OR THE FLU? HOW TO TELL

Cold symptoms restrict themselves to the upper respiratory passages. In other words, from the shoulders down, you feel pretty good. The flu comes on quickly and produces an all-over sick feeling.

Symptom	Common Cold	Flu
Onset	gradual	abrupt and dramatic
Nose	drippy	congested
Throat	scratchy	sore
Chest	slight cough as symptoms wane	cough can be severe and lingering
Heads	light headache from congestion	more pronounced headache
Muscle aches	absent	usually present
Chills/fever	absent, or low-grade fever	usually present
Sensitivity to light	absent	sometimes present
Fatigue	absent	present
Appetite loss	absent	present

The harsh, cold fact is that no pharmaceuticals—over-the-counter or prescription—can prevent or cure the common cold. Most don't even relieve symptoms and some actually make them worse. For the flu, vaccines offer limited prevention, as do a few drugs. And it's true that standard, over-the-counter pain relievers can ease some symptoms of both colds and flu.

But scientific studies show that antihistamine-decongestant combination drugs don't help colds and can produce undesirable side effects. In fact, one such study found that aspirin and acetaminophen—both common in cold drugs—actually suppressed people's immune response and increased cold symptoms such as nasal congestion. But these shortcomings don't stop Americans from using them.

The variety of cold medications you'll find in any drugstore can be dizzying—especially if you're already woozy from your cold! But herbal remedies surpass these standard drugs in a number of ways. Some enhance immune function, meaning you may escape the cold that's going around, or if you do get it, you'll fight it more effectively. Some herbs can inhibit viruses; some can alleviate symptoms. The added bonus is that traditional cold and flu herbs rarely cause adverse effects.

Of course, the very abundance of herbal cold and flu remedies is both blessing and curse. Choosing among them can be just as confusing as wandering the drugstore aisles. One suggestion: add an immune-system tonic, such as astragalus or reishi, to your daily regimen during cold and flu season. If you feel a cold or flu coming on, use immune-system stimulants, such as echinacea, and antiviral herbs to help your body marshal its own defenses. If the virus inflicts its symptoms on you, choose your herbs to relieve whatever symptoms you're experiencing. Of course, any remedy works best when you also allow yourself proper rest, increase fluids, and eat nourishing foods.

DRUG TREATMENT

Analgesics
Aspirin, acetaminophen, ibuprofen, naproxen. *Function:* reduce fever and relieve pain. Frequently used in multi-symptom drugs. *Aspirin side effects:* heartburn, indigestion, mild nausea, vomiting, irritation of the stomach lining; less commonly, aggravation of asthma. *Ibuprofen and naproxen side effects:* dizziness, nausea, stomach cramps, headache, diarrhea, skin rash.

Antihistamines
Brompheniramine, chlorpheniramine, diphenhydramine, many others (included in Comtrex, Contac, Dimetapp, Dristan, and Vicks formulas). *Function:* dry nasal secretions. *Side effects:* drowsiness, dry mouth, nose, and throat; oddly enough, nasal congestion.

Decongestants
Pseudoephedrine (Sudafed, Dimetapp Decongestant), phenyle-phrine (Dristan, Neo-Synephrine), oxymetazoline (Afrin, Dristan

A REMEDY WORTH ITS SALT

One simple remedy you'll find at the drugstore is helpful for cold and flu symptoms: saline nasal sprays and drops (such as Ocean or Ayr Non-Medicated Saline Nasal). Spraying salt water into your nose can help loosen congestion, making it easier to expel.

You can easily make your own saline solution by mixing ¼ to ½ teaspoon of table salt with 1 cup of warm tap water. Mix it fresh each day and put into a spray bottle or a dropper bottle. Use as needed. You can also try irrigating your nose with the solution, using a small pot with a spout called a neti pot available from yoga equipment suppliers.

But better yet, try irrigating your nose with a decoction of healing herbs, plus saline. The berberine-containing herbs—goldenseal, Oregon graperoot, gold thread, and barberry—act as natural antibiotics and mucous membrane tonics. Simmer ⅛ cup of herb in 1 cup of water for 10 minutes and strain. Then add this broth to the saline solution above.

12-Hour Nasal Spray, Sinex), xylometazoline (Neo-Synephrine II). *Function:* shrink swollen mucous membranes. *Oral decongestant side effects:* jitteriness, agitation, suppressed appetite, insomnia. *Nasal decongestant side effects:* overuse can lead to rebound congestion—a return of stuffiness that is often even more stubborn.

Antiviral Drugs

Amantadine (Symmetrel, Symadine); rimantadine (Flumadine). *Function:* prevent type A influenza when taken daily throughout flu season; reduce symptoms when given within 48 hours of symptom onset. *Side effects:* headache, difficulty concentrating, lightheadedness, irritability, nervousness, insomnia, nightmares; drugs may also stimulate the creation of drug-resistant viral strains. (A new flu drug, Zanamivir, is being developed; it is administered into the nose. So far studies show that it reduces the duration and intensity of flu symptoms, with far fewer side effects than other antivirals.)

The No-Good, All-Too-Common Treatment

Antibiotics have no place in the treatment of viral respiratory infections—common colds and flu—unless the illness becomes complicated by a bacterial infection. Nevertheless, studies show that doctors prescribe antibiotics to about 60 percent of their sniffling patients with colds and flu. The annual cost of unwarranted use of antibiotics for colds runs about $37.5 million. If your doctor prescribes antibiotics for your cold or flu, ask why. Ask what the side effects of such antibiotics may be. You may be able to put off using the drugs unless you develop symptoms that indicate bacterial infection—and you may learn something just by talking to your doctor.

Other Drugs

Flu shots. Immunizations can be obtained against certain strains of flu virus. Effectiveness varies and wanes quickly, depending on the type of vaccine and immune health of the recipient. *Side effects:* skin reactions at shot injection site; less commonly fever, muscle aches. (A relatively new alternative to flu shots is getting a dose of the weakened virus intranasally; so far, studies show this method is effective and has few side effects.)

Herbal Remedies

Echinacea (*Echinacea purpurea, E. angustifolia, E. pallida*)

This species is the single best-researched herb for helping the body fight colds and flu once they've begun to invade. It stimulates white blood cell activity, increases the body's production of antiviral substances such as interferon, and enhances the ability of immune cells to engulf and destroy invading microbes.

Research has shown that echinacea, when taken as soon as symptoms appear, can shorten the duration and lessen the severity of cold and flu symptoms. You'll be seeing more research about echinacea,

THE FLU-FIGHTING FUNGI

Medicinal mushrooms such as shiitake (*Lentinus edodes*) and reishi (*Ganoderma lucidum*) all possess substances called polysaccharides that stimulate the immune system. Shiitake also increases the body's production of the antiviral substance interferon. Although human trials haven't yet taken place, studies in animals show that shiitake likely offers some protection against influenza. If you're making a pot of chicken soup to help prevent a cold, throw in fresh or dried shiitakes to taste. But if you want the healing compounds in these mushrooms to help you fight a cold that you've already gotten, take them in supplement form. *Typical dosage:* 500 milligrams of standardized extract capsules or tablets, twice per day.

Meanwhile, reishi's anti-inflammatory components may help ease the respiratory-tract inflammation that often comes with colds and flu. This mushroom is a long-used and well-respected tonic in Asian medicine. *Typical dosage:* up to five 420-milligram capsules per day; or up to three 1,000-milligram tablets, up to three times per day.

because many questions remain. Which species is most effective and which parts of the plant? Which is best: tincture or capsule? Experts continue to debate the answers.

Doctors and researchers do agree on one thing: Dosage is key. You need to take enough echinacea, and take it frequently enough, to do any good. One study on treatment of flu found that a daily dose of about 1 teaspoon of a root tincture helped, but that ½ teaspoon did not. *Typical dosage:* 1 teaspoon of liquid extract; or 2 teaspoons of tincture (preferably made from the root); or 900 milligrams of solid extract in capsules per day. Divide the daily total into six doses per day for the first two days, then reduce to three to four doses per day. *Caution:* Don't use echinacea if you have multiple sclerosis, HIV infection or AIDS, or another autoimmune disease. Rarely, people with allergies to other members of the daisy family are also allergic to echinacea.

Astragalus (*Astragalus membranaceus*)

This Chinese herb possesses immune-boosting and antiviral properties. Unlike echinacea, astragalus may be taken long-term during cold and flu season; Chinese studies have found it to be an effective preventive against the common cold. Health practitioners find it particularly useful in enhancing recovery after an illness and in building resistance to infection for people who seem to catch every cold and flu virus that crosses their path. *Typical dosage:* eight or nine 400- to 500-milligram capsules per day; or 15 to 30 drops of tincture twice per day.

Asian Ginseng (*Panax ginseng*) and Siberian Ginseng (*Eleutherococcus senticosus*)

These two herbs have a strong reputation as overall health enhancers and immune-system rebuilders. Like astragalus, they are well-suited to long-term daily use. *Typical dosage for Asian ginseng*: 100 mil-

MORE HERBAL COLD COMBINATIONS

Sometimes flu or colds come with raw, irritated respiratory linings. Herbs that have demulcent qualities can help soothe inflamed throat and bronchial passages. Among these herbs are: mullein (*Verbascum thapsus*), which also has expectorant and antiviral properties; marshmallow (*Althaea officinalis*); slippery elm (*Ulmus rubra*); plantain (*Plantago lanceolata*); and licorice (*Glycyrrhiza glabra*). (For more about these herbs and their soothing actions, see Sore Throat, page 499.)

Expectorants help loosen respiratory secretions so they can be coughed up. Herbal expectorants include horehound (*Marrubium vulgare*), eucalyptus (*Eucalyptus globulus*), and thyme (*Thymus vulgaris*). Thyme is also antimicrobial and relaxes smooth muscle, a property that can help open tight airways. That's while you'll often see these herbs in combination products for colds that come with coughs.

COLDS AND FLU ◆ **183**

BASIC COLD AND FLU TEA

This blend combines herbs to soothe the symptoms of the usual cold and flu symptoms with ones that fight viruses and bacteria.

To make 1 cup of tea blend:

¼ **cup dried peppermint leaves**
¼ **cup dried lemon balm leaves**
¼ **cup dried elder flowers**
¼ **cup dried yarrow flowers**

Store in an airtight jar away from heat and light for up to a year.

To make 1 cup of tea:

1   **cup water**
1–2 **teaspoons tea blend**
½–1 **teaspoon fresh grated ginger (optional)**
Honey (optional)
Lemon juice (optional)

Bring water to a boil, then remove from heat. Add tea and ginger if using (ginger helps chase away that chilled feeling and adds a sweet/hot taste to the tea). Steep for 5 to 10 minutes. Strain; add honey and/or lemon, if desired.

ligrams of standardized products (usually standardized to 5 to 7 percent ginsenosides) one or two times per day; or up to four 400- to 600-milligram capsules per day. *Caution:* Do not use during pregnancy or nursing. Do not combine with caffeine. If you have high blood pressure, consult a doctor before taking panax ginseng. Discontinue use if you experience nervousness, irritability, insomnia, or gastrointestinal upset. *Typical dosage for Siberian ginseng*: up to nine 400- to 500-milligram capsules per day; or 20 drops of tincture up to three times per day. Take for two to three weeks, followed by a one- to two-week break.

Licorice Root (*Glycyrrhiza glabra*)

This root stimulates the production of several types of immune cells and increases the body's interferon production. It also helps reduce inflammation. Use whole-root products; the deglycyrrhizinated, or DGL, licorice (used to treat ulcers) doesn't contain the component that you want for fighting colds and flu. *Typical dosage:* up to six 400- to 500-milligram capsules per day; or 20 to 30 drops of tincture up to three times per day. *Caution:* Do not use for longer than six weeks. People with high blood pressure, diabetes, or disease of the thyroid, kidney, liver, or heart, and those taking corticosteroids should not take licorice unless advised to do so by their physician. Do not use while pregnant or nursing.

Elderberry (*Sambucus nigra, S. canadensis*)

This tree's berries are tasty flu fighters. They contain compounds that can inhibit the enzyme that flu viruses use to penetrate our cell membranes. In an Israeli study, most of the children and adults who took elderberry extract daily for flu, starting as soon as their symptoms began, got rid of it in two or three days, compared to at least six days for those who got no elderberry extract. Commercial syrups and lozenges with elderberry extract are available; follow the package directions for dosage. And don't forget about elder flowers, which have a long tradition of use in herbal tea blends to induce sweating during flu-induced fevers. *Typical dosage:* up to six 500- to 600-milligram capsules per day; or up to 40 drops of tincture every 4 hours; or up to 3 cups of tea per day (simmer 1 tablespoon of dried berries in 2 cups of hot water for 15 minutes, or steep 2 teaspoons of dried flowers in 1 cup of hot water for 10 to 15 minutes).

Elderberry

Garlic (*Allium sativum*)

This herb benefits health in myriad ways, including boosting immune function and inhibiting or killing a broad range of microbes, such as bacteria, yeast, parasites, and fungi. Studies show that garlic is active against viruses that cause colds and flus. Our bodies eliminate some of garlic's active ingredients through the lungs, putting those cold- and flu-fighters right where you want them. During cold and flu season, you might want to take garlic supplements and/or eat plenty of garlic and its cousin, the onion. Raw garlic packs the stronger antimicrobial punch. If you can't tolerate it raw, try adding minced garlic at the end of cooking to preserve active ingredients. If you're worried about garlic breath, chew parsley leaves or fennel seeds afterward. *Typical dosage:* one or more fresh cloves per day; or capsules that provide 4,000 to 5,000 micrograms of allicin per day.

St.-John's-Wort (*Hypericum perforatum*)

Usually mentioned as a remedy for mild depression, this flowering plant has many other beneficial qualities. According to studies, it can inhibit influenza A viruses and parainfluenza virus (which produces flu-like symptoms), but not cold viruses. *Typical dosage:* 300 milligrams of product standardized to 0.3 percent hypericin three times per day; or 3 cups of tea per day (steep 1 teaspoon of dried herb in 1 cup of hot water for 10 to 15 minutes); or 15 to 40 drops of tincture up to three times per day. *Caution:* May cause increased skin reactions to sun exposure.

Lemon Balm (*Melissa officinalis*)

This herb fights a host of bacteria and some viruses, including parainfluenza virus. Teas and extracts made from the leaves have a pleasant lemony, minty taste. If you enjoy gardening, consider planting lemon balm; it grows easily and prolifically in most climates. *Typical dosage:* up to nine 300- to 400-milligram capsules per day; or 1 to 3 cups of tea per day (steep 1½ to 4 teaspoons of dried herb in 1 cup of hot water for 10 to 15 minutes).

Ephedra (*Ephedra sinica*)

Chemically speaking, this herb is a near cousin to the over-the-counter drug pseudoephedrine (Sudafed). It acts as a respiratory decongestant and relaxes the airways. Unfortunately, ephedra also stimulates the cardiovascular and central nervous systems, and it has been abused for its appetite-suppressant and stimulant qualities. *Typical dosage:* 15 to 30 drops of tincture in water up to four times per day. For other products, scrupulously follow manufacturer's or practitioner's recommendations. *Caution:* Large doses can raise blood pressure and cause palpitations, nervousness, insomnia, nausea,

Herbal Steam and Bath Tea

Steam is an old-fashioned remedy for colds, coughs, and congestion. You can increase steam's effectiveness by adding herbs or their essential oils to the pot. When herbal steams are inhaled, antiseptic, decongestant, airway-relaxing herbal ingredients get right where they're needed.

4 cups water
3 tablespoons eucalyptus leaves
2 tablespoons thyme leaves
1 tablespoon rosemary leaves
1 tablespoon peppermint leaves

In a large saucepan (not a teakettle), bring the water to a boil. Remove from heat and add the herbs; allow to steep, covered, for 3 to 5 minutes. (You can substitute 3 to 5 drops of essential oil of any of those same herbs; just make sure you use a total of 3 to 5 drops, not 5 drops of each.)

Remove the pot from the burner. Carefully pour the water into a heat resistant bowl and place it on a sturdy table. Put a towel over your head and hold your face at least 12 inches away from the steam. If the temperature feels comfortable, take an experimental breath. If the steam feels good, drape a towel around your head and breathe deeply—through your nose if you have a cold or sinus infection, through your mouth if you have a cough.

After you're finished inhaling the steam, strain out the herbs and pour the solution into the bath. If you used essential oils for your steam, just run a hot bath and add 5 to 10 drops before stepping in. (Reading a steamy novel while you soak is completely optional.)

flushing, and headaches. If you use an herbal product that contains ephedra, don't exceed the manufacturer's recommended dose. Do not combine with caffeine or other stimulant herbs or drugs, nor with MAO-inhibiting antidepressants. Not recommended for people with a history of anorexia, glaucoma, thyroid disease, heart disease, high blood pressure, difficulty urinating due to prostate enlargement, or chronic insomnia. Do not use during pregnancy.

Peppermint (*Mentha × piperita*)

This herb's essential oil is often included in commercial products such as nasal decongestants, throat lozenges, cough drops, chest rubs, and inhalants. In one study, people who inhaled menthol, a component of peppermint, said they felt as if they had less nasal congestion, although the menthol didn't increase their measurable air-flow. Menthol can also relax the airways. You might try putting a few drops of peppermint or eucalyptus oil on your pillow or in an herbal steam (see "Herbal Steam and Bath Tea" on page 186). Meanwhile, essential oil, applied externally, short-circuits the nerve transmission from the pain receptors, which means you can rub diluted peppermint oil on your temples to reduce headache (just be sure to keep it away from your eyes). You can also add 5 to 10 drops of peppermint oil to a bath.

Ginger (*Zingiber officinale*)

Anti-inflammatory and analgesic, ginger also helps you cough up mucus and makes you feel warmer, which may help if you're

COLD AND FLU BREW

This traditional blend can help boost immunity and ease the discomfort of a cold or flu.

- 2¼ teaspoons echinacea leaf
- 2¼ teaspoons elder flowers
- 2¼ teaspoons yarrow leaves and flowers
- 1¼ teaspoons peppermint
- 3 cups water

Place all but the peppermint leaves in the water and simmer, covered, for 10 to 15 minutes. Remove from heat and add the peppermint. Steep, covered, for 10 more minutes. Strain herbs and discard. Drink up to 3 cups of tea per day as needed. Store in the refrigerator for up to 3 days.

COLD AND FLU VITAMINS

Research particularly supports the use of these two supplements during colds and flu.

◆ **Vitamin C.** Many, but not all, studies have found that taking vitamin C can reduce your number of colds per year. Most studies showed that vitamin C resulted in milder symptoms and reduced the duration of colds by about a third. A commonly recommended dosage during colds and flus is 500 to 1,000 milligrams every two hours. In the event of diarrhea, decrease the dose.

◆ **Zinc.** In a study of adults with colds, people who took one zinc gluconate lozenge every two hours while awake got better much quicker. They did complain of bad taste and nausea, but no serious side effects. Such lozenges are available without a prescription in most drugstores. Follow the manufacturer's directions for dosage, usually one lozenge every two hours while symptoms persist, but not longer than three or four days.

chilled. Ginger also blends well with traditional mulling spices and is an excellent condiment. (If you're feeling too warm or are running a fever, however, avoid ginger.) *Typical dosage:* ½ teaspoon dried, powdered root per day; or 1 teaspoon of the fresh ground root added to food per day; or 3 cups of tea per day (simmer 1 teaspoon of grated fresh root in 1 cup of water for 10 minutes); or up to eight 500- to 600-milligram capsules per day; or 10 to 20 drops of tincture in water three times per day.

Yarrow (*Achillea millefolium*)
This herb possesses anti-inflammatory, antispasmodic, and sweat-inducing properties. Herbalists have long included yarrow flowers in cold and flu remedies, often blended with elder flowers and peppermint. *Typical dosage:* up to 3 cups of tea per day (steep 1 teaspoon of dried flowers in 1 cup of hot water for 10 to 15 min-

utes); or 10 to 20 drops of tincture up to three times per day. *Caution*: Do not use during pregnancy.

Boneset (*Eupatorium perfoliatum*)

This herb has a long tradition of use for colds and flus. It's used to induce sweating, reduce fever, and ease body aches. In studies, it also stimulates immune cells. Whether it does so inside the human body isn't yet known. *Typical dosage:* Look for boneset in combination products and follow manufacturer's directions. *Caution:* Larger-than-recommended doses may induce vomiting.

CONSTIPATION

NORMAL BODILY RHYTHMS VARY from one person to the next. But when bowel movements become less frequent than about three per week, most health practitioners view that as a case of constipation. This is particularly true if the stools are dry, hard, or painful to pass.

Constipation usually arises from inadequate fluid and fiber intake, but it can have other causes. Many medications have a constipating effect, including codeine, tranquilizers, sedatives, iron supplements, some ulcer drugs, and some drugs used to ease spasms of the intestines, bladder, and bronchi (the airways in the lungs). General anesthesia can slow bowel movements. Constipation can also accompany abdominal conditions such as irritable bowel syndrome and bowel obstruction.

The number and types of laxatives on the market are a testament to just how common the problem of constipation is. Most of these laxatives have few side effects and many use the same ingredients as herbal remedies. The exception, as far as side effects go, are the stimulant laxatives; some herbal alternatives fall into this category. Most herbal laxatives loosen stools by adding bulk to naturally improve bowel function. For them to work, however, they require that you drink plenty of fluids. Otherwise, any bulking agent can further harden stools.

REGULAR WAYS TO STAY REGULAR

There are a few easy lifestyle changes that can help make your life more regular.

◆ **Drink more fluids.** This means eight to ten tall glasses of liquids such as water, herb tea, and juice. Vodka and white wine don't count; any form of alcohol has a dehydrating effect. The same is true of caffeinated beverages. Milk constipates some people.

◆ **Make meals fiber-rich.** Substitute whole wheat for white bread, brown rice for white. Experiment with different grains and beans. Eat lots of fresh fruits and vegetables. Foods particularly good at promoting regularity include figs, prunes, blackberries, bran, almonds, and apples. Avoid foods made from low-fiber, highly processed grains, such as grocery store cereals, crackers, and pastries.

◆ **Monitor your magnesium.** This mineral can have a laxative effect. Good food sources of magnesium include nuts, blackstrap molasses, whole grains, soy, and seafood. If you do take magnesium supplements, most nutritionists agree that you should balance them with two times as much calcium. Aim for a total daily consumption of 1,000 to 1,200 milligrams of calcium and 300 to 500 milligrams of magnesium, whether you get it from supplements or food.

◆ **Stay active.** Exercise encourages good bowel function. You don't have to run the Boston Marathon. Gentle exercises such as walking, gardening, and yoga can do the trick.

DRUG TREATMENT

Bulking Agents

Bran, malt soup extract (Maltsupex), methylcellulose (Citrucel), psyllium (Metamucil, Perdiem). *Function:* add fiber to the bowel, which gives stool bulk and makes it easier to pass. *Side effects:* brief initial bloated feeling.

Stool Softeners
Docusate (Correctol, Dioeze), mineral oil (Agoral), poloxamer 188 (Alaxin, Kondremul). *Function:* allow stool to absorb more water, making it easier to pass. *Side effects:* rare to none.

Osmotic Agents
Lactulose (Evalose, Lactulax), magnesium citrate (Citroma, Citro-Nesia), magnesium-containing laxatives (Haley's M-O, Phillips' Milk of Magnesia), others. *Function:* keep water in the intestines to soften stools. *Side effects:* rare to none.

Stimulant Laxatives
Aloe (Diocto-K Plus), bisacodyl (Bisac-Evac, Deficol), castor oil (Alphamul, Emulsoil), phenolphthalein (Ex-Lax, Feen-a-Mint), senna (Dosaflex, Fletcher's Castoria), others. *Function:* irritate the intestinal lining to prompt bowel movements. *Side effects:* cramps, diarrhea, dependence, salt imbalances.

Enemas
Phosphate solutions (Fleet). *Function:* empty the bowels. *Side effects:* may create salt imbalances with habitual use.

HERBAL REMEDIES

Psyllium Seed (*Plantago psyllium*)
These seeds and their husks are a great source of natural fiber that's easily obtainable in commercial products. You can also buy powdered seed husks at health food stores and forgo the added sweeteners, dyes, and so on. Some practitioners believe the seed husks may lodge in intestinal pockets and cause irritation, forcing the intestines to contract and expel their contents. *Typical dosage:* 1 tablespoon dissolved in an 8-ounce glass of water or juice. Drink immediately, because the seed husks swell quickly, creating a sludge that's difficult to swallow. Follow immediately with another glass of water.

Flaxseed (*Linum usitatissimum*)
This bulking agent provides a significant source of omega-3 essential fatty acids, one that is missing from the typical American diet. But its benefit for constipation stems from its fiber content. The

seeds can be ground and added to cereals or smoothies, or sprinkled directly on foods after cooking. Store the seeds in the freezer, because the oils in flax seeds spoil at even mildly warm temperatures. *Typical dosage:* 1 teaspoon of ground seeds in 1 cup of water or juice up to three times per day.

Papaya (*Papaya carica*)

This tropical fruit contains proteolytic enzymes, making it a natural digestive aid. Make a tea of the leaves, or purchase papaya enzymes in chewable tablets or capsules at a natural foods store. *Typical dosage:* Take according to manufacturer's directions.

Cascara Sagrada (*Rhamnus purshiana*)

Compounds in the bark of the cascara sagrada tree are so strong that the bark must be aged before it can be used safely. You'll see cascara sagrada as an ingredient in some over-the-counter laxatives. *Typical dosage:* up to two 400- to 500-milligram capsules per day; or ½ to 1 teaspoon of liquid extract per day. *Caution:* Do not take if pregnant or nursing. Like all stimulant laxatives, cascara sagrada can cause laxative dependency.

Senna (*Senna alexandrina*)

Among the strongest of the herbal stimulant laxatives, senna products can be derived from the seed pods or the leaves; the leaves are considered safer to use. Because the compounds in senna are so potent, this herb is best used under the advice of a doctor or other qualified practitioner. *Caution:* Do not use senna if you're pregnant or nursing, or if you're taking heart medications, licorice root, thiazide diuretics, or steroids.

Cascara sagrada

CUTS AND SCRAPES

MOST RUN-OF-THE-MILL CUTS AND SCRAPES—what doctors refer to as abrasions—usually need only a good washing with lots of tepid water and mild soap. If the wound bleeds, apply direct, steady pressure for 10 minutes. If it continues to bleed, see your doctor; you may need stitches. If foreign objects became embedded in your skin, try to remove them using a clean washcloth, sterile gauze, or tweezers. Left where they are, such invaders can lead to discomfort, infection, scarring, and, in the case of asphalt, permanent tattooing.

Wounds heal faster when left open to the air, so don't cover them with a bandage unless you plan on digging in the garden, changing the oil in your car, or doing something else to make the cut dirty.

Ointments and salves, whether conventional or herbal, can help prevent scabs from breaking open when abrasions involve areas subject to repeated stretching, such as elbows and knees. Herbs used externally in poultices, compresses, gels, or salves can speed healing and inhibit microorganisms. In the case of puncture wounds, however, do not apply herbs that hasten wound closure, such as comfrey or aloe, because rapid closure seals in microbes. Instead, choose herbs with antimicrobial properties to fight infection; let the wound gradually close.

DRUG TREATMENT

For superficial cuts and scrapes, you won't need to take any drugs by mouth—unless the wound becomes infected. In that case, it may require oral antibiotics. But there are some drawbacks to a few of the usual first-aid remedies you may have learned about.

◆ **Hydrogen peroxide.** Although a commonly used first-aid remedy, this fizzy fluid can interfere with blood clotting and is only mildly antimicrobial.

◆ **Rubbing alcohol.** This stuff stings, can actually damage tissue, inhibits blood clotting, and is not a very good antiseptic.

It's Red, It Hurts, What Is It?

Abscesses, also called boils, are tender red lumps in the skin. They typically range from one-half to one inch in diameter. They can result from a cut that becomes infected. Puncture wounds are particularly prone to infection, because they don't bleed enough to wash out bacteria. Abscesses can also result from infection in a hair follicle or skin pore. Staph bacteria (*Staphylococcus aureus*) are often to blame.

So is that what you have? The borders of a boil will feel well-defined because your body is walling off the infection that's present. After a week or so, the skin overlying the abscess becomes thinner; the abscess begins to look like a pimple. A few days later, the thinned skin ruptures and the pus drains out, relieving both the infection and the pain. Sometimes doctors hasten this process by lancing a boil, or cutting it open with a scalpel. But don't try this at home—you might make things worse.

You can hasten the healing of boils at home by applying hot herbal compresses. Make a tea of an antimicrobial herb such as Oregon graperoot or thyme leaves. Or add five drops of tea tree oil or grapefruit seed extract per cup of hot water. Wet a clean cloth in this hot-to-tolerance solution and apply to the abscess until the compress cools. Repeat three times in one session; aim for three sessions a day. Because infection is walled off in an abscess, it's unlikely that these herbs' antimicrobial properties will be absorbed deep into the skin. But the warmth will increase healing circulation to the abscess site. In addition, should the abscess begin to drain, such herbal compresses can help clear infection and prevent its spread. *Caution:* Do not squeeze an abscess or boil. This only increases the pain and spreads the infection. Once the abscess opens, it usually drains on its own, but you can gently compress the sides. If the abscess resulted from a puncture wound, is on your face, or you develop a fever or red streaks leading away from the wound, see a doctor.

◆ **Merthiolate.** It also stings and can injure tissue.

◆ **Antibiotic-containing ointments.** These include bacitracin (Baciguent), polymyxin B and bacitracin (Polysporin, Neosporin), or neomycin, polymyxin B, and bacitracin (Bactine First Aid, Mycitracin, Neo-Polycin, Neosporin Maximum Strength, Topisporin, Triple Antibiotic). These ointments are used to prevent infection (usually not necessary in minor scrapes) and keep the wound moist. Allergy to any of the component antibiotics can lead to local redness, itching, and swelling.

◆ **Topical analgesics.** These include such products as Bactine First Aid Antiseptic and many others. They often come in combination with a topical antiseptic, so they help prevent infection and relieve pain—but the pain relief is usually brief.

HERBAL REMEDIES

Aloe (*Aloe vera*)

It's not just for burns anymore. Aloe reduces inflammation and feels soothing, plus it's antibacterial. It contains allantoin, a substance that stimulates cellular proliferation; studies have shown it to hasten wound healing. Slice a fresh aloe leaf lengthwise and slather on the gel, or use a commercial preparation of pure aloe vera gel. In both cases, apply as needed.

Cayenne (*Capsicum annuum*)

This spice contains the pain-relieving component capsaicin, which speeds wound healing, inhibits bleeding, improves circulation, and fights infection. One experiment that compared capsaicin cream with other topical agents such as bacitracin, silver sulfadiazine, and aloe vera gel found that capsaicin cream produced the fastest rate of skin regrowth, making it the leader for closing wounds quickly. But cayenne burns open wounds, eyes, and sensitive genital tissues; on the other hand, a cayenne-containing cream might benefit an abscess by promoting circulation and easing pain (for more on abscesses, see "It's Red, It Hurts, What Is It?" on page 194). Whichever product you purchase, follow the manufacturer's directions on how often to apply.

Calendula (*Calendula officinalis*)

Anti-inflammatory, astringent, and antiseptic, calendula promotes new skin growth and inhibits bleeding. You can use the fresh or dried flowers in a salve or compress, or look for commercial creams or lotions that contain it. Apply them according to manufacturer's directions (usually as often as needed).

Comfrey (*Symphytum officinale*)

Another allantoin-containing herb, comfrey speeds healing. It can safely be used externally in salves, compresses, and poultices. To make a comfrey-leaf poultice, wrap fresh or dried leaves in a clean, wet cloth and apply.

Echinacea (*Echinacea purpurea, E. angustifolia, E. pallida*)

Usually discussed for its internal immune-boosting qualities, echinacea is mildly antiseptic, improves wound healing, decreases inflammation, and has a numbing effect. If you have a tincture of this herb on hand, you can use it topically, though it may sting. A glycerin extract avoids this drawback, but may be a bit sticky. If infection from a wound threatens, take the herb internally. *Typical dosage:* 1 teaspoon of liquid extract three times per day; or 2 teaspoons of tincture (preferably one made from the root) three times per day; or 300 milligrams of solid extract in capsules three times per day. *Caution:* People allergic to ragweed may also be allergic to echinacea. Those with autoimmune disorders should not take it internally.

Garlic (*Allium sativum*)

Try applying a crushed clove of this microbe-fighter to a boil or abscess; tape it in place for an hour or two. Bear two things in mind: one, the antibiotic components may not penetrate to the heart of an abscess; two, the garlic may irritate your skin. If irritation occurs, discontinue. Garlic's near relative, onion, can be used in a similar way.

Gotu Kola (*Centella asiatica*)

Extracts of this herb have become popular in Europe for both internal and external use in the healing of wounds. The active compound, asiatic acid, is particularly effective in stimulating synthesis of collagen, a prominent component of the deeper layers of skin. *Typical dosage*: up to eight 400- to 500-milligram capsules per day; or 20 to 40 drops of tincture up to two times per day.

Grapefruit Seed Extract
With broad antimicrobial action against bacteria such as strep, staph, and tetanus, this extract is available as a concentrate, skin cleanser, ointment, and antiseptic spray. Follow the manufacturer's recommendations for dosage.

Honey
Though it's a bee product, not an herb, honey is a time-honored wound healer. Scientific studies confirm that it speeds healing and fights infection. In an Israeli study, health care workers applied fresh, unprocessed honey to the open, infected wounds of infants that had failed to heal with conventional treatment. After five days of twice-daily honey applications, all infants were much improved. Three weeks later, all wounds had healed. Of course, this can be a messy remedy; it's likely to attract both pets and pests! To keep them away, cover the wound with gauze and tape in place.

Oregon Graperoot (*Mahonia aquifolium*)
Like its relatives barberry and goldenseal, this herb is anti-inflammatory and infection fighting. Its liquid extract can be applied to abrasions, and if infection threatens, the extract can be taken internally. There's not much research yet to support a typical internal dose, so follow manufacturer's or practitioner's recommendations.

Plantain (*Plantago* spp.)
This weed contains antimicrobial and anti-inflammatory substances and the tissue-knitting substance allantoin. Tear a leaf and you'll see it's also mucilaginous, or gooey. You can mash a few leaves into a poultice and apply to a wound. Herbalist Sunny Mavor, coauthor of *Kids, Herbs, and Health,* calls plantain "a backyard bandage."

Tea Tree Oil (*Melaleuca alternifolia*)
This oil from an Australian shrub is a good antiseptic, particularly useful for treating or preventing bacterial skin infections. Simply apply the undiluted oil to a scrape or cut, as needed.

Thyme (*Thymus vulgaris*)
Smell that pungent, clean scent? Thyme contains volatile oils with potent antimicrobial action. You can wash a wound with a tea made of the leaves (steep 1 teaspoon in 1 cup of hot water for 10 minutes) or with a cup of water containing three to five drops of thyme essential oil.

DANDRUFF

IN INFANTS, IT'S CALLED CRADLE CAP, but in adults it goes by a harsher name—dandruff. Either way, it refers to flaking pieces of skin on the scalp, which can be noticeable.

Dandruff is an inflammation of the skin, which is why it produces redness along with those telltale flakes. Although it typically occurs on the head, it can also appear on the face, back, stomach, and folds of the body. Psoriasis is a similar disease; it's often confused with dandruff. Unfortunately, dandruff can be a chronic disorder that lasts a lifetime.

Nobody knows exactly what causes dandruff. It may be inherited. It may be related to an infection of the skin by a fungus similar to the one that causes athlete's foot. It may even be caused by an allergic reaction to the fungus itself. Stress, fatigue, weather extremes, oily skin, infrequent hair or skin cleaning, obesity, and alcohol-containing skin lotions can trigger outbreaks of dandruff. The elderly and patients with AIDS and Parkinson's disease tend to develop dandruff more frequently than other people.

DRUG TREATMENT

Shampoos
Shampoos containing tar (Denorex, T-Sal), zinc pyrithion (Head and Shoulders), or selenium (Selsun Blue). *Function:* remove the outer layer of dead cells from the skin. *Side effects:* irritation and inflammation of the hair follicles, allergic reactions.

HEALTHY SCALP RINSE

The herbs in this hair and scalp rinse have antifungal and soothing properties. The vinegar helps restore the hair's correct pH.

2 cups apple cider vinegar
¼ cup dried sage, rosemary, or thyme leaves, or any combination

Heat the vinegar just to the boiling point. Remove from heat and add the herbs. Cover and steep for 10 minutes. Strain; discard the herbs. Pour into empty shampoo bottles and label. Use about ¼ cup in 2 cups of water as a rinse after shampooing.

Ketoconazole shampoos (Nizoral). *Function:* block the growth of fungus that can be associated with dandruff. *Side effects:* stinging, itching, and redness of the skin.

Internal Drugs

Corticosteroids or hydrocortisone (Medrol, Hexadrol, Benisone). *Function:* decrease the inflammation and itching associated with dandruff. *Side effects:* redness, acne, and thinning of the skin.

HERBAL REMEDIES

Evening Primrose (*Oenothera biennis*)

The oil from this plant's seeds is commonly used to treat allergic rashes, but it may help if you have dandruff. Evening primrose contains gamma-linolenic acid, or GLA, which is converted by the body to anti-inflammatory prostaglandins. *Typical dosage:* 8 to 12 capsules per day; or try rubbing evening primrose oil into the scalp.

Flaxseed (*Linum usitatissimum*)

Another beneficial seed oil, flaxseed, with its high levels of omega-3 fatty acids, turns up in lists of remedies for many inflammatory conditions. *Typical dosage:* 1 teaspoon per day internally; you can also use flaxseed oil as a scalp rub.

Tea Tree (*Melaleuca alternifolia*)

The essential oil of this tree is a potent antifungal agent. It's also very strongly drying, so your best bet is to add a few drops of tea tree oil to one of the above-mentioned oils. Rub the mixture into the scalp before bedtime. In the morning wash it out.

DEPRESSION

ALMOST EVERYONE EXPERIENCES depression at some time in his or her life. Depression is that sad, hopeless, middle-of-the-winter, dark night of the soul place where one feels trapped in despair. But depression is more than just a feeling—it is a profound psychological and physical experience.

The American Psychiatric Association defines depression as a condition in which a number of symptoms persist for at least one month. If you have four of the following symptoms, you are probably depressed; if five, you are definitely depressed.

◆ Feelings of worthlessness, self-reproach, or inappropriate guilt

◆ Recurrent thoughts of death or suicide

◆ Poor appetite with weight loss, or increased appetite with weight gain

◆ Insomnia or hypersomnia (sleeping more than usual)

◆ Physical hyperactivity or inactivity

◆ Loss of interest or pleasure in usual activities, or decrease in sexual drive

◆ Loss of energy and feelings of fatigue

◆ Diminished ability to think and concentrate

Along with these symptoms, many physical functions in the body can become unbalanced as well. Constipation and changes in the

WHEN DEPRESSION IS SERIOUS

Depression can be painful. If you are seriously considering suicide as a solution to your depression, please get help now. Call your primary care physician or a local crisis line; if you can't do either of these, go to the emergency room of your local hospital or a nearby psychiatric clinic.

menstrual cycle are common. You may feel cold, weak, and sluggish. Depression may occur as a transient, brief event or it may be a lifelong struggle. When depression results from a life event such as the death of a loved one, the end of a relationship, or the loss of a job, the feelings may be appropriate and normal. In fact, a period of grief and sadness is essential. Treatment is generally not needed unless the depression is unusually prolonged, is severe enough to make someone nonfunctional, or is resulting in serious suicidal thoughts.

Some people experience lifelong or recurrent depressions not necessarily related to outside events. In these people, current scientific theory holds that there is an imbalance in neurotransmitters—compounds that transmit information to and from nerve cells. Among the neurotransmitters involved in depression are serotonin (a mood-controlling brain chemical), melatonin, dopamine, adrenaline, and noradrenaline. These compounds can be affected to some extent by most treatments that help ease depression, including drugs, herbs, and nutrients.

Most people with depression should seek a thorough medical evaluation. Symptoms that look like depression might be caused instead by a specific medical condition, such as thyroid disease, hypoglycemia, hormonal imbalances, or a drug side effect. These conditions need their own treatment. Also, whatever the cause of the depression, various types of therapy can be extremely helpful. Look for a therapist who has experience in working with depression. Support groups are also helpful.

WORK WITH YOUR DOCTOR

If you are already taking antidepressant drugs and wish to try herbs instead, it's mandatory to work with your doctor to develop a schedule for making this transition. Don't try it alone. Some herbs for depression can have harmful interactions with commonly prescribed antidepressants; others take time to show their full effects.

Drug Treatment

Selective Serotonin Reuptake Inhibitors (SSRIs)

Fluoxetine (Prozac), sertraline (Zoloft), paroxetine (Paxil), fluvoxamine (Luvox), others. *Function:* prevent the metabolism of the mood-controlling brain chemical serotonin, thus increasing the amount of this neurotransmitter available to the brain. *Side effects:* agitation, anxiety, insomnia, tremors, headaches, nausea, sexual dysfunction; less commonly, paradoxical sedation.

Tricyclic Antidepressants

Amitriptyline (Elavil, Limbitrol), imipramine (Tofranil), doxepin (Adapin, Sinequan), others. *Function:* adjust norepinephrine metabolism; some also affect serotonin, the mood-controlling brain chemical, and dopamine. *Side effects:* sedation, dry mouth, constipation, low blood pressure.

Monoamine Oxidase Inhibitors (MAO Inhibitors)

Phenelzine sulfate (Nardil), tranylcypromine sulfate (Parnate). *Function:* inhibit an enzyme that breaks down various neurotransmitters. *Side effects:* serious interactions with some drugs and some foods; headache, dry mouth, drowsiness, weight gain.

Sedatives

Trazodone (Desyryl), nefazodone (Serzone). *Function:* ease nighttime insomnia due to depression. *Side effects:* sedation, dry mouth, constipation, low blood pressure.

Other Drugs

Bupropion (Wellbutrin). *Function:* affect serotonin, norepenephrine, and dopamine. *Side effects:* agitation, anxiety, insomnia, tremors, headaches, nausea, appetite suppression.

Venlafaxine (Effexor). *Function:* affect serotonin, norepinephrine, and dopamine. *Side effects:* insomnia, anxiety, weight loss, increased blood pressure.

HERBAL REMEDIES

St.-John's-Wort (*Hypericum perforatum*)

For mild to moderate depression, this herb lives up to its hype. More than 40 scientific studies have verified the traditional use of this herb for depression. Studies have compared St.-John's-wort with placebos (fake pills) and with antidepressant drugs. All showed that this herb is effective in the treatment of mild to moderate depression, appearing to work in about 70 percent of cases. It works as well as prescription drugs and has significantly fewer side effects.

In all the studies, however, St.-John's-wort took at least two

BITTERS MAKES IT BETTER

Here's an irony: Something nasty tasting can help you recover your taste for life's sweetness. A preparation called bitters, often made from such herbs as gentian, wormwood, and mugwort, can help ease depression's effects on the body because of the stimulating and enlivening effect of bitters on the digestive system. Remember that depression is not just a state of mind; it affects the entire body's physiology. Bitters improve endocrine and digestive processes, lift energy, and help to treat constipation, a common symptom in depression. Bitters are readily available in herb stores in a variety of liquid extract forms. Take the extract with meals, at a dose of 1 dropperful to ½ teaspoon in water three times per day; or follow the manufacturer's or practitioner's instructions.

The Ultimate Mood-Lifter: Movement

There is no question that exercise can improve mood and lift depression. Exercise stimulates the body and may increase some of those important neurotransmitters. It is especially good to exercise outdoors at least some of the time; fresh air, sunshine, and proximity to nature are all mood-lifters. Although you might find it hard to initiate an exercise program when you are already depressed, only the first steps are the hardest. So consider asking someone else to exercise with you; having company can encourage you to get going and reduce the isolation that is common in depression. You don't need to do anything elaborate, expensive, or strenuous; just going for a walk will do the trick.

weeks to have any effect. In some people it can take up to one month. *Typical dosage:* 900 milligrams of capsules standardized to 0.3 percent hypericin per day in divided doses, with meals (including a dose at bedtime if you suffer from insomnia); or ¼ to 1 teaspoon of tincture three times per day. (A simple tea made from the dried herb won't help depression; the herb loses its potency when it dries.) *Caution:* St.-John's-wort may cause mild stomach upset, rashes, restlessness, insomnia, or sensitivity to sun exposure.

Oats (*Avena sativa*)
This is the same plant that goes into your morning oatmeal. It is a wonderful tonic for the nervous system, having generalized nourishing and soothing qualities. The plant is traditionally used not only for depression but also for anxiety, stress, fatigue, and debility. The seeds have the strongest medicinal qualities, especially when harvested at what is called the milk stage. If you squeeze the fresh green seeds, a little drop of milky fluid emerges. When buying dried oats for tea, look for pale green to yellow seeds, rather than something that looks like chopped straw. *Typical dosage:* 3 cups of tea per day (steep 1 tablespoon of dried seeds in 1 cup of

THE MOOD-FOOD CONNECTION

Almost any nutritional deficiency can contribute to depression. So it is especially appropriate to correct possible deficiencies of vitamin C and the B vitamins (biotin, B_{12}, folic acid, niacin, pantothenic acid, pyridoxine, and thiamin). Other factors that can promote depression are food allergies, excess caffeine and sugar, and rich, heavy, nutrient-poor diets.

hot water for 10 to 15 minutes); or ½ to 1 teaspoon of tincture three times per day.

Lavender (*Lavandula angustifolia*)

This beautiful, fragrant herb has a gentle relaxing and nourishing effect on the nervous system, while lifting the spirits and easing depression. It promotes refreshing sleep as well. Just the smell of lavender has an antidepressant effect. Its essential oil can be applied to the body, inhaled, or added to bath water. *Typical dosage:* 1 cup of tea three times per day (steep 1 teaspoon of flowers in 1 cup of hot water for 5 minutes); or ⅛ to ½ teaspoon of tincture three times per day. *Caution:* Do not take essential oil internally.

Vervain (*Verbena officinalis*)

This is another herb traditionally used in treatment of depression, though such use is not scientifically backed. Vervain has nourishing and balancing effects on the entire nervous system. It's also a gently relaxing remedy. Herbalists consider it especially helpful when depression is related to chronic illness. As an added benefit, it can help to heal any damage that has occurred to the liver. *Typical dosage:* 1 cup of tea three times per day (steep 1 teaspoon of dried herb in 1 cup of hot water for 5 to 10 minutes); or ⅛ to 1 teaspoon of tincture three times per day.

Vervain

Ginkgo (*Ginkgo biloba*)

This amazing herb is beneficial for treatment of diseases of the cardiovascular and nervous system. It increases blood supply to the brain and improves nerve cell function. It enhances memory and other intellectual functions. Ginkgo can be an excellent treatment for depression, especially in the elderly, where it may counteract age-related decreases in the receptors for serotonin. It can be exceptionally helpful in treating depression in two groups: older adults who have mild decreases in intellectual functioning, and those with histories of stroke or other diseases of the nervous system. In younger people, it might help if problems with memory or concentration are prominent. *Typical dosage:* 40 to 60 milligrams of standardized extract capsules three times per day; or ¼ to ½ teaspoon of tincture three times per day.

Kava-Kava (*Piper methysticum*)

Especially appropriate for daytime use, this herb has been shown to alleviate the anxiety that can accompany depression without causing sedation or decrease in mental functioning. Scientific studies of kava actually show that it may improve memory and mental functioning. *Typical dosage:* up to six 400- to 500-milligram capsules per day; or 15 to 30 drops of tincture up to three times per day.

(For more herbal sedatives that work well in cases of insomnia or anxiety related to depression, see Anxiety, page 84.)

DIABETES

MOST PEOPLE THINK OF SUGAR as a sweet, white powder we stir in our coffee or tea. But if you are among the 10 million to 12 million or more Americans with adult-onset diabetes mellitus—many of whom are undiagnosed—this sweet stuff is a source of danger.

The problem is not so much sugar as insulin, a human protein hormone that's critical in helping the body use sugar. In Type I diabetes, the type that usually becomes evident in childhood or young adulthood, the pancreas cannot produce insulin or cannot produce nearly enough. Symptoms include intense thirst, frequent urination, and rapid weight loss. Type I diabetes can eventually damage the eyes, kidneys, heart, and nerves, and lead to coma and death. It can be controlled by regular doses of insulin in the proper amounts. Keeping the precarious balance between insulin dosage and sugar intake is one of the major challenges faced by people with Type I diabetes.

Type II diabetes, also known as diabetes mellitus or adult-onset diabetes, is a bit more complex. It usually doesn't appear until the early to mid forties, although the stage may be set for the disease many years earlier. In some cases it can resemble Type I diabetes and stem from inadequate production of insulin in the pancreas. In most cases, however, the problem is not a simple lack of insulin, but a defect in the receptors for insulin in the cell walls of fat and muscle tissue and the liver.

Basically, the usual transfer of glucose—a major energy source for the body—into these organs just doesn't work right. Doctors call this problem insulin resistance. And it means you can have elevated blood glucose despite normal or elevated levels of insulin. Symptoms of Type II diabetes may not appear for years or decades. When insulin deficiency or resistance increases, it results in increased thirst and urination that may worsen over a period of weeks. If blood-sugar levels zoom, someone with diabetes may develop severe dehydration, which can lead to confusion, drowsiness, and seizures.

Long-term complications of Type II diabetes are similar to those of Type I, but include a high incidence of heart disease, high blood pressure, and stroke. So it's worth it to have your doctor monitor your blood-sugar levels as you age.

It's interesting that before the advent of insulin and oral hypoglycemics, herbal medicines were often used to help treat diabetes. Goat's rue (*Galega officinalis*), which had been used by European herbalists for centuries, contains guanidine, which is now used as a chemical precursor to the modern drug metformin. Unfortunately, goat's rue itself is too toxic for regular use.

There are, however, many safe botanical medicines that are helpful in managing Type II diabetes or the blood-sugar problems that can lead up to the condition. They don't mean that you can discontinue insulin or other drugs without consulting your doctor.

Diabetes is a serious condition that affects all of the body's sys-

Getting Off the Sugar Roller-Coaster

For both types of diabetes, diet is an important part of treatment—perhaps the most important. But it's also quite complex and individualized. Foods that cause blood-sugar problems in one person may provoke different reactions in others. In addition, experts disagree about what constitutes an optimal diet. There are shelves of books that discuss recommended and forbidden foods for diabetes in great detail.

For a person with Type I diabetes who is dependent on insulin, meals must be eaten on a regimented schedule. Food portions and calories must be monitored in a precise fashion so the proper dose of insulin can be determined. Blood glucose must also be measured frequently to assess the adequacy of control. For some people, known as "brittle diabetics," a few extra bites of food can make the difference between a normal level of blood sugar and one that is out of control.

For many years, conventional wisdom targeted dietary fat as the biggest "hidden" health risk for people with Type II diabetes. Dietary carbohydrates weren't considered as important. Because ingestion of sugars and starches immediately raises blood sugar, doctors and nutritionists reasoned that people with diabetes could safely eat all the

tems. The wisest course is to incorporate herbal medicines with your doctor's approval and monitor your responses carefully.

Drug Treatment

Insulin

Many types and many trade names. *Function:* control blood sugar levels in people with Type I diabetes and some with Type II diabetes. *Side effects:* overuse can raise cholesterol and blood pressure and increase body fat.

carbohydrates they wanted as long as they compensated by taking more insulin. Another assumption was that complex carbohydrates (starches) are preferable to simple sugars because they are absorbed more slowly, causing a slower rise in blood sugar.

Newer research is showing that insulin is not a benign substance. In excessive amounts, insulin can raise cholesterol, increase body fat, and raise blood pressure. If this is true, it means people who have diabetes must not only restrict dietary fat, but also closely monitor their intake of both simple and complex carbohydrates.

Dietary recommendations for people with non–insulin-dependent, Type II diabetes are even more controversial. For many years, the standard advice given was to eat a low-fat, high-starch, moderate-protein diet. But several studies indicated that the large amounts of starch in this type of diet can raise insulin levels above normal, worsening the condition. This tends to be confirmed by anthropological studies that suggest pre-agricultural, hunter-gatherer humans had fewer cases of diabetes and heart disease. They consumed much higher amounts of protein, obtained from wild game and nuts, healthful fats from the same sources, and minimal amounts of grains and other carbohydrates. Of course, the usual sources of "junk" calories in the typical Western diet find a place in neither group's recommendations; you won't find double-chocolate-chip cookies on either list.

Oral Hypoglycemic Agents (Sulfonylureas)

Tolbutamide (Orinase), tolazamide (Tolinase), chlorpropamide (Diabenese), glyburide (Diabeta, Micronase), glypizide (Glucotrol). *Function:* lower blood sugar by stimulating cells in the pancreas to release more insulin. *Side effects:* with long-term use, increased risk of death from heart disease.

Biguanides

Metformin hydrochloride (Glucophage). *Function:* increase insulin's activity in muscle and fat tissue and prevent the liver from

THE BODY FAT CONNECTION

Since obesity clearly contributes to the majority of chronic health problems experienced by people with diabetes, experts do agree on the importance of maintaining a healthy weight and monitoring your total percentage of body fat. They recommend between 22 percent and 24 percent in women and 15 percent to 17 percent in men. The best method for doing so is a program of regular exercise.

releasing extra glucose into the bloodstream. *Side effects:* nausea, diarrhea, loss of appetite, and abdominal discomfort.

Thiazolidinediones
Pioglitazone (Acts), aosiglitazone (Arandia). *Function:* counteract insulin resistance by increasing the activity of receptors in liver, muscle, and fat cells. *Side effects:* none common.

Glucosidase Inhibitors
Acarbose (Precose). *Function:* prevent blood glucose from rising after ingestion of complex sugars when used with a starchy, high-fiber diet. *Side effects:* gas, bloating, and malabsorption of nutrients.

HERBAL REMEDIES

Gymnema (*Gymnema sylvestre*)
This Ayurvedic remedy is probably one of the most common herbs used to treat diabetes. Gymnemic acid, a component of the herb, acts directly on the tongue to block its ability to sense sweetness. This action can help you forgo the sweet treats that may be aggravating the condition. But it occurs only when the herb is chewed or placed on the tongue before eating, not when gymnema is taken in pill or capsule form.

Gymnema also appears to stimulate the pancreas to produce more insulin and to enhance the activity of insulin. Consequently, it can be helpful in both Type I and Type II diabetes. It can be taken along with hypoglycemic medication; some patients find they can eventually stop taking the drugs. *Typical dosage:* 400 milligrams of capsules per day.

Fenugreek (*Trigonella foenum-graecum*)
Ancient Greek and Roman herbalists used this spice to treat diabetes. Modern research has shown that fenugreek seeds not only lower blood glucose but also reduce insulin levels, total cholesterol, and triglycerides while increasing HDL (the "good" cholesterol). Fenugreek seeds also contain up to 50 percent fiber, which is a clue to how they work in diabetes: the fiber in the seed slows down the rate at which food is emptied from the stomach. This in turn delays absorption of glucose from the small intestine, resulting in lower blood sugar. Many nutritional experts believe that all people with diabetes should make fenugreek seeds a regular part of their diets. *Typical dosage:* for non-insulin-dependent diabetes, as little as 5,000 milligrams of powdered seed per day. For severe or insulin-dependent diabetes, up to 50,000 milligrams (50 grams) twice per day. *Caution:* May produce flatulence.

Bitter Melon (*Momordica charantia*)
Also known as bitter gourd or balsam pear, this fruit is cultivated in many tropical countries, where it is widely used as a folk remedy for diabetes. Clinical studies in India have verified bitter melon's benefits. It contains several phytochemicals that appear to act in ways similar to sulfonyurea drugs, without the side effects. Bitter melon also contains compounds that are close chemical relatives of insulin. *Typical dosage:* 3 tablespoons to 6 fluid ounces per day. For those who can't tolerate the juice, a standardized extract may soon be available. *Caution:* The seeds and fruit rind are poisonous. Excessive amounts of the juice (more than double the recommended dosage) may cause delayed nausea, vomiting, diarrhea, and hypoglycemia. It's best to use bitter melon under the guidance of a licensed professional.

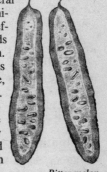
Bitter melon

Bilberry (*Vaccinium myrtillus*)
The fruit of this bush is a rich source of the bluish pigments called anthocyanidins and proanthocyanidins, two of the many types of

flavonoids. Flavonoids are well-known for their beneficial effects on capillaries. Since one of the main complications of long-term diabetes is damage to the small blood vessels of the eyes, the kidneys, and the tips of the toes and fingers, bilberry and other proanthocyanidin-containing herbs are often recommended for diabetes. *Typical dosage:* 80 to 160 milligrams of capsules standardized to contain 25 percent anthocyanidins per day.

Grapeseed Extract (*Vitis vinifera*)

Another rich source of anthocyanidins and proanthocyanidins, grapeseed extract has the same benefits for people with diabetes as bilberry. *Typical dosage:* 100 to 300 milligrams of proanthocyanidin content per day.

Diarrhea

Food poisoning. Overeating. Antibiotics, stimulant laxatives, and other drugs. Viruses, bacteria, and parasites. Megadoses of vitamin C. An attack of nerves. Any one of these things can send you running for the nearest toilet.

The good news is, many types of diarrhea go away on their own. Regardless of the cause, the best way to manage diarrhea is to drink plenty of fluids. If you don't, you'll become dehydrated, which will make you feel much worse.

Drug Treatment

Antibiotics

Erythromycin (E-Mycin, Erybid, Ery-Tab, others), trimethoprim-sulfamethoxazole (Bactrim, Cotrim, Protrin, Trisulfam, others). *Function:* eliminate bacteria such as campylobacter, salmonella, shigella, *Vibrio cholerae* (the cholera bacteria), or *Escherichia coli.* *Side effects:* mild nausea, vomiting, and diarrhea; vaginal yeast infection.

REASONS TO CALL YOUR DOCTOR

Make an appointment to see your doctor as soon as possible if you develop the following symptoms. If none of these apply to you, you can probably manage your diarrhea at home.

◆ Your diarrhea lasts longer than a week or becomes recurrent.

◆ You have fever, bad abdominal cramps, or blood, mucus, or pus in your stools.

◆ You think you've become dehydrated as evidenced by dry lips and mouth and a failure to urinate for eight hours.

◆ You recently traveled to a foreign country or were in close contact with someone who did.

◆ You recently drank water directly from a stream, river, or lake.

Other Drugs

Loperamide (Imodium, Apo-Loperamide, Maalox Anti-Diarrheal, Pepto Diarrhea Control). *Function:* slow intestinal contractions to halt diarrhea. *Side effects:* none common.

Attapulgite (Diar-Aid, Diasorb, Fowlers Diarrhea Tablets, Rheaban, Parepectolin). *Function:* absorb gasses, irritants, toxins, and some bacteria and viruses. *Side effects:* none common.

Kaolin and pectin (Donnagel-MB, Kao-Con, Kaolin, Kaopectate, Kapectolin, K-Pek). *Function:* make loose stools less watery and may also help absorb toxins. *Side effects:* none common.

Bismuth subsalicylate (Pepto-Bismol, Helidac). *Function:* bind the toxins of some bacteria, stimulate the absorption of fluids from the intestines into the blood, and decrease intestinal inflammation and motility. *Side effects:* black stools and dark tongue, which cause no harm and cease after the medicine is stopped.

WHAT TO DO WHEN THE RUNS ARE RUNNING

Here's how to care for a mild or brief case of diarrhea at home.

◆ Hold off on solid foods for 12 to 24 hours. Or if the diarrhea isn't severe, avoid only whole-grain cereals, raw fruits, and vegetables.

◆ Drink lots of clear liquids. Diarrhea can quickly lead to dehydration. Good beverage choices include water, herbal teas, sports drinks (Recharge, Gatorade, and others), and diluted vegetable and fruit juices. Full-strength fruit juice can aggravate diarrhea. And milk is best avoided because you'll likely have trouble digesting it.

◆ Eat cooked fruits and vegetables, particularly cooked carrots and applesauce. Bananas, active-culture yogurt, and low-fiber grains such as white rice and flour are also good choices.

HERBAL REMEDIES

Agrimony (*Agrimonia eupatoria*)
Agrimony contains astringents, which have a drying action in the bowel. *Typical dosage:* 1 to 3 cups of tea per day (steep 1 teaspoon of dried leaves in 1 cup of hot water for 10 minutes).

Apples (*Malus domestica*)
Pectin, which apple peels are packed with, is a common antidiarrhea remedy and a prime ingredient in over-the-counter medications such as Kaopectate. Pectin is a soluble fiber that adds bulk to watery stools. Just make applesauce or bake an apple with the peel on (preferably using organic apples). Stay away from apple juice, however; it tends to further loosen stools.

Blackberry and Raspberry (*Rubus* spp.)
The roots and leaves of both berry plants act as astringents to help relieve diarrhea. *Typical dosage:* about 3 cups of tea per day

(steep 2 teaspoons of dried leaves in 1 cup of hot water for 10 minutes).

Bilberry (*Vaccinium myrtillus*)
This shrub's fruits contain both tannins and pectin. *Typical dosage:* 2 or 3 capsules or tablets, standardized to 25 percent anthocyanosides, per day.

Carob (*Ceratonia siliqua*)
This chocolate substitute also contains tannins and provides a safe approach to treating diarrhea for all ages. Simply add carob powder to applesauce or other easy-on-the-bowels foods.

Carrots (*Daucus carota*)
In cooked form, these veggies are an age-old remedy for diarrhea. One study found that carrot soup actually prevented bacteria, including *E. coli,* from sticking to the small intestines of patients with severe diarrhea. Carrots are also rich in carotenes, an essential ingredient for immune function. All you need do is steam sliced carrots until soft and blend into a soup.

Tea (*Camellia sinensis*)
No matter where you are, you can usually find a tea bag. Simply dunk it in hot water, wait five minutes, and drink.

Oregon Graperoot (*Mahonia aquifolium*)
This herb and its berberine-containing cousins, goldenseal (*Hydrastis canadensis*), gold thread (*Coptis chinensis*), and barberry (*Berberis vulgaris*), fight a broad range of microbes. Studies have found berberine effective in diarrhea caused by bacteria such as shigella, salmonella, *E. coli,* and *V. cholerae*, and by the parasite giardia. *Typical dosage:* 60 drops (about 2 dropperfuls) of tincture three times per day; or up to six 500- to 600-milligram capsules per day. *Caution:* Do not use herbs containing berberine during pregnancy.

Garlic (*Allium sativum*)
The "stinking rose" kills a variety of viruses, bacteria, and parasites. *Typical dosage:* one or two raw, minced cloves of garlic a day; or up to three 500- to 600-milligram capsules per day (look for a product that delivers 4,000 to 5,000 micrograms of allicin per day).

Putting "Good" Bacteria to Work

Lactobacilli are a type of bacteria normally found in the intestines. Studies show that taking various strains of lactobacilli can help prevent cases of, and improve recovery from, diarrhea caused by a virus called rotavirus. They work in several ways: by out-competing undesirable bacteria and preventing "bad" bacteria from clinging to the intestinal lining, by strengthening local immune response in the gut, and by stimulating white blood cells.

You can ingest these bacteria when you eat active-culture yogurt or kefir (a yogurt drink). Just make sure the fine print on the label says the product contains live cultures. You can also take a supplement, usually in the form of *Lactobacillus acidophilus*.

Peppermint (*Mentha × piperita*) and Catnip (*Nepeta cataria*)

These two mint family herbs have antispasmodic action, a quality you'll appreciate if you have intestinal cramping. *Typical dosage:* 3 cups of tea per day (steep 1 to 2 teaspoons of dried leaf in 1 cup of hot water for 10 minutes). *Caution:* Do not use catnip if pregnant; do not use peppermint if you have heartburn or esophageal reflux.

Grapefruit Seed Extract

Made from the seed, pulp, and inner rind of grapefruit, these products can be helpful in fighting both bacterial and parasitic infections. Studies show they can kill salmonella, shigella, *V. cholerae*, and candida. They can also inhibit the growth of giardia. Some people take grapefruit seed extract as a preventive when they travel to areas where the water is questionable. It comes in liquid or tablet form; follow manufacturer's directions on dosage.

DIVERTICULOSIS

IMAGINE SQUEEZING A SMALL balloon with your hand and watching parts of it protrude between your fingers. That's similar to what happens in the colon of a person with diverticulosis. Little pockets form as a result of consuming a low-fiber diet, straining for bowel movements, or having a weakness in the colon or large intestine wall. These pockets, or diverticula, are somewhat common in anyone over age 40. They occur in as many as 40 percent of people over age 50 and in almost all people over age 90. Diverticula might produce no symptoms, but they can divert digestive contents. If intestinal contents remain inside them, the result is inflammation, infection, bleeding, and pain—a condition known as diverticulitis.

If inflammation in these pockets progresses, infection can develop, producing fever, nausea, vomiting, painful bloating, rectal bleeding, and severe abdominal tenderness, especially in the lower left side. Diverticulitis has much in common with appendicitis—either can cause a surgical emergency if a rupture occurs. For this reason, it is crucial that diverticulitis be evaluated by a doctor.

DRUG TREATMENT

Antispasmodics
Hyoscyamine (Levsin), dicyclomine (Bentyl), hyoscyamine combined with atropine, scopolamine, and phenobarbital (Donnatal). *Function:* block the action of acetylcholine, a chemical involved in bowel cramping. *Side effects:* dry mouth, nausea, blurry vision, dizziness, difficulty with urination.

Anti-Inflammatories
Aspirin, ibuprofen, naproxen, indomethacin (Indocin). *Function:* relieve the pain that accompanies inflamed diverticula. *Side effects:* allergic reactions, bleeding stomach ulcers, fluid retention.

Antibiotics

Cephalexin (Keflex), cephadroxil (Duricef), ciprofloxaxin (Cipro), oflaxaxin (Floxin). *Function:* kill a broad spectrum of infectious bacteria, indicated when elevated white blood cells or fever are present. *Side effects:* allergic reactions, diarrhea.

EATING FOR DIGESTIVE HEALTH

To prevent diverticulosis, there's one simple change you can make: Eat more fiber. It prevents constipation and the resultant straining to produce a bowel movement, which weakens the bowel walls and creates these painful pockets.

The best sources of dietary fiber are whole grains, legumes, crisp vegetables, and fruits with the skins on.

Once diverticulosis begins to cause symptoms, however, you'll want to avoid specific types of fiber in your diet. Insoluble fiber—the kind that does not dissolve in water—can still be beneficial, but it is also more prone to collect in the narrow necks of diverticuli. Examples of insoluble fiber are nuts, seeds, corn, and the skins of apples, cucumber, and tomatoes.

Soluble fiber dissolves in water to form a soft gel and is less likely to plug up diverticuli. This type of fiber is found in oat bran, flaxseed meal, barley malt, gelatin, peeled apples, brown rice, and psyllium seed husks. Such fibers are an essential part of the diet to prevent recurrent attacks of diverticulitis.

Because poor digestion aggravates symptoms, chew your food thoroughly. Some people find it very helpful to supplement their diets with digestive enzymes, such as bromelain from pineapple stem and papain from papaya (follow manufacturer's recommended dosages). Caffeine and alcohol can irritate the digestive tract, so avoid them whenever possible.

HERBAL REMEDIES

Psyllium (*Plantago ovata*)

Cultivated in Iran and India, this plant has seed husks rich in mucilage, the soluble fibers similar to those found in oat bran, flaxseed meal, and guar gum. The husks have a long history of use by both herbalists and medical doctors to treat constipation and diverticulosis. *Typical dosage:* up to 1 teaspoon of the husks or 2 teaspoons of ground husks stirred into a glass of water per day (drink immediately because the mixture thickens rapidly); or up to six 660-milligram capsules with one full glass of water per day. Psyllium is also available in commercially produced energy bars. *Caution:* May cause gas, bloating, and diarrhea; avoid by starting with lower doses and building up slowly. Allergic reactions can occur in some people.

Peppermint (*Mentha × piperita*)

This menthol-containing herb has many benefits, including relieving pain, cooling inflammation, and fighting yeasts and other microbes. Most important, it has potent antispasmodic properties that make peppermint useful for alleviating cramps. In using peppermint for this purpose, take an enteric-coated capsule so the active ingredient is released in the intestines and not the stomach. *Typical dosage:* 1 to 2 capsules containing 0.2 milliliter of the oil two or three times per day as needed; to apply topically to relieve stomach discomfort, dilute peppermint essential oil with an equal quantity of vegetable oil, such as olive, sesame, or almond, and apply directly above the painful spot. Peppermint can be used topically and internally at the same time. *Caution:* Some people are very sensitive to peppermint oil and experience a burning sensation in the rectum after ingesting it; allergic reactions to topical use of the oil are rare but possible.

Aloe Vera (*Aloe barbadensis*)

The gel from inside the leaves of this plant has benefits appreciated by anyone who has used it to treat sunburn. Aloe gel as a topical application has anti-inflammatory effects soothing to the intestinal wall and mild antibacterial activity. (Be aware that only the gel is useful for this condition; the yellow substance from the outside of the leaves is a potent cathartic that can cause diarrhea.) Oral preparations of aloe are increasingly being used by physicians to treat a wide variety of gastrointestinal ailments, including diverticulosis. *Typical dosage:* two to eight capsules per day; or ¼ to ½ cup of reconstituted juice four times per day (use a product specifically intended for oral use and with a guaranteed amount of aloe vera mucopolysaccaride). *Caution:* Some people have allergic reactions to aloe juice.

Cat's Claw (*Uncaria tomentosa*)

This picturesquely named herb has a long history of use as part of South American folk medicine. It was used to treat infections, arthritis, and a wide range of intestinal disorders, including diverticulosis and diverticulitis. Despite its popularity, there are no good medical studies that confirm its effectiveness. But cat's claw is reasonably safe to use, so it may well be worth a try. *Typical dosage:* 20 to 60 milligrams of standardized extract per day; or 15 drops of tincture two to three times per day; or 3 cups of tea per day (simmer 1 tablespoon of root bark in 1 cup of water for 10 to 15 minutes; cool and strain). *Caution:* May interfere with fertility or lower blood pressure. Do not use if pregnant or nursing.

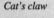
Cat's claw

Wild Yam (*Dioscorea villosa*)

This tuber is known by pharmacists as the source of raw materials used to make numerous hormones, such as progesterone. Without chemical processing, wild yam has little hormonal activity, but it does possess antispasmodic and anti-inflammatory effects that make it very useful for diverticulosis. *Typical dosage:* 1 to 2 dropperfuls of tincture three or four times per day; or 1 to 2 capsules or tablets of powdered root three times per day. *Caution:* Some people experience mild nausea at the high end of the dosage range.

EAR INFECTIONS

IF YOU'RE A SWIMMER, THEN you probably know about the type of outer ear infection that involves the ear canal, typically resulting from swimming; hence the common name "swimmer's ear." Inner ear inflammation is not nearly as common, but it does happen. It's caused by viral upper respiratory infections that extend to the inner ear.

If you do get this kind of infection, take all the normal precautions you would for any other viral illness. Be prepared to seek medical attention, because the symptoms of such infections can be dramatic: severe dizziness, nausea, vomiting, and sometimes difficulty maintaining a fixed gaze.

Other things that can make adult ears ache are traumatic injuries, foreign bodies lodged in the ear canal, and referred pain from swollen lymph nodes in the neck caused by sore throats.

DRUG TREATMENT

Antibiotic or Antifungal Eardrops

Polymyxin B neomycin hydrocortisone (Cortisporin Otic, Otocort), chloramphenicol (Chloromycetin), colistin, neomycin, hydrocortisone (Coly-Mycin S), clotrimazole. *Function:* eliminate active outer ear infections. *Side effects:* allergies to neomycin resulting in local swelling and redness.

Oral Antibiotics

Amoxicillin (Amoxil), erythromycin-sulfisoxazole (Pediazole), trimethoprim-sulfamethoxazole (Septra, Bactrim), cefprozil (Cefzil), cefaclor (Ceclor). *Function:* eliminate bacterial infections of the middle and inner ear. *Side effects:* nausea, vomiting, diarrhea, sore mouth or tongue, thrush (white patches in the mouth due to fungal infection), fungal diaper rash in infants and toddlers, and vaginal infection in teens and women.

Antinausea Drugs

Prochlorperazine (Compazine), promethazine hydrochloride (Phenergan), meclizine (Antivert). *Function:* help reduce vertigo

A Healing Helping of Heat

Ear infections can hurt—especially middle and outer ear infections. You can reduce discomfort by applying a hot water bottle or warm washcloth or by putting warm olive oil into the ear canal. You can also try an herbal ear oil. Look for commercial products that contain garlic, mullein, or St.-John's-wort. *Caution:* Do not put anything in the ear canal if you have signs of a perforated eardrum (any drainage from the ear), or if you are going to see a doctor soon.

that accompanies inner ear infection. *Side effects:* drowsiness; dryness of mouth, nose, and throat; for prochlorperazine, dizziness, blurred vision, constipation, difficulty urinating, low blood pressure.

Other Drugs
Acetic acid eardrops (VoSoL, Swim-EAR). *Function:* keep the ear dry to discourage subsequent outer ear infection. *Side effects:* none known.

Herbal Remedies

Echinacea (*Echinacea angustifolia, E. purpurea, E. pallida*)
This powerful immune-booster is the one to reach for when fighting an acute infection. *Typical dosage:* up to nine 300- to 400-milligram capsules per day; or 60 drops of tincture three times per day. Some herbalists recommend taking a dose every hour or two while you have symptoms. *Caution:* If you're allergic to other members of the aster family, such as ragweed, you may be allergic to echinacea. Do not use if you have autoimmune disease.

Astragalus (*Astragalus membranaceus*)
This herb, revered in Traditional Chinese Medicine, is the one to take long-term if you or a child seems to be prone to recurring in-

fections. *Typical dosage:* Eight or nine 400- to 500-milligram capsules per day; or 15 to 30 drops of tincture twice per day.

Oregon Graperoot (*Berberis aquifolium*)

Berberine-containing herbs such as Oregon graperoot act as natural antibiotics. Studies show that berberine kills many types of bacteria; you can substitute other berberine-containing herbs such as goldenseal (*Hydrastis canadensis*), barberry (*Berberis vulgaris*), or gold thread (*Coptis* species). *Typical dosage:* 1 teaspoon of tincture in water three times per day; or up to six 500- to 600-milligram capsules per day. *Caution:* Do not use during pregnancy.

Garlic (*Allium sativum*)

Compounds in this familiar bulb kill many organisms, including bacteria and viruses. Studies show that garlic is active against some of the viruses that cause the colds and flu, which make conditions ripe for ear infections. *Typical dosage:* one or more fresh cloves per day; or up to three 500- to 600-milligram capsules per

---

Swimmer's Eardrops

If you have a tendency to get swimmer's ear or feel the beginnings of an infection, you can make your own antibiotic eardrops or irrigation solution.

¼ cup white vinegar
¼ cup rubbing alcohol

One of the following:

2–3 drops grapefruit seed extract
3 drops of garlic tincture
3–5 drops echinacea tincture

Sterilize a 4-ounce bottle by immersing it in boiling water for 10 minutes. Mix all ingredients in the bottle. Cap tightly; store out of light. To use, put a few drops into the ear with a sterile eyedropper. Allow to run out of the ear.

day (look for products that deliver a dose of 4,000 to 5,000 micrograms of allicin per day).

Lemon Balm (*Melissa officinalis*)

This pleasant-tasting herb is antiviral, antibacterial, and calming. If an ear infection has you feeling on edge, it may be just what the herbalist ordered. *Typical dosage:* 3 to 4 cups of tea per day (steep 1 to 2 teaspoons of dried leaves in 1 cup of hot water for 10 minutes); or up to nine 300- to 400-milligram capsules per day.

Licorice (*Glycyrrhiza glabra*)

Antiviral and anti-inflammatory, licorice may help tame an infection while fighting the viruses that caused it. *Typical dosage:* up to six 400- to 500-milligram capsules per day; or 20 to 30 drops of tincture up to three times per day. *Caution:* Do not take licorice for more than six weeks. Do not take it at all if you have high blood pressure, diabetes, disease of the thyroid, kidney, liver, or heart; or if you're taking diuretics; or if you are pregnant or nursing. If you are taking other corticosteroids, consult your doctor.

Ginger (*Zingiber officinale*)

Studies have found ginger effective in relieving motion sickness and other causes of nausea. *Typical dosage:* ½ to 1 teaspoon of dried powder made into a tea or taken in capsules; or 10 to 20 drops of tincture diluted in water three times per day; or up to eight 500-milligram capsules per day. You can also suck on ginger candies (as long as the flavoring comes from real ginger) or crystallized ginger.

ECZEMA

THEY'RE RED, ITCHY, SOMETIMES weepy patches of skin—and they show up on more than 10 percent of Americans. Scratching worsens them; the patches become scaly, thickened, and infected. They're the calling card of eczema.

Although the medical name for eczema, atopic dermatitis, means allergic skin inflammation, researchers have not yet nailed down the precise role that allergies play in this condition. They do know that eczema seems to occur along with other allergic conditions, such as asthma and hay fever.

DRUG TREATMENT

Topical Corticosteroids

Many types (Kenelog, Cortaid, Cortef, others). *Function:* suppress skin inflammation; usually used topically, but in rare, severe cases, used internally. *Side effects of topical drugs:* thinning skin, linear streaks on the skin, suppression of body production of steroids. *Side effects of oral drugs*: acne, nausea, vomiting, indigestion, headache, insomnia, dizziness, increased appetite, weight gain, poor wound healing, immune system suppression; with long-term use, muscle loss, cataracts, and osteoporosis.

Sedating Antihistamines

Diphenhydramine (Benadryl), clemastine (Tavist), hydroxyzine (Atarax, Vistaril). *Function:* decrease itching by blocking body chemicals called histamines. *Side effects:* drowsiness; dizziness; dry mouth, nose, and throat.

Nonsedating Antihistamines

Astemizole (Hismanal), loratadine (Claritin), cetirizine (Zyrtec). *Function:* decrease itching by blocking histamines. *Side effects:* dry mouth, nose, and throat; astemizole can cause heart-rhythm disturbances.

Other Drugs

Topical creams containing coal tar (Aquaphor, Fotar, others). *Function:* decrease itching and inflammation when corticosteroid creams fail, or when the potency of topical corticosteroids needs to be reduced. *Side effects:* inflammation of hair follicles, increased skin reactions to sun exposure.

Aluminum acetate solution (Burow's solution). *Function:* help relieve skin irritation. *Side effects:* usually none.

Herbal Remedies

Licorice (*Glycyrrhiza glabra*)

This herb has potent anti-inflammatory properties, just what you want in an herbal remedy for eczema. It seems to act similarly to corticosteroids, but without the negative side effects of such drugs. Licorice also inhibits the breakdown of cortisol, the body's own corticosteroid.

In a British study, children with eczema who drank a tea made from 10 Chinese herbs—one of which was licorice—showed marked improvement over those who received a placebo tea that didn't contain the herbs. Typical dosage: up to two 400- to 500-milligram capsules three times per day; or 20 to 30 drops of tincture three times per day; or up to 3 cups of tea per day (simmer 2 teaspoons of dried root in 3 cups of hot water for 10 to 15 minutes). Because licorice is intensely sweet, you might want to include other herbs in your tea.

To use licorice externally, make a tea by simmering 2 tablespoons of ground dried root in 2 cups of water for 15 minutes. Strain, cool, and apply to eczema patches with a clean washcloth. Or you can look for natural skin products that contain licorice or glycyrrhetic acid, one of licorice's active ingredients. *Caution:* Do not take internally for more than six weeks. Do not use if you're pregnant or have high blood pressure, heart or liver disease, diabetes, or severe kidney disease.

Burdock (*Arctium lappa*)

Taken internally, this root decreases inflammation. Herbalists consider it a traditional remedy for many kinds of skin disorders, including eczema. Rich in minerals, burdock also contains inulin, which stimulates an immune pathway to destroy the skin bacteria that can worsen eczema. *Typical dosage:* 1 to 4 cups of tea per day

ALLERGIES AND ECZEMA

Research indicates that three types of allergens may contribute to eczema.

◆ **Food allergens.** Although food allergies can be a factor for some people with eczema, so far no simple, bulletproof tests accurately diagnose all food allergies. Many experts think the best test is removing the common culprits—especially milk, eggs, and peanuts—from the diet for at least four days and watching for changes in your skin and overall health. Then reintroduce the suspect foods one at a time, no sooner than every three days. If a food re-creates or worsens your symptoms, you've solved at least part of your itchy mystery.

◆ **Airborne allergens.** Whether they're inhaled or they come in contact with your skin, these fly-abouts may be part of an eczema problem. The most common culprit is the very common household dust mite. Others are plant pollens, animal danders, and molds.

◆ **Microbes.** Bacteria and yeast can aggravate skin allergies. Many people with eczema also have more bacteria, such as *Staphylococcus aureus,* on their skin than people without the condition. People with eczema are also more likely to develop fungal skin infections and allergic reactions to these fungi. Cleaning with antibiotic or antifungal products can help.

(simmer 2 teaspoons of dried root in 3 cups of hot water for 10 to 15 minutes); or two 400- to 500-milligram capsules three times per day; or 10 to 25 drops of tincture three times per day. To use externally, simmer 1 tablespoon of dried root in 2 cups of water for 10 to 15 minutes. Strain, cool, and apply with a clean cloth.

Dandelion (*Taraxacum officinale*)

Like burdock, this common plant contains inulin, which improves the body's ability to dispose of unwanted bacteria. Dandelion also stimulates digestion and liver function. And it's chock full of vitamins and minerals, many of which help maintain healthy skin. You can eat the young, fresh leaves raw in salads or steamed as a vegetable. *Typical dosage:* 1 to 4 cups of tea per day (simmer 2 to 3 teaspoons of dried root in 2 cups of hot water for 15 minutes); or two 400- or 500-milligram capsules three times per day.

Gotu Kola (*Centella asiatica*)

This versatile herb can be used externally and internally to help heal wounds and reduce skin inflammation. *Typical dosage:* 1 cup of tea per day (steep 1 teaspoon of dried herb in 1 cup of hot water for 10 minutes); or up to eight 400- to 500-milligram capsules per day; or 20 to 40 drops of tincture twice per day. For external use, cool the tea above and apply it to eczema patches using a clean cloth. You can also find gotu kola as an ingredient in herbal creams.

Echinacea (*Echinacea purpurea, E. angustifolia, E. pallida*)

This American wildflower contains substances that fight infection, decrease inflammation, and stimulate the formation and repair of connective tissue. A German study found that a salve made from the juice of the above-ground parts of *E. purpurea* was effective in treating several types of inflammatory skin conditions, including eczema. In addition to using echinacea salves, you can apply an echinacea tea as a cool compress. Simmer 1 ta-

HOW TO KEEP THE MOISTURE IN

Because eczema is generally a dry skin condition, you want to keep your skin moist. Although baths hydrate the skin, turn down the hot water, which often aggravates itching. And don't soak too long or bathe too frequently; you're depleting your skin's natural oils. On the few parts of your body that need soap (most do not), use a mild variety. Finally, when you're done bathing, pat excess water rather than rub dry. Immediately slather on a body lotion or cream to hold the moisture. Avoid products with alcohol, synthetic fragrances, or lanolin; use products that incorporate skin-soothing herbs.

THE FATTY-ACID CONNECTION

Some people with eczema have fatty acid imbalances. Basically, they need more of the omega-3 fatty acids (the kind found in cold-water fish and flaxseeds) and more of an omega-6 fatty acid called gamma-linolenic acid (found in borage, black currant, and evening primrose seeds).

Some studies—not all—have found that medicinal oils rich in gamma-linolenic acid, such as evening primrose oil, improve the condition. One suggested dose for evening primrose oil is 3,000 milligrams in capsules per day.

Other studies show benefits from fish oil, a rich source of omega-3 fatty acids. Flaxseed oil contains alpha-linolenic acid, which the body can convert to the omega-3 fatty acids that occur in fish oil. But if you really want to boost your overall health along with your skin's health, incorporate into your diet foods rich in omega-3's: cold-water fish (mackerel, salmon, herring, sardines, anchovies, bluefin), ground flaxseeds, pumpkin seeds, walnuts, and dark green leafy vegetables.

blespoon of dried, minced root in 2 cups of water for 15 minutes. Strain, cool, and apply to inflamed skin with a clean cloth.

Comfrey (*Symphytum officinale*)
This traditionally revered herb contains allantoin, an ingredient in many skin lotions. Allantoin soothes the skin and speeds healing by promoting the growth of skin cells. To use, apply comfrey as either a salve or a compress. Simmer 2 teaspoons of dried root in 2 cups of water for 10 minutes, strain, and cool; use a clean cloth to sponge on the solution. *Caution:* Do not apply to broken or abraded skin. If you're pregnant or nursing, avoid applying comfrey or comfrey products to large areas of skin.

Coleus (*Coleus forskohlii*)
This Indian variety of coleus should not be confused with the common houseplant. The medicinal coleus can reduce the release

of histamine and other inflammatory chemicals by increasing levels of a substance called cyclic adenosine monophosphate (cAMP) within cells. So far, studies have focused on its use for asthma, but researchers are currently looking at new eczema drugs that also work to prevent the breakdown of cAMP. If drug companies are willing to bet research funds on cAMP's role in eczema, then herbs that affect cAMP may be worth a try for your eczema. Michael T. Murray, N.D., author of *The Healing Power of Herbs,* recommends that people with eczema take 50 milligrams of an extract standardized to contain 18 percent of the active ingredient forskolin two or three times per day.

Oregon Graperoot (*Berberis aquifolium*) and Goldenseal (*Hydrastis canadensis*)

These herbs have a place in the treatment of eczema for two reasons. First, they promote good digestion and liver function, thereby helping the body get rid of minor toxins that may promote inflammation. Second, the berberine that both herbs contain is a potent antimicrobial substance. It fights bad bacteria such as streptococcus and staphylococcus that can complicate eczema. *Typical dosage:* up to six 500- or 600-milligram capsules per day in divided doses; or 10 to 20 drops of tincture three times per day. To use externally, simmer 2 teaspoons of dried root of either herb in 2 cups of water for 10 to 15 minutes, strain, cool, and use as a wash. *Caution:* Do not take either herb internally during pregnancy.

Oats (*Avena sativa*)

This familiar breakfast grain soothes and moistens skin. There are three great ways to use oats for eczema. Method 1: Boil 2 to

ONE GOOD EXCUSE TO SUNBATHE

Sunlight often helps clear up eczema. To reduce the risk of sunburn, either keep sun exposure short or wear a hypoallergenic sunblock. Go indoors if you start to feel hot and sweaty, which can aggravate itching.

3 quarts of water, toss in 2 handfuls of oatmeal, and simmer for 10 to 15 minutes. Strain into a bathtub of water, or cool the solution and apply to your skin with a clean cloth. Method 2: Put 1 to 2 handfuls of oatmeal in an athletic sock or tie into a piece of muslin. Drop the oat sock in the bath as the hot water is running. You can then use the oat bundle as a sponge on itchy areas. Method 3: Buy a commercial colloidal oatmeal mix such as Aveeno. These products are designed to be poured directly into the bathtub. The one method to avoid is pouring whole oats directly into the bath. This creates a giant cleaning project and isn't good for your plumbing.

Avocado (*Persea americana*)

Avocado is good to eat because it contains vitamins A, D, and E. The same vitamins make avocado good for the skin. To help reduce the itching, dryness, and inflammation, apply the mashed fruit directly to patches of eczema, or (if green's not your color) apply the oil.

Avocado

ENDOMETRIOSIS

AMONG THE HEALTH PROBLEMS that affect women, endometriosis is the most mysterious. It occurs when uterine tissue migrates outside the uterus to the ovaries, fallopian tubes, cervix, bowel, or bladder. Sometimes this tissue even grows outside the pelvic region—in the lungs, for example.

The problem is not where the tissue ends up, but what it does. It

THE DIFFERENCE DIET CAN MAKE

Fats and dairy products can stimulate estrogen production, aggravating symptoms of endometriosis. Stick to low-fat, high-fiber foods, including abundant amounts of vegetables and fruits. Avoid partially hydrogenated oils, including margarine, and increase your intake of essential fatty acids from salmon, nuts, and seeds.

Phytoestrogens found in soy-based foods and other beans can help prevent natural or synthetic estrogens from overstimulating body tissues. Eat these foods regularly, daily if you can.

And cut down on those lattes, sodas, and chocolate binges—caffeine can dramatically worsen symptoms of endometriosis.

swells and bleeds monthly, directed by hormones that cause the same changes in normal uterine tissue.

The symptoms of endometriosis vary greatly from one woman to another. Sometimes they're severe; other times they're virtually nonexistent. In fact, some women don't even realize they have the disease until their doctors diagnose it while looking for the cause of some other disorder—infertility, for example.

Perhaps the most common symptoms of endometriosis are abdominal pain, severe menstrual cramps, excessive bleeding, irregular periods, or painful sexual intercourse. These same symptoms can also indicate pelvic inflammatory disease, irritable bowel syndrome, or a growth on the ovaries. That's why diagnosing endometriosis is difficult.

Women usually learn they have endometriosis between the ages of 25 and 35, yet the problem is thought to start near the time menstruation begins. While theories abound as to the cause, the condition is known to be stimulated, in part, by estrogen and other menstrual-cycle hormones. When these hormones are kept in balance, endometriosis symptoms often disappear, thus rendering the disease inactive.

There are surgical options for treating endometriosis. One such procedure is called laparascopy. Using a small, flexible viewing instrument called a laparoscope, doctors first locate the afflicting spots. Sometimes surgical tools or lasers are attached to the laparascope for removing the endometrial tissue and any surrounding scar tissue. After such surgery, however, endometrial tissue can regrow in the same spot.

DRUG TREATMENT

Oral Contraceptives
Ethinyl estradiol norethindrone acetate (Loestrin), others. *Function:* prevent ovulation in women with mild endometriosis. *Side effects:* dizziness, headache, stomach upset, bloating, nausea.

Synthetic Progesterone
Medroxyprogesterone—oral (Provera), medroxyprogesterone acetate—injection (Depo-Provera). *Function:* stop ovulation and control estrogen levels. *Side effects:* nausea, vomiting, headache, dizziness, depression, sleeplessness, irritability, weight gain, others.

Natural Progesterone
Creams (ProGest, PhytoGest, FemGest), capsules, vaginal or rectal suppositories. *Function:* stop ovulation and control estrogen levels. *Side effects:* rare to none. *Note*: Natural progesterone is synthesized from wild yam (*Dioscorea villosa*), but creams containing *only* wild yam extract—though helpful for some

SUPPLEMENTS FOR ENDOMETRIOSIS

Antioxidants can help prevent tissue damage and reduce inflammation and scarring. Try the following daily regimen:

◆ Vitamin E: 400 to 800 IU

◆ Vitamin C: 2,000 milligrams

◆ Grapeseed or green tea extract: 200 to 400 milligrams

◆ Magnesium: 500 milligrams

women—are not the same as those containing adequate amounts of natural progesterone. Ask your pharmacist or doctor to recommend a product if you find this distinction confusing.

Testosterone Derivatives

Danocrine (Danozol). *Function:* reduce the size of endometrial areas and decrease pain. *Side effects:* weight gain, unwanted hair growth, hot flashes, vaginal dryness, deepening of the voice, acne, fatigue, water retention, decreased sexual drive.

GnRH Agonists

Nafarelin (Synarel), leuprolide (Lupron). *Function:* relieve pelvic pain and shrink extensive areas of abnormal tissue before surgery. *Side effects:* cessation of normal periods accompanied by menopause-like symptoms.

HERBAL REMEDIES

Valerian (*Valeriana officinalis*)

This herb has been used for centuries to treat conditions associated with pain, including menstrual difficulties. Experimental studies have shown it acts as a mild sedative and relieves cramping. *Typical dosage:* 300 to 400 milligrams in capsules standardized to 0.5 percent essential oil per day; or 20 to 60 drops of tincture per day.

Chamomile (*Matricaria recutita*)

A popular calming herb with antispasmodic properties, chamomile may help quell cramps. It also soothes a mildly upset stomach, a symptom some women experience along with abdominal cramps. *Typical dosage:* up to six 300- to 400-milligram capsules per day; or 3 to 4 cups of tea per day (steep ½ to 1 teaspoon of dried flowers in 1 cup of hot water for 10 to 15 minutes); or 10 to 40 drops of tincture three times per day. *Caution:* Some people experience allergic reactions to chamomile.

Cramp Bark (*Viburnum opulus*)

Native Americans regarded cramp bark as a uterine sedative and tonic. By relaxing uterine muscles, the herb has been beneficial in treating menstrual cramps, discomfort during pregnancy, and in the prevention of miscarriage. *Typical dosage:* up to 3 cups of tea per day (steep 1 teaspoon of bark in 1 cup of water for 10 to 15 minutes). *Caution:* Do not use if you have kidney stones.

Wild Yam (*Dioscorea villosa*)
Various yams are used in Ayurvedic and Traditional Chinese Medicine. The root of this particular species of wild yam has anti-inflammatory properties that may be helpful in relaxing uterine spasms. *Typical dosage:* up to two 400-milligram capsules per day; or 20 to 40 drops of tincture up to five times per day.

Motherwort (*Leonurus cardiaca*)
Chinese researchers have found that motherwort increases the volume of blood circulation and stimulates uterine activity. The herb can help with such endometrial symptoms as late periods and clotted or sluggish menstrual flow. *Typical dosage:* 3 cups of tea per day (steep ½ to 1 teaspoon of dried herb in 1 cup of hot water for 10 to 15 minutes); or 20 to 50 drops of tincture up to five times per day. *Caution*: Do not use during pregnancy or attempts to become pregnant.

ENDOMETRIOSIS TEA

Drink 2 cups of this tea per day for 2 weeks for a single course of treatment.

- 1 teaspoon vitex berries
- 1 teaspoon red clover blossoms
- 1 teaspoon wild yam root
- 1 teaspoon cramp bark
- ½ teaspoon horsetail
- ½ teaspoon red raspberry leaves
- ½ teaspoon motherwort
- 1 quart water

In a medium saucepan, combine the herbs and water and bring to a boil. Turn down the heat and simmer for about 5 minutes. Remove from the heat, cover, and let steep an additional 15 minutes. Strain and discard the herbs.

Feverfew (*Tanacetum parthenium*)

A proven remedy for migraines, feverfew also has a 2,000-year history as a folk medicine for regulating women's menstrual cycles. How it works isn't known, but it may be worth a try. *Typical dosage:* up to 400 milligrams in standardized capsules per day; or two average-sized fresh leaves per day; or 15 to 30 drops of tincture per day. *Caution:* Do not use during pregnancy.

Yarrow (*Achillea millefolium*)

More than 40 active ingredients have been isolated in yarrow. It can reduce inflammation, relax cramps, and arrest excessive bleeding. *Typical dosage:* ¾ teaspoon of tincture in a little water three times per day, starting 10 days before menstruation; discontinue for two weeks after your period ends. *Caution:* Do not use during pregnancy.

Vitex (*Vitex agnus-castus*)

Also called chaste berry, vitex normalizes and stimulates the pituitary gland functions, particularly those regulating female sex hormones. *Typical dosage:* up to three 650-milligram capsules per day; or 15 to 40 drops of tincture per day; or 1 cup of tea per day (steep 1 scant teaspoon of dried ground berries in 1 cup of hot water for 10 to 15 minutes). *Caution:* Do not use during pregnancy or with hormone replacement therapy.

Vitex

Black Cohosh (*Actaea racemosa*)

Another hormone balancer, black cohosh is approved in Germany for several conditions associated with female hormonal irregularities. Because hormonal imbalances are thought to be the cause of endometriosis, this herb is worth a try. *Typical dosage:* three 500- to 600-milligram capsules per day; or 10 to 25 drops of tincture as often as every four hours. *Caution*: Do not use during pregnancy or attempts to become pregnant.

Dang Gui (*Angelica sinensis*)

One of the more frequently prescribed herbs in Traditional Chinese Medicine, dang gui is used to tone and regulate the female repro-

TWO TREATMENTS WORTH A TRY

Many herbalists use castor oil packs for any kind of pelvic pain. Preliminary studies suggest that they improve immune system functioning. To make a castor oil pack, saturate a piece of flannel or wool folded in four thicknesses with cold-pressed castor oil at room temperature. Put the flannel directly on your lower abdomen. Cover it with a plastic bag, and then place a hot water bottle or a heating pad on top of the plastic. Try using the pack for an hour at a time, three times a week, for at least three months. If you find that it relieves symptoms of endometriosis, scale back to once a week.

Acupuncture has been shown to greatly reduce and sometimes eliminate menstrual pain. One preliminary study indicates it may also be effective in treating infertile women who have endometriosis.

ductive system. *Typical dosage:* up to six 500- to 600-milligram capsules per day; or 5 to 20 drops of tincture up to three times per day. *Caution*: Do not use during pregnancy.

Red Raspberry (*Rubus idaeus*)
This herb is recommended by many modern-day herbalists for toning the uterus during pregnancy and facilitating childbirth. Some women swear by this herb's ability to relieve heavy periods. *Typical dosage:* up to six 430-milligram capsules per day; or up to 10 cups of tea per day (steep 1 teaspoon of dried leaves in 1 cup of hot water for 10 to 15 minutes). *Caution:* If you're pregnant, use red raspberry only under the supervision of a health practitioner.

Dandelion (*Taraxacum officinale*)
Widely used in Europe, dandelion helps the liver break down excess hormones that may encourage endometrial growth. *Typical dosage:* 2 cups of young leaves eaten raw or lightly cooked; or 3 to 9 teaspoons of dried herb three times per day; or 30 to 60 drops of liquid extract three times per day; or 2 cups of tea per day (steep

½ teaspoon of sifted dry root in 1 cup of hot water for 10 to 15 minutes).

Burdock (*Arctium lappa*, *A. minus*)

Burdock is another herb that helps the liver break down excess hormones such as estrogen. *Typical dosage:* up to six 400- or 500-milligram capsules per day; or 3 cups of tea per day (steep 1 teaspoon of dried root in 1 cup of hot water for 10 to 15 minutes); or 25 to 40 drops of tincture three times per day.

Yellow Dock (*Rumex crispus*)

Traditionally used for chronic skin ailments, jaundice, and constipation, yellow dock is also considered a cleansing herb, though solid research confirming its use is lacking. *Typical dosage:* up to four 500-milligram capsules per day; or 20 to 40 drops of tincture up to two times per day. *Caution:* Avoid during pregnancy.

EYESTRAIN

FOR MOST OF US, VISION IS the most important sense. Much of the information we receive about the world around us passes to our brains through our eyes.

Because our eyes are in use most of our waking hours, they naturally get tired. But eyestrain tends to be ignored because of the seriousness of other eye diseases, and perhaps because we assume we can't do anything about it.

Although eyestrain doesn't permanently damage our vision, it does cause headaches, pain, blurry vision, difficulty focusing, and in extreme cases dizziness, nausea, twitching of the facial muscles, and migraines.

Eyestrain can have a number of causes other than simple overuse: a strain or weakness in the ciliary or eye muscles, improper lighting, or overall tension or anxiety. Overuse can occur whether our focus is close (computer screens, for example) or far (driving long distances). But a constant close focus tends to cause more eyestrain.

There is no scientific proof that herbs help to treat eyestrain—and don't look for any in the near future. Because it's such a temporary problem, the search for cures has taken a backseat to finding treatments for more serious eye problems such as glaucoma and macular degeneration. Nevertheless, many herbs have a history of use in soothing the irritation associated with eyestrain. The most common way of using herbs is as a compress. (For instructions on how to prepare one, see "Herbal How-To's for Eyestrain".)

Drug Treatment

Though there is no medical treatment for eyestrain, if it becomes a chronic problem, you should see an ophthalmologist to rule out the possibility of other eye diseases such as glaucoma. In many cases, eyestrain indicates a need for a new eyeglass prescription. If that's true for you, new lenses alone can help alleviate the problem.

Herbal Remedies

Eyebright (*Euphrasia officinalis*)
This herb has a tradition of use for a variety of eye troubles, specifically watery eyes. Eyebright is both anti-inflammatory and astringent; it helps relieve both swelling and irritation. *Typical dosage:* drink 1 to 3 cups of tea per day (steep 2 to 3 teaspoons of dried herb in 1 cup of hot water for 10 to 15 minutes); or strain and cool the tea to apply in a compress as needed.

Bilberry (*Vaccinium myrtillus*)
The berries of this shrub are respected in many cultures as a treatment for the eyes and a boost to vision. The anthocyanosides in bilberry fruit can strengthen capillaries, which may relieve the bloodshot appearance of strained eyes. Although bilberry gets more attention, the more common blueberry, cranberry, and huckleberry contain similar compounds. Their possible eye benefits give you a great excuse to include them regularly in your

Eyebright

Herbal How-To's for Eyestrain

One of the best ways to use herbs for eyestrain is in a compress. Because eyestrain usually involves irritation and inflammation of the eyes, a compress both soothes and cools. Plus, a compress is safer than an eyewash, because an eyewash risks introducing bacteria that may cause infection.

Whichever herb you choose, make a strong tea or infusion (steep 1 to 2 teaspoons of dried herb in 1 cup of hot water for 10 to 20 minutes). Use the tea to dampen a soft cloth, put the cloth over your eyelids, and lean back with your eyes closed for at least 10 minutes.

To pamper sore eyes even more, follow the herbal compress by applying a couple of cold cucumber slices to your eyelids.

diet. *Typical dosage:* 2 or 3 standardized capsules or tablets per day.

Goldenseal (*Hydrastis canadensis*)

This astringent can be used for tired, irritated, and itching eyes. Goldenseal contains berberine, which constricts the blood vessels, helping to decrease the bloodshot appearance of strained eyes. It also has slight anesthetic properties, which can relieve pain. Other berberine-containing herbs that would be just as effective include barberry (*Berberis vulgaris*) and Oregon graperoot (*Berberis aquifolium*). Use any of these herbs in a compress as needed.

Witch Hazel (*Hamamelis virginiana*)

The bark of the witch hazel tree is widely used to relieve body aches and pains. An infusion of the bark contains astringent tannins that act as anti-inflammatory agents. Although the majority of the commercial witch hazel products are clear-colored and do not contain tannins, they usually are soothing and refreshing. At one time, the American Medical Association listed witch hazel as a treatment for eye inflammations. You can use witch hazel alone in

MONITOR THAT COMPUTER SCREEN

Although modern computer screens do not emit enough radiation to harm the eyes, they do cause significant eyestrain. How can you tell? If you see black-and-white objects tinged with color after working on the computer, you've probably been working too long.

You can help decrease computer-related eyestrain by adjusting the arrangement of your workstation. Most people tend to have their computer screens too low, which causes shoulder and back strain in addition to eyestrain. The top of your screen should be at eye level or slightly below so that the middle of the screen is about 6 to 8 inches below eye level. The distance between your eyes and the screen should be about arm's-length, or 20 to 28 inches. Keep in mind that if you wear trifocals, bifocals, or reading glasses, they may need to be changed to compensate for this positioning.

Minimize glare on your screen by adjusting the lighting in the room or adding a glare filter to the screen itself. Another way to reduce glare is to decrease the amount of white paper on the desk surrounding the computer. Remember to wipe dust off the screen periodically to make it easier to see. Also, make sure the screen is properly focused to reduce straining.

Because you tend to blink less often while your eyes are fixed, it is important to consciously remind yourself to blink frequently or to periodically close your eyes for a few seconds while at the computer. This bathes the eyes in fluid and keeps them from drying out. Finally, remember to take mini-breaks every hour or so, and to change your body position after them. That helps your back, too.

a compress or combine it with an infusion of the other herbs in this chapter.

Chamomile (*Matricaria recutita*)

This anti-inflammatory herb is often used for symptoms associated with tension. Its anti-spasmodic and soothing qualities would work well for eyestrain, and it has a history of use in treating conjunc-

PUSH-UPS FOR YOUR EYES

Since a fixed gaze causes most eyestrain, the best way to avoid such strain is to do eye exercises. Industrial hygienist George Wahl suggests taking frequent mini-breaks from your workstation.

◆ Every 10 minutes: Simply look away from the computer screen at something at least 20 feet away.

◆ Every hour: Do additional eye exercises and stand up to move your neck and shoulders. Repeatedly change your focus from a near point to a far point. If you are able to see mountains, trees, or any other variable-height horizon, trace the outline with your eyes. If you are without a window, at minimum trace the corners of the room with your eyes. Then, without moving your head, look far to the right and far to the left, up to the ceiling and down to the floor.

Reading can also cause significant eyestrain, so if you read a lot, remember to use these exercises.

tivitis. Chamomile can relieve pain and swelling as well as act as a mild sedative. *Typical dosage:* 1 cup of tea taken internally as needed (steep ½ to 1 teaspoon of dried flowers in 1 cup of hot water for 10 to 15 minutes); or use in a compress as needed. *Caution:* Those allergic to ragweed may be allergic to chamomile.

Calendula (*Calendula officinalis*)

Sometimes called pot marigold, this plant produces a yellow flower traditionally used to soothe watery and irritated eyes. *Typical dosage:* 1 cup of tea taken internally up to three times per day (steep 1 heaping teaspoon of dried flowers in one cup of hot water for 10 to 15 minutes); or use the tea in a compress as needed.

FATIGUE

EVERYONE EXPERIENCES FATIGUE from time to time. The cause is usually obvious: from staying up until 2 A.M. to finish a project, to not sleeping well because of a late-night encounter with a pepperoni pizza.

But lately, doctors have been noticing that complaints of chronic, ongoing fatigue are becoming more common among their patients. In some practices, fatigue may in fact be the most common complaint. Modern Americans are experiencing an epidemic of fatigue.

In most cases, a reason can be found for ongoing fatigue—and it's not usually a disorder. Most of us are working too hard, not getting enough rest, and not paying attention to what our bodies need. Our days are spent rushing around from job to grocery store to picking up the kids to making dinner and cleaning the house—and we rarely find time for the nurturing, self-renewing time-out we all need.

The first step in treating fatigue is always nonmedical: Look at what's going on in your life and be willing to change what's making

ABOUT USING HERBS FOR FATIGUE

There are two categories of herbs that you need to know about if you're fighting fatigue: adaptogens and adrenal tonics. Both types of herbs help the body adapt to stress; adrenal tonics support overworked adrenal glands, the organs that respond to changing demands and general stress. They're good for both chronic, long-term stress that results in fatigue and the kind of short-term, intense stress that gives you that wiped-out feeling.

Adaptogens, meanwhile, have a broad-spectrum but gradual effect on many of the body's symptoms. They're best for building your health back up after long-term stress or serious health challenges.

you drained and depleted. Leave the briefcase at work this weekend and spend a day on the couch with a novel, take a nap, go for a brisk walk in the woods, have lunch with a good friend, or treat yourself to a warm bath before bed. Imagine that you have an energy checkbook: If you only spend energy and never make any deposits, you'll naturally wind up overdrawn. Listen and your body will tell you which of your activities are deposits and which are like writing a big fat check.

Sometimes, however, it's not just how you live. Occasionally, fatigue may be caused by a specific medical problem, such as anemia, thyroid disease, a drug side effect, undiagnosed depression, or a sleep disorder like sleep apnea. It can also be a side effect of certain medications. If your fatigue is particularly persistent, consider getting a medical evaluation to rule out an underlying problem.

Even if you don't have a specific medical condition, fatigue is a red flag warning you that you are stressing your body. When you feel fatigued, you are more vulnerable to diseases of all kinds. Ignoring ongoing fatigue may also predispose you to chronic fatigue syndrome, a specific disease in which profound, ongoing fatigue is the prominent symptom. If your fatigue is present whether or not you exert yourself, is not alleviated by rest, is worsened by exercise, or is associated with chronic muscle and joint pain, sore throat, tender, swollen lymph nodes, or problems involving memory and concentration, you may already have chronic fatigue syndrome.

DRUG TREATMENT

There are no specific drug treatments for everyday fatigue. The remedy most doctors recommend is simple: rest! They also tend to warn against over-the-counter pick-me-ups such as Vivarin. These drugs work because they contain caffeine, a nervous system and adrenal gland stimulant. Take too much of these drugs and you may exerience their side effects: anxiety, irritability, rapid heart rate, increase in blood pressure, gastritis, and insomnia.

HERBAL REMEDIES

Siberian Ginseng (*Eleutherococcus senticosus*)
This favorite, tried-and-true fatigue-buster is safe for long-term use in most people. A large body of scientific evidence shows that Siberian ginseng improves performance in all kinds of activ-

MUSHROOM ENERGY TEA

In Traditional Chinese Medicine, practitioners often make a strong tea of reishi as a remedy for fatigue.

⅛ ounce chopped or powdered reishi mushroom
3 cups water

Combine the water and mushroom in a pot with a lid. Bring to a boil. Reduce the heat, cover and simmer for 30 minutes. Strain. Drink in divided doses throughout the day; refrigerate for up to three days.

ities under stressful conditions. It also reduces the incidence of diseases, such as viral infections. Because the quality of Siberian ginseng products varies significantly, buy the best quality product available and follow package directions. *Typical dosage:* up to nine 400- to 500-milligram capsules per day; or 10 drops to ¼ teaspoon of tincture three times per day. *Caution:* In rare cases this herb may be too stimulating. It occasionally causes breast tenderness in women. If you experience either side effect, discontinue use.

Chinese Ginseng (*Panax ginseng*)

The properties of this herb are similar to those of Siberian ginseng. It has a long and venerable history in Traditional Chinese Medicine. Depending on the type used and the quality of the product, Chinese ginseng can sometimes be too strong or too stimulating and is not recommended for long-term use by most people. White ginseng—the dried root of *Panax* ginseng—is gentler and less stimulating than red ginseng, the steamed root. *Panax* ginseng is probably best used under supervision of an experienced practitioner. *Typical dosage:* up to four 500- to 600-milligram capsules per day; or 100 milligrams of standardized product one or two times per day. Start with lower dosages and work up

Chinese ginseng

gradually. *Caution:* Do not use if you have high blood pressure or are pregnant.

Licorice (*Glycyrrhiza glabra*)

Licorice is an adrenal tonic and increases energy. It also has anti-inflammatory and antiviral properties. It adds a pleasant taste to tea blends and can also be taken in tincture form. *Typical dosage:* 1 to 3 cups of tea per day (steep 1 to 2 teaspoons of dried root in 1 cup of hot water for 10 to 15 minutes); or ⅛ to ½ teaspoon of tincture three times per day. *Caution:* Do not take internally for more than six weeks. Do not use if you're pregnant or have high blood pressure, heart or liver disease, diabetes, or severe kidney disease.

Schisandra (*Schisandra chinensis*)

This mild adaptogen, or tonic herb, is also thought to support the health of the lungs and kidneys. Practitioners of Traditional Chinese Medicine feel it helps maintain energy and strengthen tissue. It has a subtle calming effect, improves sleep, balances blood sugar, is good for the liver, and may increase memory. *Typical dosage:* 3 cups of tea per day (simmer 1 teaspoon of dried fruit in

NATURAL STIMULANTS TO AVOID

Your local health food store is likely to carry a variety of products advertised as energy boosters. They may be natural, but that doesn't mean they're good for you. In general, avoid herbal stimulants containing ephedra (ma huang) or caffeine (kola nut, guarana, or yerba maté). Unfortunately, that includes those double lattes you've been using to get over the mid-afternoon need for a nap! Ephedra- and caffeine-based stimulants may give you a temporary boost, but in the long run they increase fatigue by overstimulating the body and exhausting the adrenal glands. Chronic health problems, including symptoms that resemble chronic fatigue syndrome, have been observed in people who use these products long-term.

GREEN MEANS MORE GIDDY-UP

Green energy drinks can give you a natural boost that's good to your system. Some people get a quick energy lift from nutrient-rich green drinks containing blue-green algae, spirulina, chlorella, wheat grass, or barley greens. Often available at health food stores or juice bars in powder form, these products can be mixed with a glass of juice or made into a smoothie. Wheat grass can be juiced and taken straight or mixed with other fresh juices. Stinging nettle (*Urtica dioica*) is another energy-lifting herb that works because of its high nutrient and mineral content.

When you can get or make these types of teas and juices, it can't hurt to drink several cups per day. And don't forget to boost the amount of green, leafy vegetables and herbs in your diet; they're all great for maintaining your energy level.

1 cup of hot water for 10 to 15 minutes); or ⅛ to ½ teaspoon of tincture three times per day.

Reishi (*Ganoderma lucidum*)

One of the most important herbs in Traditional Chinese Medicine, reishi is useful for so many conditions that it would take a whole book to describe them all. Besides increasing energy and supporting the immune system, reishi has a calming but not sedative effect on the body and improves sleep. *Typical dosage:* up to six 580-milligram capsules per day; or ¼ to 1 teaspoon of tincture three times per day; or as a tea (see "Mushroom Energy Tea" on page 245). *Caution:* May cause gastrointestinal upset in some people.

Astragalus (*Astragalus membranaceus*)

Another traditional energy tonic, astragalus strengthens the immune system and is good for both digestion and lung function. Sometimes this root is available in bulk in health food stores; long and flat, it looks like a tongue depressor. These sticks can be added to soups, stews, rice, or any food that simmers for at least 30 minutes. When cooking is complete, remove the wilted stick and discard. The medicine has gone into your food! Astragalus has a neutral, somewhat pleasant taste. *Typical dosage:* 3 cups of tea per day (simmer ⅓ to ½ ounce of the dried herb in 3 cups of water for 30 minutes); or ¼ to 1 teaspoon of tincture three times per day; or eight or nine 400- to 500-milligram capsules per day.

Codonopsis (*Codonopsis pilosula*)
A gentle energy tonic, this herb is also soothing to the digestive tract. *Typical dosage:* 3 cups of tea per day (simmer ⅓ to ½ ounce of the dried herb in 3 cups of water for 30 minutes); or ¼ to 1 teaspoon of tincture three times per day.

Herbal Bitters
A group of herbs that pack a bitter taste—usually including gentian (*Gentiana* species), wormwood (*Artemesia absinthium*), mugwort (*A. vulgaris*), and others—can help boost overall energy. Bitter herbs increase endocrine function and improve digestive processes; many people experience a temporary increase in energy after a dose. Bitters preparations are available in a variety of forms and combinations in natural products stores, usually in liquid extract form. *Typical dosage:* between 1 dropperful and ½ teaspoon three times per day, taken with meals.

Peppermint (*Mentha × piperita*)
This pleasant-tasting herb makes a wonderful, refreshing tea. It is mildly stimulating but also eases anxiety and tension, and it eases

FIRING THE ENERGY ENGINES

Any spice that you perceive as hot, such as ginger, cinnamon, cardamom, hot peppers, mustard, and horseradish, is likely to help increase your circulation. When you're fatigued, you often feel cold and tense; such herbs counteract those physical sensations. Look for these energy-stoking spices in teas or as seasoning in foods, unless you're experiencing infection, fever, or other "hot" conditions, such as hot flashes.

any gastrointestinal upset that may be present along with the stress that's causing fatigue. *Typical dosage:* 1 cup of tea as often as needed (steep 2 to 4 teaspoons of dried leaf in 1½ to 3 cups of hot water for 15 minutes). *Caution:* Avoid peppermint if you have esophageal reflux or heartburn.

Rosemary (*Rosemarinus officinalis*)

Another aromatic herb, rosemary has a gently stimulating effect on both the nervous and circulatory systems. It tends to lift the spirits if depression is present, soothe digestive complaints, and is reputed to improve memory. *Typical dosage:* 1 cup of tea up to three times per day (steep 1 teaspoon of dried leaves in 1 cup of hot water 10 to 15 minutes); or a few dropperfuls of tincture three or four times per day.

FIBROIDS

DON'T LET THE TERM FIBROID TUMOR scare you. Uterine fibroids, or leiomyomas, are called tumors because they are solid masses, not because they are cancerous. In fact, almost all are benign.

These slow-growing masses, composed of muscle and fibrous tissue, develop in the muscle layers of a woman's uterine wall. Most fibroids never cause problems. But the ones that do can cause symptoms such as heavy menstrual bleeding, bleeding between periods, a sensation of heaviness in the pelvis, frequent urination, sudden severe cramps, or infertility. The excessive bleeding that some fibroids cause may lead to fatigue and anemia.

In addition, fibroids may prevent pregnancy by blocking the pathway of sperm or preventing implantation of an embryo. During pregnancy, fibroids may increase the chance of miscarriage or heavy postpartum bleeding. A large fibroid may obstruct delivery or interfere with uterine contractions.

Fibroids occur most frequently in women between the ages of 35 and 45 who have never been pregnant. Most women who get one fibroid develop others, sometimes 100 or more. Overall, nearly half

UTERINE FIBROID TEA

This tea blend combines hormone-balancing herbs with those that ease cramps.

- 2 **teaspoons vitex berries**
- 1 **teaspoon black cohosh root**
- ½ **teaspoon dandelion root**
- ½ **teaspoon prickly ash bark**
- ¼ **teaspoon cramp bark**
- ¼ **teaspoon cinnamon bark**
- 4 **cups water**

Combine the herbs in the water and bring to a boil. Lower heat and allow the tea to simmer for a few minutes. Remove from the heat and steep for 20 minutes. Strain and drink at least 2 cups of tea per day for 3 to 4 months.

of all women develop fibroids by age 40. These masses rarely occur before age 20 and tend to shrink after menopause.

The cause of fibroids remains a mystery, but the tumors seem to respond to changes in levels of the hormone estrogen. When estrogen is plentiful, such as during pregnancy or while a woman is taking oral contraceptives, fibroids grow. Other factors may make a woman more prone to developing fibroids, including obesity, alcohol use, a high-fat diet, vitamin B deficiency, and high levels of the hormone progesterone.

The most common treatment for fibroids is hysterectomy, the surgical removal of the uterus. Women who want a less drastic measure or who want to remain fertile may be candidates for myomectomy, a surgery that removes only the fibroid masses themselves.

DRUG TREATMENT

Gonadotropin-Releasing Hormone (GnRH)

Leuprolide (Lupron), gonadorelin (Factrel), nafarelin (Synarel). *Function:* inhibit release of hormones that stimulate the growth of fibroids. *Side effects:* hot flashes, brittle bones, increased risk of heart disease, other physical changes associated with menopause.

EASY PAIN RELIEF

Try these simple methods to ease the discomfort of uterine fibroids.

♦ **Hot sitz baths.** Water as hot as you can stand it will increase circulation in the pelvis, relax tight muscles, and relieve discomfort.

♦ **Essential oils.** Add several drops of rosemary, lavender, or juniper essential oils to the sitz bath to stimulate pelvic circulation.

♦ **Castor oil.** The skin absorbs warm castor oil's active constituents, lectins, which stimulate the immune response to help shrink fibroids. Five drops of lavender essential oil added to a castor-oil pack encourages relaxation. To make a pack, soak a clean cloth in castor oil, then place it on the abdomen or on any painful areas. Cover the cloth with plastic wrap, then another clean cloth. Finally, apply a heat source—a hot water bottle, a heating pad, or a cloth bag of lentils, corn, or rice that's been microwaved for a few minutes. Leave on for about an hour.

HERBAL REMEDIES

Milk Thistle (*Silybum marianum*)

Traditional Chinese Medicine attributes fibroids to liver problems. Because the liver breaks down excess circulating estrogen, taking milk thistle to help shrink fibroids makes sense. Many studies have shown that silymarin, a compound in milk thistle seeds, stimulates liver repair, blocks toxins from entering the organ, and protects it from free radicals. *Typical dosage:* 140 milligrams of standardized silymarin three times per day for three months, then 90 milligrams three times per day; or 10 to 25 drops of tincture up to three times per day for three to four months.

Burdock (*Arctium lappa, A. minus*)

In addition to treating liver conditions, burdock root has shown antitumor capabilities in animal studies. *Typical dosage:* up to six

400- to 500-milligram capsules per day; or 1 cup of tea three times per day (1 teaspoon of dried root steeped in 1 cup of hot water for 10 to 15 minutes); or 10 to 25 drops of tincture three times per day. Whichever form you take, continue for three to four months.

Vitex (*Vitex agnus-castus*)

One of the most widely known women's herbs, vitex was recommended by Hippocrates in 450 B.C. Researchers believe that vitex works by regulating the pituitary gland, the one that tells other glands how much of each hormone to make. The hormone in question here is estrogen, on which vitex has a regulating effect. Vitex needs to be taken for six months for its full benefits to be felt. *Typical dosage:* 2,000 to 5,000 milligrams in capsules per day; or 1 to 2 dropperfuls of tincture two times per day. *Caution:* Do not take during pregnancy. Vitex may lessen the effectiveness of oral contraceptives.

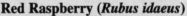

Red Raspberry (*Rubus idaeus*)

This herb is useful if your fibroids cause excessive bleeding during menstruation. Herbalists believe that it gradually improves the tone of the uterus. (If you believe that fibroids are causing other menstrual symptoms, see Menstrual Problems, page 408). *Typical dosage:* 1 to 2 cups of tea two or three times per day (steep 1 teaspoon of dried leaves in 1 cup of hot water for 10 to 15 minutes). *Caution:*

Red raspberry

DIETARY SUPPLEMENTS

To help shrink fibroids, try taking the following supplements once daily for 3 to 4 months:

◆ Vitamin C: 1,000 to 2,000 milligrams

◆ Beta carotene: 150,000 IU

◆ Selenium: 400 micrograms

◆ Zinc: 30 milligrams

If you are pregnant, use only under the supervision of an experienced practitioner.

Poke Root (*Phytolacca americana*)

When fibroids cause tenderness in the lower abdomen, topical application of poke root oil can help. Rub the oil on the area twice a day, morning and evening, as long as discomfort persists. *Caution:* If skin irritation occurs, discontinue use. Do not take this herb internally; it is highly toxic even in small doses.

FIBROMYALGIA

FIBROMYALGIA IS BECOMING well-known as a condition that researchers believe may be related to chronic fatigue syndrome. Possibly in response to stress, lack of sleep, an injury or infection, or another trauma or disease, your muscles begin to ache. Pain might develop gradually and affect a wide area, or it may come on suddenly and sharply in specific areas. You might feel burning, stiffness, shooting pain, or an overall throbbing sensation. The soreness can center on the shoulders, the hip or upper thigh muscles, or the elbows and knees.

Perhaps fibromyalgia's most distinguishable feature is that the aches are often accompanied by anxiety, depression, fatigue, or an inability to sleep. Doctors often call the sleep disturbances nonrestorative sleep—you may be able to drop off, but when you wake you don't feel rested. In fact, you may be even more fatigued.

Symptoms of fibromyalgia may worsen during periods of stress, overexertion, trauma, extreme temperature, infection, or emotional crisis. Although the disorder isn't dangerous or life-threatening, it can be very disruptive. Curiously, it is seldom seen outside of Western industrialized countries, leading researchers to theorize that lifestyle or dietary factors may play a role. But theories are all that's available so far; no one yet knows what causes this disease.

Unfortunately, fibromyalgia is easily mistaken for other kinds of pain. But anti-inflammatory drugs such as naproxen and ibuprofen seldom lessen fibromyalgia pain. Pharmaceutical sleep aids can further diminish the quality of sleep and they can cause dependence. Low doses of antidepressants may help relieve some sleep disturbance symptoms and decrease pain. Occasionally, doctors may administer injections of local anesthetics or corticosteroids directly into the painful spots.

DRUG TREATMENT

Tricyclic Antidepressants

Amitriptyline (Endep, Elavil, Halcion), imipramine (Tofranil, Janimine). *Function:* relieve muscle pain and promote sleep. *Side ef-*

EATING TO EASE THE PAIN

Many holistic practitioners believe that diet plays a role in causing fibromyalgia, though they're not quite sure how or why. Their recommendations:

♦ Drink plenty of fluids, especially freshly squeezed vegetable and fruit juices, for their antioxidant content. Carrot juice is highly recommended because it's particularly packed with beta carotene.

♦ Eat plenty of green leafy vegetables.

♦ Eat small meals throughout the day rather than large infrequent ones.

♦ Keep your digestive system moving by eating high-fiber foods or taking a fiber supplement.

♦ Avoid red meats, shellfish, fatty foods, and acidic foods such as tomatoes and vinegar. Also avoid white potatoes, green peppers, and eggplant. Limit or completely avoid foods that are high in hydrogenated or saturated fats.

♦ Eliminate caffeine and alcohol and greatly reduce sugar consumption.

♦ Investigate your own food allergies. If you think certain foods may worsen your symptoms, try doing without them and note what happens.

fects: sleepiness, tremor, blurred vision, constipation, weight gain, and withdrawal symptoms.

Selective Serotonin Reuptake Inhibitors (SSRIs)
Fluoxetine (Prozac), sertraline (Zoloft), paroxetine (Paxil). *Function:* prevent the metabolism of the mood-controlling brain

SUPPLEMENTS FOR FIBROMYALGIA

The following supplements are designed to nourish muscle cells and enable them to use energy more efficiently through better oxygenation. They also control inflammation and depression and promote more restful sleep.

◆ **NADH (Nicotinamide adenine dinucleotide-hydrogen).** This compound helps control pain and muscle spasms. *Typical dosage:* 5 to 10 milligrams each morning on an empty stomach; take with 6 to 8 ounces of water.

◆ **Malic acid and magnesium.** These two chemicals help muscles use glucose properly. Together, they may help reduce fibromyalgia symptoms. *Typical dosage:* 300 milligrams of malic acid and 200 to 300 milligrams of magnesium, both three times per day.

◆ **5-HTP (5-Hydroxy-tryptophan).** Studies have found this compound helps decrease the pain and insomnia of fibromyalgia by increasing serotonin levels. *Typical dosage:* 50 to 300 milligrams per day.

◆ **SAM-e (S-adenosylmethionine).** This new compound is being hailed as a natural antidepressant. But clinical studies show that it can also reduce fibromyalgia pain and elevate mood. Because depression can occur with fibromyalgia, this supplement may be worth a try. *Typical dosage:* 200 to 1,600 milligrams per day.

◆ **Coenzyme Q$_{10}$.** This enzyme helps boost oxygen supplies to muscle tissue, helping it to flush inflammatory chemicals more quickly. *Typical dosage:* 60 to 400 milligrams per day.

chemical serotonin, thus increasing the amount of this neurotransmitter available to the brain and reducing pain symptoms. *Side effects:* anxiety, nervousness, insomnia, gastrointestinal distress, blunting of emotional response.

Herbal Remedies

Grapeseed Extract (*Vitis vinifera*)

From the seeds of wine grapes come powerful antioxidant and natural anti-inflammatory compounds called procyanidins. They've been used to treat everything from varicose veins to poor night vision. For people with fibromyalgia, these compounds help to inhibit the inflammatory response, the chemical reactions responsible for pain and soreness. *Typical dosage:* 50 to 300 milligrams of oligomeric procyanidins (OPCs) per day. You may want to start with a higher dose to saturate cells and then taper down to a lower dose.

Devil's Claw (*Harpagophytum procumbens*)

The analgesic and anti-inflammatory properties of this herb make it a favorite for fibromyalgia. It also boosts digestion, helping your body absorb nutrients better, which improves overall health. *Typical dosage:* 200 to 800 milligrams per day of a root extract containing 1.5 percent harpagoside content. *Caution:* Do not use devil's claw if you have gastric or duodenal ulcers, or if you're pregnant or nursing. If you have heart disease, use the herb only under a doctor's supervision.

White Willow Bark (*Salix alba*)

This bark has been used for over a thousand years to relieve pain. Salicin, aspirin's forerunner, is white willow's active constituent. Apart from its ability to ease pain, salicin reduces inflammation, but unlike aspirin, it will not thin the blood or irritate the stomach. *Typical dosage:* up to six 400-milligram capsules per day; or 3 cups of tea per day (steep ½ to 1 teaspoon of powdered bark in 1 cup of hot water for 10 to 15 minutes); or follow the manufacturer's recommendations.

Willow

Ginkgo (*Ginkgo biloba*)

This best-selling medicinal herb brings more oxygen to muscle cells when they're under stress. Ginkgo is also a powerful antioxidant. Compounds called ginkgolides inhibit a specific body chemical involved in inflammatory disorders. *Typical dosage:* 60 to 180 milligrams per day of product standardized to 24 percent flavone glycosides.

Cayenne (*Capsicum* spp.)

Creams containing capsaicin, the stuff that makes peppers hot, can help relieve pain and boost circulation to tender muscles. Such creams work because the capsaicin is a counterirritant, meaning the heat you feel distracts your brain from the pain signals that other nerves are sending. *Typical dosage:* capsaicin creams vary in their strength; read the labels carefully and compare percentages of capsaicin content. Begin with a medium to low strength (depending on your own sensitivity) and work up; follow the manufacturer's recommendations on how frequently to apply. *Caution:* Do not apply close to the nose, mouth, eyes, or other sensitive areas; thoroughly wash your hands with soap after each application.

St.-John's-Wort (*Hypericum perforatum*)

Studies have found that this herb, now famous for easing mild to moderate depression, can also help treat sleep disorders. It is especially good at promoting longer periods of deep sleep, which is exactly what people with fibromyalgia need most. *Typical dosage:* up to 900 milligrams of an extract containing 0.3 percent hypericin per day, in divided doses. *Caution:* If you are already taking other antidepressants, consult your doctor before beginning to take St.-John's-wort. May cause increased skin reactions to sun exposure.

Flatulence

G AS PRODUCTION IS A NORMAL part of digestion—and a frequent target of adolescent humor. When gas is odoriferous, excessive, or noise-producing, it's uncomfortable as well as embarrassing. If it builds up, it can contribute to abdominal discomfort.

What causes gas? It's made by the intestinal bacteria that ferment food in the colon, or large intestine. Generally, the fermentation of most carbohydrate products is odorless, while the fermentation of proteins has an odor caused by hydrogen sulfide. On the other hand, certain foods have reputations as gas-producers, including broccoli, potatoes, dairy products, and beans.

Sometimes it's not what you eat or drink, but how fast: Swallowing air while eating or drinking too quickly can set the stage for gaseous episodes. Carbonated beverages can cause problems as well.

If you are prone to flatulence, it is important not to overeat. Eat your meals slowly and enjoy your food. Adding yogurt or other fermented foods to your diet can also help by maintaining a healthful level of bacteria in the intestines. Finally, if there are certain foods that seem to give you gas—and you don't want to give them up— try eating just small amounts of them regularly to build a tolerance.

Gas is not a new ailment. And people have used herbal remedies to cure it for centuries. Agents that prevent or relieve gas formation in the intestines, whether they are pharmaceuticals or herbs, are called carminatives. Conventional medicine has used herbal carminatives for years; doctors still sometimes tell their patients to take a few drops of peppermint oil in a glass of warm water to calm excess gas. Meanwhile, many nonherbal, over-the-counter drugs (and a few prescription ones) are sold to relieve gas—but their effectiveness is questionable.

Drug Treatment

Antacids
Simethicone (Mylanta II, Di-Gel, Extra Strength Gas-X). *Function:* combine small gas bubbles to form larger ones. In theory the gas is easier to expel; in practice that has not proven to be true.

Side effects: allergic reactions, bloating, constipation, diarrhea, gas, heartburn.

Prokinetic agents such as cisapride (Propulsid) and metoclopramide (Reglan). *Function:* help move the contents of the stomach and the intestines. Although these drugs rarely help gas, they are sometimes prescribed for this purpose. *Cisapride side effects:* dizziness, vomiting, sore throat, chest pain, fatigue, back pain, depression, dehydration, diarrhea, abdominal pain, constipation, flatulence, runny nose. *Metoclopramide side effects:* fatigue, apathy, depression, rash.

Other Drugs

Activated charcoal (Carcocaps, Charcoal plus, Flatulex). *Function:* bind to intestinal gases such as sulfur and methane. Although there is no evidence that gas volume is reduced, charcoal may minimize the odor. *Side effects:* upset stomach, vomiting, constipation, diarrhea, black stools; also, charcoal should not be taken with other drugs as their absorption will be blocked.

HERBAL REMEDIES

Peppermint (*Mentha × piperita*)

Why do restaurants offer these little candies at the door? Because peppermint contains menthol, which stimulates the flow of bile into the intestines, promoting digestion. Peppermint also helps relax the esophageal sphincter, allowing gas to be released from the stomach via burping. Moreover, mint can help relieve the nausea that may accompany excessive gas. If you don't want to eat candy, a cup of hot peppermint tea is something to enjoy after dinner. *Typical dosage:* 6 to 12 drops of essential oil in water three times per day; or up to 3 cups of tea per day (steep ½ teaspoon of dried herb in 1 cup of hot water for 15 minutes); or 10 to 20 drops of tincture in water after meals. *Caution:* Do not use peppermint if you have heartburn or esophageal reflux.

Chamomile (*Matricaria recutita*)

This tension-easing herb also helps dispel gas and can increase the flow of bile, which aids digestion. The flavonoids from chamomile have been shown to relax the muscle of the intestines, decreasing spasms. Chamomile is also an anti-inflammatory. It is best used as an after-dinner tea, perhaps mixed with peppermint. *Typical dosage:* 3 to 4 cups of tea per day (steep ½ to 1 teaspoon of dried flowers in 1 cup of hot water for 10 minutes). *Caution:* Those allergic to ragweed may be allergic to chamomile.

Aniseed (*Pimpenilla anisum*)

This aromatic little seed has been shown in human studies to dispel gas. *Typical dosage:* up to 3 cups of tea per day (steep ½ teaspoon of dried, crushed seed in 1 cup of hot water for 5 to 10 minutes).

Ginger (*Zingiber officinale*)

This root's fame for its ability to quell nausea often overshadows its usefulness for simple indigestion and gas. Ginger also increases bile secretion and tones the bowel. Try pouring boiling water over a teaspoon of fresh crushed root and adding maple syrup for a delicious dessert tea.

Aniseed   Drink it after a meal that might upset the stomach. *Typical dosage:* up to eight 500- or 600-milligram capsules per day; or ½ to 1 teaspoon fresh ground root per day; or 10 to 20 drops of tincture in water per day.

Fennel (*Foeniculum vulgare*)

Mentioned in most European medical texts, fennel has a time-honored history as a digestive herb. The gas-dispelling qualities of fennel seeds have been known for hundreds of years; additionally they ease bloating and digestive spasms. *Typical dosage:* up to three 400- or 500-milligram capsules per day; or 1 cup of tea per day (simmer 1 teaspoon of crushed seeds in 1 cup of water for 10 to 15 minutes); or 30 to 60 drops of tincture in water up to four times per day.

FUNGAL SKIN INFECTIONS ·

F UNGI ARE PLANTLIKE ORGANISMS that like to grow in dim, dank
places and feed off dead tissues. Think of mushrooms on the
forest floor. Then again, maybe you'd rather not, because fungi can
also grow on our bodies and live off the dead tissue of hair, nails,
and skin.

You might be host to the fungi that cause athlete's foot, ringworm, ringworm of the scalp, or jock itch. The rashes that these
fungi produce are itchy and mildly contagious. Most can be han-
dled with over-the-counter or herbal remedies. Call your doctor if
you're not sure whether your rash is fungal, if home treatments

AN OUNCE OF FUNGUS PREVENTION

If you're prone to fungal infections, here are a few strategies for keeping them away.

◆ Keep skin clean and dry.

◆ Because fungal infections can spread, don't share
combs, brushes, hats, towels, clothes, or shoes with
others.

◆ To reduce the risk of getting athlete's foot, have a spare
pair of socks handy and change into them if your feet
become sweaty. Better yet, wear sandals.

◆ Disinfect shower stalls and tubs frequently.

◆ To prevent jock itch, change into dry clothes after exercising; choose loose clothing that improves air circulation and wear fabrics that breathe or that wick away
perspiration.

CURE FROM THE CUPBOARD

Vinegar is a simple antifungal treatment. Apply plain white, distilled, or apple cider vinegar with a cotton ball or clean cloth, or soak the affected area in vinegar for two minutes. Do this two times a day until itching is gone and continue for one week afterward.

fail to relieve it in two to four weeks, or if the rash is severe or becomes infected with bacteria (if this happens, you'll see increased redness and yellow discharge). Also see your doctor for fungal infections of the scalp or nails, because these infections can be difficult to treat. In the case of progressive scalp infections, they can produce scarring and permanent hair loss.

DRUG TREATMENT

Topical Antifungal Drugs
Miconazole (Monistat), clotrimazole (Lotrimin), tolnaftate (Tinactin, Desenex, Absorbine), undecylenate (Cruex). *Function:* kill the fungus that creates the rash. *Side effects:* not common.

Selenium-sulfide-containing shampoos (Selsun Blue, Head and Shoulders Intensive Treatment). *Function:* reduce shedding and spread of the fungus in scalp ringworm. *Side effects:* not common.

Oral Antifungal Drugs
Griseofulvin (Fulvicin, Grifulvin, Gris-PEG, Grisactin, Grisovin-FP). *Function:* cure scalp ringworm, nail fungus, or more severe, extensive, or stubborn skin infections. *Side effects:* headache.

HERBAL REMEDIES

Tea Tree Oil (*Melaleuca alternifolia*)
This potent antifungal oil can kill several types of organisms. In a study of people with toenail fungus (which is extremely hard to get rid of), 100 percent tea tree oil performed as well as a 1 percent solution of clotrimazole. *Typical dosage:* apply undiluted oil to clean, dry feet or ringworm lesions two or three times per day.

Continue for 7 to 10 days after fungal rash clears. *Caution:* Some people find tea tree oil mildly irritating. If you do, dilute it with an equal amount of vegetable oil. If you experience an allergic reaction to the diluted product, discontinue use. Do not take tea tree oil internally.

Garlic (*Allium sativum*)

This herb can kill many microbes, including the fungi that infect the skin. Because straight garlic can irritate skin, dilute it in olive oil. Mash or blend a clove with 1 or 2 teaspoons of olive oil and apply this paste to the skin. Remove after an hour. You can also make a garlic-infused oil by adding 4 crushed cloves to a jar containing ¼ cup of olive oil. Let stand at room temperature for three days, strain, and store in the refrigerator for up to six months. Apply the oil to the skin two to three times a day. For persistent infections and scalp ringworm, you might also want to take garlic internally. *Typical dosage:* 1 to 2 raw, minced garlic cloves mixed into food, or three 500- to 600-milligram capsules per day (look for a daily dose of 4,000 to 5,000 micrograms of the active ingredient allicin per day).

Grapefruit Seed Extract

This extract is made from the seed, pulp, and inner rind of grapefruit. Studies show the extract fights several types of fungi, including those that infect the skin. You can apply the liquid concentrate to the skin three times a day until the infection clears, then two times a day for another week.

Cinnamon (*Cinnamomum verum*) and Clove (*Syzygium aromaticum*)

These two common spices are antifungal, according to the German Commission E, that country's version of the Food and Drug Administration. Studies show that both herbs inhibit fungi that commonly infect the skin. An easy way to use them is to dab the diluted essential oil of either plant on the rash three times a day. Or apply a diluted blend of geranium, cinnamon, clove, and tea tree essential oils. To dilute the oils, mix ⅛ teaspoon of essential oil with 1¼ teaspoons of a neutral vegetable oil, such as almond, olive, or sesame. *Caution:* Try a patch test of these oils first, applying the diluted blend to a very small area of skin unaffected by the rash. If irritation occurs, do not use. Do not take these essential oils internally.

Geranium Essential Oil (*Pelargonium* spp.)
This flower oil is both antifungal and anti-inflammatory. Its anti-inflammatory properties relieve itching. Adults can use this oil undiluted. Apply two or three times per day; continue for several days after the rash clears. *Caution:* Do not take essential oils internally.

GALLSTONES

FOR A SMALL SAC OF FLUID IT SURE has a long, funny name: gallbladder. And it takes not the slightest bit of attention from you as it does its work of holding the fat-digesting fluid with another funny name—bile—and dispensing it after meals.

But when bile becomes oversaturated with cholesterol or, more rarely, calcium, the extra compounds may crystallize, forming gallstones. Such stones can vary in size from smaller than a pea to as large as an egg. Many times, you won't even know you have them; one-third to one-half of the people with gallstones experience no symptoms.

The problem arises when a gallstone gets stuck in the bile duct—one of the tubes through which bile flows on its way to the small intestine. When that happens, you feel severe pain in the upper right section of your abdomen, often with nausea, vomiting, bloating, or belching. Sometimes the pain subsides; that means the stone may have fallen back into the gallbladder or been forced into the intestines. Rarely, an infection may develop because of the obstruction, resulting in fever, chills, or jaundice.

Approximately 20 million people in the United States have gallstones and at least one million new cases are diagnosed each year. More than 300,000 people have their gallbladders surgically removed each year just because of gallstones.

Diet plays a major role in the development of gallstones because bile is secreted when fatty substances are digested. Eating foods high in fat, protein, or sugar can make you more prone to stones.

You're also more likely to get gallstones if your cholesterol is high, you have food allergies, or you've experienced rapid weight loss.

Obese women over 40 who have had children are more likely to suffer from gallstones; in fact, with each pregnancy, a woman increases her chances of developing gallstones because pregnancy upsets the balance between cholesterol and bile acids.

Doctors tend to prefer surgery rather than drug treatment for gallstones. The usual procedure is removal of the gallbladder. New laser surgery techniques involve only a small incision and allow rapid recovery. A new treatment called lithotripsy is also available; it uses sonic shock waves to break up the stones. Another technique involves placing a tube into the gallbladder through which a strong solution capable of dissolving the stone is administered. Doctors and researchers are still evaluating the effectiveness and safety of these last two methods.

The gallbladder and the liver work together as an efficient team. Hence, the herbs that support the liver often help with gallstones.

DRUG TREATMENT

Bile Salts
Chenodiol (Chenix), ursodiol (Actigall). *Function:* dissolve gallstones by dilution. *Side effects:* diarrhea.

HERBAL REMEDIES

Dandelion (*Taraxacum officinale*)
The root of this common lawn weed has traditionally been used to treat both liver and gallbladder obstructions, improve overall liver function, and promote bile production. More bile means there's less chance of it becoming oversaturated with cholesterol or calcium, and that means it's less likely gallstones will form. *Typical dosage:* 1,000 to 2,000 milligrams of powdered root per day.

Milk Thistle (*Silybum marianum*)
A superior herb for liver support, cleansing, repair, and protection, milk thistle also reduces the concentration of cholesterol in the bile. That means fewer gallstones. *Typical dosage:* 200 to 400 mil-

SUPPLEMENTS FOR GALLBLADDER SUPPORT

You can't just take a pill to fight your body's tendency to form gallstones. But there are a few nutrients that can be solid allies.

◆ **Vitamin C.** Deficiencies in vitamin C have been linked to gallstone formation; taking C in supplements may prevent more from forming. *Typical dosage:* 1,000 to 3,000 milligrams per day, with meals.

◆ **Vitamin E.** So you gave in to temptation and ordered the French fries anyway. Well, vitamin E helps to scavenge free radicals, the damaging molecules that eating oxidized fats—like those fried foods—creates. Clinical studies also indicate that it may prevent gallstone formation. *Typical dosage:* 200 to 800 IU per day.

◆ **Lecithin.** Some research suggests that low levels of lecithin in the bile may cause gallstones. Lecithin, a type of nutrient called a phospholipid, also helps to break up fats, which is important to proper cholesterol digestion. It may also increase the capacity of bile to dissolve cholesterol. *Typical dosage:* 1,000 milligrams three times per day with meals.

◆ **Essential fatty acids.** These wonder chemicals help the body control cholesterol and digest other fats. Look for a product that offers a combination of omega-3 and

ligrams of product standardized to 80 percent silymarin per day, in divided doses.

Turmeric (*Curcuma longa*)

Curcumin, which gives turmeric its yellow pigment, is antioxidant, anti-inflammatory, and most important, cholesterol-lowering. Studies have shown that it also increases the ability of bile to dissolve cholesterol and calcium. Again, the bottom line is less likelihood that gallstones will form. *Typical dosage:* 300 to 1,000 milligrams of capsules standardized to 95 percent curcumin per day.

omega-6 fatty acids; you'll find both in fish, flaxseed, borage seed, black currant seed, and evening primrose oils. *Typical dosage:* 1,000 to 4,000 milligrams per day. Keep these oils refrigerated.

◆ **Taurine.** Studies of people who took supplements of this amino acid found that they secreted more bile—the magical fat-digesting fluid—and that the bile they secreted was able to dissolve more cholesterol. *Typical dosage:* 500 to 3,000 milligrams per day.

◆ **Hydrochloric acid.** Think it's odd for this dangerous acid to appear on a list of supplements? This hydrochloric acid is the kind that your stomach uses to digest food. People who lack sufficient amounts of this acid may be prone to developing gallstones. *Typical dosage:* 1 to 5 capsules with meals; start with one and build up, following the recommendations of the manufacturer or your doctor.

◆ **Fiber.** Psyllium, pectin, and guar gum can decrease cholesterol levels and keep the bile acid pool active, which discourages disease and stone formation. In studies on animals, the ones who ate the least fiber had the highest incidence of gallstones. And new evidence suggests that non-obese women whose digestive systems move slowly are prone to gallstones. So they need to be sure of getting enough fiber, especially if they have a family history of gallbladder disease. Follow manufacturer's recommendations for dosage.

Artichoke (*Cynara scolymus*)

This herb is one of the group known as bitters, because that's how they taste. Bitters jumpstart the whole digestive system before a meal; they prime the bile pump, so to speak. Studies have shown that artichoke leaf can effectively lower cholesterol; it especially helps facilitate the digestion of fats. *Typical dosage:* 800 to 1,200 milligrams per day.

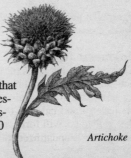

Artichoke

The Stone-Zapping Diet

If you have gallstones, you've probably heard people urging you to change your diet. They're right: Minimizing your intake of saturated fat (cutting fatty red meats, fried foods, and hydrogenated fats) does work wonders. Here's what else you can do:

◆ Emphasize a low-fat diet high in raw foods. Eat plenty of broiled fish, carrots, apples, lemons, oranges, grapes, celery, garlic, onions, tomatoes, dates, melons, and fiber-rich foods.

◆ Learn to love beets. Seriously. In addition to the foods mentioned above, beets are a great food for cleansing the blood and liver. Try beet juice, or a carrot-apple-beet combo juice.

◆ Avoid fried foods, fatty foods, animal fat, margarine, commercial oils, chocolate, and coffee. Minimize your consumption of sugar and refined carbohydrates.

Peppermint (*Mentha × piperita*)

Several studies suggest that this essential oil, when taken in an enteric-coated capsule, may dissolve gallstones. An enteric coating is one that passes through the stomach's digestive fluids intact to deliver its healing properties lower in the digestive tract. Studies suggest peppermint oil can help keep gallstone blockage from occurring. *Typical dosage:* 0.2 to 0.4 milliliter in enteric-coated capsules two times per day between meals.

GENITAL WARTS

T HEY'RE NOT EXACTLY A SUBJECT for polite conversation. But genital warts are the most common viral sexually transmitted disease. About 50 million people in the United States have had an encounter with them. Women between the ages of 22 and 30 are the most commonly affected.

These small, painless, flat or mushroom-shaped growths appear singly or in clusters on the genitals. Or they don't appear at all. That's their special hazard: Only 30 percent of people infected actually develop warts. And the 70 percent of cases in which no warts appear are most often linked to cervical dysplasia, abnormal cells on a woman's cervix that can be a precursor to cervical cancer.

Genital warts are caused by specific strains of the human papillomavirus—the same virus that causes less worrisome common warts. These strains are transmitted by skin-to-skin contact, usually during intercourse. Four weeks to nine months after exposure, blistery and perhaps itchy sores with a red base appear first on the genitals, then the anus and buttocks. The warts may stay the same, grow larger, or completely disappear, but the virus remains in the body and may recur months or even years later.

Risk factors for genital warts include multiple sex partners, cigarette smoking, and immune weakness. If you are female and test positive for a genital warts virus, be sure to get regular Pap smears and pelvic exams to keep an eye on the health of your cervix. This is especially important if you also have genital herpes, another risk factor for cervical dysplasia.

Genital warts are a condition you do not want to treat on your own. Be sure to consult your doctor, who can give you more information about risk factors and treatment options. It's especially important for your doctor to monitor the progress of the condition.

DRUG TREATMENT

No known drugs can eliminate the human papillomavirus. The warts themselves can be removed by freezing, surgery, laser or electric burning, or toxic chemicals. And they recur in up to 75 percent of cases.

Genital Wart Oil

This oil is potent—which it must be to destroy warts—so use it carefully.

½ teaspoon castor oil
¼ teaspoon thuja essential oil
¼ teaspoon tea tree essential oil
800 IU vitamin E oil (2 opened 400 IU capsules)

Combine all of the ingredients. Protect the skin around the wart with salve, leaving only the wart exposed. Carefully apply the mixture to the wart with a cotton swab two to four times per day for no more than one week. *Caution:* Do not take essential oils internally.

Herbal Remedies

Garlic (*Allium sativum*)

Amazing garlic not only fights viruses but also is good for the heart and treats bacterial infections. Allicin, a sulfurous compound in garlic, appears to encourage healing. *Typical dosage:* one or more fresh cloves, raw or only slightly cooked, per day; or up to three 500- to 600-milligram capsules per day (look for at least 5,000 micrograms of allicin per day).

Garlic

St.-John's-Wort (*Hypericum perforatum*)

Well-known for its usefulness in treating mild to moderate depression, this herb is also antiviral. It's known to help in cases of herpes, so it's worth a try with genital warts. *Typical dosage:* 450 milligrams in capsules two times per day for three days, then skip a day, repeating for nine months or longer; or ¾ teaspoon of tincture two times per day for the same time period.

GLAUCOMA

G LAUCOMA CAN BE A SILENT THIEF: Probably half the people who have it develop no symptoms. Meanwhile, their vision is slowly being stolen by pressure that gradually damages the optic nerve in the eye. Others who have glaucoma experience blurred vision, loss of side vision, colored rings or halos around lights, or eye pain.

What's happening inside the eye? A liquid referred to as the aqueous humor flows around the parts of the eye, bringing them nourishment and carrying away wastes. If the fine vessels supplying this liquid deliver too much fluid or don't drain well enough, pressure builds up in the eye.

This pressure can damage the optic nerve, resulting in vision loss. And such damage is irreversible, making early detection critical.

Glaucoma can occur because of trauma, tumors, diabetes, high blood pressure, heredity, or use of corticosteroid eyedrops. If you have any type of disease involving the circulatory system, you might also be at risk for developing glaucoma. Luckily, optometrists can measure pressure inside the eyes to detect early stages of glaucoma, although increased pressure doesn't always mean glaucoma exists.

WHEN GLAUCOMA SYMPTOMS ARE AN EMERGENCY

Although most cases of glaucoma develop gradually, a rare type called acute closed-angle glaucoma develops rapidly and requires immediate attention by a medical professional. If you have pain and redness in the eyes, hazy vision, nausea and vomiting, and headaches accompanied by a marked loss of vision, see a doctor immediately. This disorder can cause permanent loss of vision in two to five days if left untreated.

VITAMINS FOR YOUR EYES

Vitamin C has been shown to reduce pressure inside the eyes. If you are at risk for glaucoma, use either vitamin C supplements or herbs and foods that are high in vitamin C.

Other antioxidants may also help to prevent glaucoma, but little research has been done. If you're at risk for this thief of vision, it's worth making part of your routine a daily cup of antioxidant tea. Look for teas that contain rosemary, shepherd's purse, or turmeric.

It's also a good idea to make sure you get a variety of antioxidants in your diet. Eat lots of fruits and vegetables, especially the colorful ones.

Sources of Vitamin C

◆ Bell peppers
◆ Citrus fruits
◆ Parsley
◆ Strawberry leaves and fruit
◆ Turmeric

Herbs High in Antioxidants

◆ Rosemary
◆ Shepherd's purse
◆ Turmeric

There are three levels of treatment for glaucoma: drugs, laser therapy, and surgery. Five different groups of drugs are used to treat glaucoma, each having a slightly different way of working. If drug treatment is ineffective, laser therapy or surgery is then used to reduce the pressure in the eye.

DRUG TREATMENT

Beta Blockers

Timolol (Timoptic), betaxolol (Betoptic). *Function:* decrease the amount of fluid made inside the eye. *Side effects:* tiredness, confusion, decreased heart rate, bronchial spasms similar to asthma (potentially life-threatening).

Prostaglandins
Latanoprost (Xalatan). *Function:* reduce pressure in the eye by allowing more fluid to leave. *Side effects:* allergic reactions of the skin, muscle and joint pain, occasionally a change in eye color, thickening of eyelashes.

Adrenergics
Apraclonidin (Iopidine). *Function:* allow less fluid to enter the eye. *Side effects:* dry mouth, decreased blood pressure, tiredness.

Carbonic Anhydrase Inhibitors
Acetazolamide (Diamox), dichlorphenamide (Daranide). *Function:* decrease flow of sodium and water into the eye, thus decreasing pressure. *Side effects:* tiredness, weight loss, depression, anorexia, decreased sexual appetite, nausea, intestinal cramps, diarrhea, heartburn, possibly kidney damage. These drugs have fewer side effects when used as eyedrops.

Cholinergics
Pilocarpine (Isopto Carpine, Ocusert). *Function:* allow more fluid to leave the eye. *Side effects:* constriction of the pupil, myopia (nearsightedness).

HERBAL REMEDIES

Bilberry (*Vaccinium myrtillus*)
Traditionally used for all problems concerning the eye, the fruits of this shrub contain anthocyanosides. These compounds can help prevent the breakdown of vitamin C, which in turn can reduce pressure inside the eye. Blueberries, cranberries, and huckleberries also contain anthocyanosides. *Typical dosage:* 2 or 3 capsules or tablets standardized to 25 percent anthocyanosides per day.

Ginkgo (*Ginkgo biloba*)
An extract made from the leaves of this tree contains bioflavonoids called ginkgolides, which may be beneficial for glaucoma. *Typical*

An Herb to Avoid

You may have heard about treating glaucoma with jaborandi (*Pilocarpus* spp.). This South American herb contains pilocarpine, a standard glaucoma drug. Although the drug was originally made from the plant, today pilocarpine is manufactured synthetically. This fact is not merely interesting trivia, however, because using the herb itself is not considered safe. An overdose can cause death due to fluid buildup in the lungs.

dosage: three capsules per day (containing at least 40 milligrams of extract standardized to 24 percent flavone glycosides and 6 percent ginkgolides).

Gout

It's the stuff of legend, an old-fashioned disease that supposedly afflicts only the elderly, the rich, and the over-indulgent. But gout isn't humorous—it's painful. Imagine shards of ground glass inside your joints. Only the shards aren't glass, but crystals of uric acid, a byproduct of the breakdown of old cells and the construction of new ones.

Uric acid is usually filtered out of the body by the kidneys. But when there's too much of the acid in the bloodstream, it begins to accumulate in the joints.

Uric acid crystals inflict intense joint pain, often in nighttime attacks that come without warning. The big toe is most often affected, but other joints, including knees, ankles, elbows, and fingers, can be involved. Swelling, inflammation, a sensation that the joint is on fire, and chills or fever can also result.

Nine out of ten people with gout are middle-aged men; over half of those with gout have a genetic predisposition to the ailment.

SUPPLEMENTS TO EASE THE PAIN

You can take a number of supplements to alleviate the pain of gout and help ward off future attacks. But be aware that they aren't a substitute for improving your diet. (Also be aware that niacin supplements may precipitate an attack of gout, as nicotinic acid competes with uric acid for excretion from the kidneys. If you're currently taking niacin for heart disease, high cholesterol, or other conditions, ask your doctor about gout and this supplement.)

◆ **Folic acid.** This nutrient is important in the breakdown and metabolism of proteins; it also inhibits the action of an enzyme responsible for the production of uric acid. *Typical dosage:* 200 to 400 milligrams per day.

◆ **Alpha lipoic acid (ALA), vitamin E, and selenium.** This terrific trio helps to suppress the production of leukotrienes, chemicals that play a role in joint inflammation. ALA and selenium help vitamin E fight damaging free radicals more effectively. *Typical dosage:* 50 to 800 milligrams of ALA per day; 200 to 400 IU of vitamin E per day; and 200 micrograms of selenium per day.

◆ **Omega-3 and omega-6 fatty acids.** You can get these in fish oil, flaxseed oil, or evening primrose oil, but the source doesn't matter. What matters is that these fatty acids inhibit the production of the inflammatory agents released in gout in several ways. *Typical dosage:* 1,200 to 2,000 milligrams of fish oil per day plus 500 to 1,500 milligrams of omega-6 fatty acids per day (sunflower, safflower, olive, and soy oils contain omega-6 fatty acids).

◆ **Broïmelain.** This enzyme is found in the pineapple plant and functions as an effective anti-inflammatory. *Typical dosage:* 500 to 1,500 GDUs (gelatin digestion units) per day; or just eat plenty of fresh pineapple.

Get a Doctor's Diagnosis

Because several other disorders can mimic the symptoms of gout, it is important to see a doctor for an accurate diagnosis of any persistent joint pain. Blood and urine tests may or may not show a high level of uric acid. Your doctor may want to take x-rays or draw fluid from the synovial sac that cushions the joint to find out if what's ailing you is really gout or some other disease.

Those who are overweight and those prone to high blood pressure, heart disease, or diabetes are likely candidates.

Gout has traditionally been thought of as a disease of the affluent who dine on fatty meats, wines, and rich dairy products. But newer research points to a different culprit: beer. One study found that the major dietary difference between 61 men with gout and a group of men who didn't have it was that 41 percent of the gout group drank more than a dozen cans of beer—two and a half liters—a day.

A Gentler-on-Joints Diet

Gout is among the most food-instigated disorders described in this book. Luckily, mild cases are also easily treated by changes in diet. And at least you know the enemy: uric acid.

But how do you fight it? One way is to withhold compounds that the body breaks down into uric acid. One of these compounds, purine, occurs in many foods. A low-purine diet is essential in treating and preventing gout.

Try to avoid the following foods.

- Alcohol
- Anchovies
- Asparagus
- Cauliflower
- Dried beans and lentils
- Herring
- Lunch meats
- Oatmeal
- Organ meats
- Mushrooms

Suds imbibers aside, the reason certain people are prone to gout remains somewhat of a mystery. Researchers have linked the disease to prior joint injuries, periods of stress, and alcohol or drug consumption. Certain diuretics and antibiotics can trigger gout; studies have also shown that gout can result from the presence of tumors, kidney disorders, lead poisoning, and enzyme deficiencies. Mild cases of gout may be completely controlled by dietary changes. But continuing attacks may need more intensive care because they can cause permanent joint and kidney damage.

DRUG TREATMENT

Nonsteroidal Anti-Inflammatories (NSAIDs)

Indomethicin (Indocin), ibuprofen, naproxen (Naprosyn, Alleve). *Function:* decrease inflammation and pain. *Side effects:* abdominal pain, indigestion, dizziness, stomach ulcers, stomach bleeding, nausea, nightmares.

- ◆ Mussels
- ◆ Peas
- ◆ Poultry
- ◆ Sardines
- ◆ Saturated fat
- ◆ Spinach
- ◆ White flour
- ◆ White sugar
- ◆ Yeast products

After that list, you might ask what's left? Try eating plenty of the following foods.

- ◆ Fresh vegetable juices (carrot, celery, parsley)
- ◆ Grains, seeds, and nuts
- ◆ High-fiber foods and complex carbohydrates
- ◆ Plenty of water to facilitate excretion of uric acid
- ◆ Raw fruits and vegetables
- ◆ Vegetable broths

Other Drugs

Colchicine (many products). *Function:* inhibit inflammation and decrease pain. *Side effects:* diarrhea.

Allopurinol (Zyloprim). *Function:* reduce the formation of uric acid. *Side effects:* nausea, vomiting, diarrhea, numbness, skin rashes, cataracts, drug interactions.

Probenecid (Benemid, Probalan), sulfinpyrazone (Anturane). *Function:* decrease the amount of uric acid in the body by acting on the kidneys. *Side effects:* stomach and intestinal irritation, skin rash.

HERBAL REMEDIES

Grapeseed (*Vitis vinifera*)

You've likely seen commercial products that include grapeseed or pine bark extracts. These contain powerful antioxidants called procyanidins that neutralize damaging free radicals in joints and work as natural anti-inflammatory agents. *Typical dosage:* 50 to 200 milligrams of procyanidins per day.

Turmeric (*Curcuma longa*)

This spice, familiar to anyone who enjoys Indian food, contains a compound called curcumin. Like grapeseed, turmeric is antioxidant and anti-inflammatory. It's also effective at easing the stiffness and pain that come with gout. Turmeric is especially effective when combined with boswellia (see below). *Typical dosage:* 300 to 900 milligrams per day of a product standardized to 95 percent curcumin.

CHEER FOR CHERRIES AND BERRIES

Not all good things are off limits to people with gout. In studies, cherries (especially black cherries), blueberries, and strawberries have proven their ability to reduce levels of uric acid in studies. Black cherry juice is probably the most effective. Use it in pure juice form and drink ⅛ to ¼ cup per day.

Boswellia (*Boswellia carterii*)

This resin, also known as Indian frankincense, contains an acid that in animal studies has shown an ability to control arthritis. It also inhibits inflammation and improves circulation to affected joint tissues. *Typical dosage:* 300 to 400 milligrams per day of an extract containing 65 percent boswellic acid, two times.

Devil's Claw (*Harpagophytum procumbens*)

This herb has an extensive history of use as an anti-inflammatory, pain reliever, and digestive stimulant. Because improper digestion of protein plays a role in gout, causing the uric acid buildup that leads to those shard-like crystals, this is a remedy tailor-made for people with gout. *Typical dosage:* 600 to 800 milligrams per day of product standardized to 1.5 percent harpagoside. *Caution:* Do not use if you have gastric or duodenal ulcers. Do not use during pregnancy or nursing. If you have heart disease, use only with a doctor's supervision.

Yucca (*Yucca schidigera*)

Another digestion-improving herb, yucca has been found in some studies to treat arthritis pain, swelling, and stiffness. Although those studies were controversial, yucca has seen continued use for joint pain. *Typical dosage:* 1,000 to 1,500 milligrams two or three times per day.

Celery Seed (*Apium graveolens*)

If you like this seed as a seasoning, here's another reason to appreciate it. An extract of celery seed has the ability to calm inflammation and neutralize the harmful effects of uric acid. *Typical dosage:* 2 to 4 tablets of celery seed extract per day.

Gum Disease

Do your gums bleed—even a little? Are they red, sore, or puffy? Have you ever had bad breath, or has your dentist ever told you that you need to brush and see the hygienist more frequently? If you answer "yes" to any of these questions, you may have some form of periodontal or gum disease.

According to the American Dental Association, approximately three in four people over age 20 have some stage of gum disease. It might be gingivitis, the earliest and most treatable stage, when careful brushing, flossing, and regular dental cleanings can reverse the damage. Or it might have progressed to the point where tooth loss can occur.

Teeth are not embedded in the jaw like fenceposts in concrete. They are surrounded by living tissue called the periodontal membrane. This tissue acts as a shock absorber for the tooth. Thousands of tiny fibers connect to the tooth and to the bones of the jaw.

In a normal, healthy mouth, a slight space called a pocket exists between the tooth and the periodontal membrane. It usually measures one to two millimeters, or about an eighth of an inch. When food particles and bacteria remain trapped in this space, they form plaque, a sticky goo that clings to the teeth. Plaque hardens into tartar, which settles into this pocket in layers, eventually deepening it. Over time, the gums lose their normal pink color, get puffy and red, and may bleed when brushed.

Left untreated, layers of tartar continue their progress down the roots of the tooth, eventually penetrating the periodontal membrane and eroding the bones that hold the tooth in place. The teeth involved loosen and eventually fall out.

Why do some people get gum disease and not others? For one thing, the bacteria that cause it are contagious; they can be spread by kissing. For another, there seems to be a link between gum disease and adult-onset diabetes. Vitamin C deficiency may also play a role, allowing greater passage of the bacteria into the tissues that surround the teeth.

Researchers are now investigating why many of the same people who suffer from gum disease also have cardiovascular disease. It's possible that the same dietary habits or deficiencies promote both problems. And although gingivitis may seem minor, the bacteria that cause it can be aspirated into the lungs, causing pneumonia. Finally, gingivitis is one of the early signs that the immune system may be having problems and it should not be ignored.

The best way to prevent gum disease is to brush and floss regularly. Also, see a dentist periodically to remove the plaque that builds up. If you tend to get a lot of plaque, see a dentist at least twice a year.

Treatment for periodontal disease usually involves some sort of mechanical procedure in which a dental hygienist deep-cleans the gums and removes plaque from the area of the tooth under the gum. This is often accompanied by antibiotic treatment; more and more, antibiotic treatment alone is being used. There are no drugs, however, that can be taken internally to reverse the progress of gum disease. In advanced cases, surgical procedures are performed.

DRUG TREATMENT

Antibiotics
Penicillin, penicillin V (Pen-Vee K, V-Cillin). *Function:* kill the bacteria responsible for gum infection. *Side effects:* development

BACTERIA-FIGHTING GUM RINSE

Although this rinse isn't especially tasty, it will help heal inflamed gums.

- **5 drops goldenseal tincture**
- **5 drops myrrh tincture**
- **2 cloves crushed garlic**
- **1 dash of cayenne**
- **2 cups water**

Combine all ingredients. Swish in the mouth for 2 to 3 minutes, three or four times per day.

of penicillin-resistant bacteria, excitability, skin rash, yeast infections, and alteration of intestinal bacteria, which may cause intestinal irritation, nausea, vomiting, and diarrhea.

Other Drugs

Doxycycline (Doryx, Vibramycin). *Function:* kill the bacteria responsible for gum infection. *Side effects:* development of antibiotic-resistant bacteria; alteration of intestinal flora, which causes intestinal irritation, nausea, vomiting, diarrhea; anorexia; yeast infections; less commonly, liver and kidney toxicity.

Metronidazole (Flagyl). *Function:* kill anaerobic bacteria that may cause gingivitis. *Side effects:* nausea, headache, dry mouth, metallic taste in the mouth, weakness.

HERBAL REMEDIES

Echinacea (*Echinacea purpurea, E. angustifolia, E. pallida*)

Just as it fights the bacteria and viruses that cause colds, flu, and minor infection, echinacea fights gum bacteria by enhancing the functioning of the body's immune system. Use it as a mouth rinse or swab it onto sore or swollen gums. You can also take it internally. *Typical dosage:* up to nine 300- to 400-milligram capsules per day; or up to 60 drops of tincture three times per day.

Goldenseal (*Hydrastis canadensis*)

One of this root's compounds, berberine, is a potent antibacterial substance. Goldenseal also stimulates digestion and the secretion of bile, which helps you get more nutrients from the foods you eat— a good thing in case nutritional deficiencies have made you more prone to gingivitis. In addition, goldenseal is astringent, which helps tone gum tissue. *Typical dosage:* up to six 500- to 600-milligram capsules per day; or 20 to 50 drops of tincture per day. *Caution:* Goldenseal has not been proven safe for pregnant or nursing women. If you have heart problems, consult your doctor before using it.

Calendula (*Calendula officinalis*)

Well-known for its healing properties, calendula benefits gums with its antiviral, anti-inflammatory, and immune-stimulating compounds. It may also help treat ulcers and sore throats. *Typical dosage:* apply tincture to the affected area up to three times per day.

Aloe (*Aloe vera*)

Aloe is a proven healer of skin injuries. Because it has the same effect on the gums, a number of mouth rinses and other dental products include aloe. Look for it in herbal dental products, or mix pure aloe vera gel with tinctures of the herbs in this chapter. Swab this paste on sore gums as needed.

Bilberry (*Vaccinium myrtillus*) and Hawthorn (*Crataegus* spp.)

Both of these berries contain procyanidins, substances that are powerfully anti-inflammatory and may help strengthen gum tissue. To use them against gingivitis, buy a few ounces of the powdered version of either herb. Mix the powder with enough water to make a paste and swab onto the infected gums. Leave on 5 to 10 minutes, then rinse and floss.

HANGOVER

IF YOU WAKE UP WITH A HEADACHE, dizziness, fatigue, and nausea the morning after a big celebration, chances are you remember exactly what caused those symptoms, because they're familiar: You have a hangover. The best advice medical experts can give you is to monitor your alcohol intake, but occasionally even one drink can be too much. That's because tolerance for alcohol varies widely from person to person, from drink to drink, and from occasion to occasion. You may be able to knock back a six-pack at a weekend football gathering with no ill effects, but wake up woozy and in pain after a few glasses of wine at a relative's wedding.

Generally, the more you weigh, the more you can drink without getting a hangover. Also, if you drink regularly, your production of the enzymes that metabolize alcohol increases and so does your tolerance. This doesn't mean that consuming high quantities of alcohol is good for you—it simply means that if you *don't* drink regularly, you're more likely to feel ill effects from those occasional nights on the town, as unfair as that seems.

When you drink, the alcohol is metabolized in your liver. There, it forms toxic byproducts, which then circulate through the body, causing the pain that you feel as a hangover. The kidneys filter these waste products of alcohol out of the blood, but they must remove water while they're doing it. That causes dehydration, one of the major hangover symptoms. Your body also uses many vitamins and nutrients to break down alcohol, especially the B vitamins. This results in a slight state of malnutrition that can worsen if your occasions for indulging occur every weekend—a good reason to make extra sure to take your vitamins during the holiday party blitz.

Eating lots of sugar can make a hangover worse, as can mixing different types of alcohol; both of these actions make the liver work harder. Generally speaking, light-colored alcoholic beverages, such as white wine or vodka, are less likely to produce a hangover than, say, red wine or scotch.

If you are planning a night out or a celebration where you know you will be drinking, eat a well-balanced wholesome meal beforehand and make sure you drink plenty of water. After the celebration, drink a large glass of water before going to bed, take a B-complex supplement that supplies at least 50 milligrams of niacin, and take a liquid bitters preparation (look for products that contain dandelion, gentian, mugwort, or Angostura bitters) in water with a little honey. This may lessen the pain of the hangover you'll feel the next day.

DRUG TREATMENT

Analgesics

Aspirin, acetaminophen, ibuprofen. *Function:* relieve headache and other pain. *Aspirin side effects:* gastritis; at very high doses, vomiting, ringing in the ears. *Acetaminophen side effects:* dizziness, excitement, disorientation, liver damage. *Ibuprofen side effects:* gastrointestinal irritation and bleeding, rash; with high doses, blood, liver, and kidney damage.

DON'T JUMP THE GUN WITH PAINKILLERS

You're thinking, well, might as well wash my analgesics down with my last slug of beer and beat my hangover to the punch? Think again. Pain relievers should *not* be taken with alcohol. Aspirin and alcohol are both stomach irritants; combining them can damage the stomach lining.

Acetaminophen and ibuprofen are metabolized by the liver, as is alcohol. Combining booze and one of these drugs can overload the liver. In fact, just such a combination has been in one case the cause of a liver transplant—not exactly the way you'd want to remember a celebration.

HERBAL REMEDIES

Willow (*Salix* spp.)

The bark of this group of trees contains the same pain-relieving ingredient found in aspirin in much smaller amounts, so it may be less stressful on your stomach. You'll also find similar pain-relieving compounds in wintergreen. To make a tea, use the bark of willow or the leaves and flowering tops of wintergreen. *Typical dosage:* 1 to 3 cups of tea per day (steep ¼ to ½ teaspoon of powdered bark or wintergreen leaves and flowers in 1 cup of hot water for 10 to 15 minutes).

Dandelion (*Taraxacum officinale*)

This bitter herb's root may help with hangovers by gently relieving constipation and stomachaches. It also stimulates the liver, which may have a beneficial effect on alcohol metabolism. And dandelion is a good source of antioxidants, such as vitamin A, that may help repair some of the damage the festive activities wreaked on

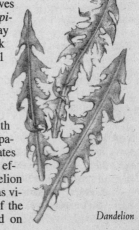

Dandelion

your body. *Typical dosage:* 2 cups of tea per day, morning and evening (steep 1 to 2 teaspoons of dried root in 1 cup of hot water for 10 to 15 minutes); or 30 to 60 drops of tincture three times per day for the day or two that symptoms persist.

SUPPLEMENTS FOR THOSE WHO IMBIBE

So you travel a lot with your job—and such travel involves a lot of social imbibing with potential clients. What can you do? First off, keep monitoring your alcohol intake and switch to club soda after a certain number of drinks. Second, try taking the following supplements to minimize alcohol's effect on your overall health.

♦ **Zinc.** The enzymes that break down alcohol need this mineral to do their work. People who drink frequently are often deficient in zinc; if you want to take a supplement, take 15 milligrams. Or you can try eating a piece of whole-grain toast or some rice before imbibing. This not only supplies zinc but also soaks up alcohol in the stomach, allowing it to be absorbed more slowly.

♦ **B vitamins.** The whole complex of these nutrients tends to be depleted in those who drink frequently. Like zinc, B vitamins are used by the enzymes that metabolize alcohol. Take a product that supplies at least 50 milligrams of each B vitamin (thiamine, niacin, B_6, B_{12}) and 100 micrograms of folic acid after drinking.

♦ **Vitamin C.** This antioxidant may help in the breakdown and removal of alcohol from the body. Take 1,000 milligrams of vitamin C as soon as possible after drinking a lot.

♦ **Vitamin A.** Excessive drinking depletes this important vitamin. Morning-after Bloody Marys, made with tomato juice, may help hangovers because of their high levels of lycopene, a vitamin A relative. Just make your Mary a virgin—meaning blend it without the alcohol—and you've got a very healthful drink.

SWEET CURE FOR A SPLITTING HEAD

Honey contains as much as 40 percent fructose, a form of sugar that may speed the metabolism of alcohol and decrease the effects of a hangover. So if tea and toast is all your dicey stomach can handle, you can amply sweeten the tea with honey. High amounts of fructose can also be found in most fruits.

Ginkgo (*Ginkgo biloba*)

Typically used to improve circulation, improve memory, and decrease dizziness, ginkgo may help with hangover. In Japan, the seeds of this tree are served at cocktail parties to prevent drunkenness and hangovers. *Typical dosage:* three 40-milligram capsules of standardized extract per day.

Red or Chili Peppers (*Capsicum* spp.)

Hot peppers contain the pain-relieving compound capsaicin. Try dried, ground peppers or powdered cayenne in a glass of tomato juice the morning after. But keep this Bloody Mary a virgin: Fighting a hangover with another drink only delays your body's recovery. *Typical dosage:* a pinch or so in food.

Milk Thistle (*Silybum marianum*)

This herb's seeds have a long history of use in protecting the liver. It contains silymarin, which has been shown to protect the liver against a number of toxins, including alcohol. A frequent drinker or recovering alcoholic should take milk thistle extract on a daily basis. *Typical dosage:* 70 to 120 milligrams three times per day. If you are planning a rare, no-holds-barred celebration, take 70 to 120 milligrams once before drinking to help protect your liver.

Hay Fever

Most people love spring and summer—the sight of pink blossoms, the sound of birdsong, the scent of fresh-mown grass. But those who suffer from hay fever think of spring and summer as Big Sneeze Seasons—the sight of used tissues, the sound of sniffling and blowing, the distress of watery, itchy eyes. Such allergy symptoms plague some people year-round; doctors call this phenomenon perennial allergic rhinitis.

Hay fever has become more common worldwide than ever before, particularly among children and young adults. Among all ages, one in five now gets hay fever.

Drug Treatment

Traditional Antihistamines
Diphenhydramine (Benadryl), brompheniramine, clemastine, chlorpheniramine, others (many trade names). *Function:* block the action of histamine, a chemical released during allergic reactions, thereby relieving symptoms such as itching, sneezing, and mucus production. *Side effects:* sedation, dizziness, dry mouth, nose, and throat; less commonly agitation, irritability, nightmares, weakness, fatigue; for antihistamines used as nasal sprays, bitter taste, nose irritation, increased secretions.

Nonsedating Antihistamines
Astemizole (Hismanal), fexofenadine (Allegra), cetirizine (Zyrtec, Reactine), loratadine (Claritin). *Function:* block the action of histamine; these new drugs also fight inflammation. *Side effects:* dry mouth, nose, and throat; astemizole may cause heart-rhythm disturbances.

Oral Decongestants
Phenylpropanolamine (in combination remedies Contac, Dimetapp, many others), phenylephrine (Nasahist, Nalgest, many others), pseudoephedrine (Sudafed, combination drugs). *Function:* relieve stuffiness (but no other allergy symptoms) by constricting

the small blood vessels in the respiratory mucous membranes. *Side effects:* nervousness, irritability, insomnia, suppressed appetite, heart palpitations, rapid heart rate.

Nasal Spray Decongestants
Phenylephrine (Dristan, Neo-Synephrine), oxymetazoline (Afrin, Sinex), xylometazoline (Neo-Synephrine II). *Function:* relieve stuffiness (but no other allergy symptoms) by constricting the small blood vessels in the respiratory mucous membranes. *Side effects:* rebound congestion (the return of more stubborn congestion after use is discontinued); risk of dependency and abuse.

Intranasal Corticosteroids
Beclomethasone (Vancenase, Beconase), budesonide (Rhinocort), fluticasone (Flonase), triamcinolone (Nasacort), mometasone (Nasonex). *Function:* help control the allergic response to prevent symptoms. *Side effects:* burning or drying of the nose, sneezing; less commonly nosebleed, sore throat, ulcers in the nose.

Other Drugs
Cromolyn sodium (Nalcrom, Nasalcrom). *Function:* block the release of inflammatory chemicals such as histamine when used preventively. *Side effects:* burning or stinging inside nose, increased sneezing.

  Immunotherapy. Also called hyposensitization, desensitization injections, or allergy shots; involves repeated injections of allergens into the skin. Usually reserved for people whose symptoms don't respond adequately to avoidance and drug therapy.

HERBAL REMEDIES

Stinging Nettle (*Urtica dioica*)
One study found that nettle may offer some relief to people with hay fever. Of the 69 patients who completed the study, 58 percent rated the freeze-dried preparation of nettle effective; 48 percent said it worked as well or better than their conventional medications. *Typical dosage:* 300 milligrams of freeze-dried nettle in capsules two or three times per day.

Ephedra (*Ephedra sinica*)
Also known as ma huang, this herb acts as a decongestant just like its chemically synthesized counterpart, pseudoephedrine. It's

Salt for the Sneezes

Here's a simple home remedy for relieving hay fever: wash out your nose with salt water, with or without herbs. To make your own salt solution, add ½ teaspoon salt or baking soda to 1 cup of warm, clean water. You can also make an herbal tea and add the salt to that. Good candidates include herbs with astringent and anti-inflammatory action, such as eyebright, and those that act as mucous membrane tonics and antimicrobials, such as Oregon graperoot or goldenseal. Put your saline or herb solution into one of the following containers: a creamer with a long spout, an eyedropper, or a neti pot (a small pot designed for this purpose available at yoga equipment stores).

To use, turn your head to one side and lower it over the sink. Keeping your forehead slightly higher than your chin, gently pour the solution into your uppermost nostril. The solution will drain out your other nostril. (Some of it may run down the back of your throat, so don't breathe while you're doing this.) This form of nasal irrigation helps flush out pollens, molds, and other allergens. It also helps thin mucus, making it easier to expel by gently blowing into a tissue.

available dried in teas, capsules, tablets, and liquid extracts. Dosage guidelines for ephedra vary, which is cause for some concern, because overdoses of this herb can cause serious side effects. Abuse of ephedra compounds in combination with caffeine has even caused deaths. Ephedra offers a good example of why herbal dosages are both tricky and controversial: An amount that has little effect on one person may be too much for another whose body size is smaller or whose metabolism is faster. *Typical dosage:* 15 to 30 drops of tincture in water up to four times per day; or follow manufacturer's or practitioner's instructions. *Caution:* Do not exceed the recommended dose. May cause high blood pressure, palpitations, nervousness, insomnia, nausea, flushing, appetite loss, headache. Not recommended for people with a history of anorexia, glaucoma, thyroid disease, heart disease, high blood pressure, difficulty urinating because of prostate enlargement, or chronic insomnia. Do not use during pregnancy or in combination with other central nervous system stimulants such as caffeine, theophylline, MAO-inhibiting drugs, and amphetamines.

Peppermint (*Mentha × piperita*)

Inhaling peppermint's volatile oils makes you feel as if you can breathe easier, even when airflow is not actually increasing. One study found that both menthol oil extracted from peppermint and peppermint essential oil have anti-inflammatory effects. The researchers called for clinical trials to see if mint could help relieve

SUPPLEMENTS FOR PEOPLE WITH HAY FEVER

The following vitamins and other supplements may help make allergy season a bit more manageable.

◆ **Vitamin C and bioflavonoids.** Although antihistamine drugs inhibit histamine after its release, these supplements prevent its formation. Foods rich in the bioflavonoid quercetin include onions, garlic, and cayenne peppers. The recommended dose of vitamin C is 2,000 to 3,000 milligrams per day in divided doses; for quercetin, it's 500 milligrams two or three times per day.

◆ **Omega-3 fatty acids.** Abundant in flaxseed, flaxseed oil, and cold-water fish (salmon, herring, mackerel, and others), these acids can affect chemical pathways in the body in a way that eases allergy symptoms. Gammalinolenic acid, an omega-6 fatty acid contained in evening primrose, borage, and black currant seed oils, has a similar effect. On the other hand, the saturated fats found in animal-derived foods tend to increase chemicals that promote inflammation. Some practitioners recommend a dose of up to a tablespoon of flaxseed oil per day to ensure adequate omega-3 intake. But don't cook with flaxseed oil, as heat—even storage at room temperature—causes it to turn rancid.

such conditions as hay fever and asthma. Until the results are in, go ahead and drink mint tea (steep 1 teaspoon of dried herb in 1 cup of hot water for 15 minutes) as needed if it helps your hay fever. You can also use essential oil of peppermint in steam inhalation. Simply boil a pot of water, pour it carefully in a heat resistant bowl, and add three to five drops of the essential oil. Cover your head with a towel. Holding your face at least 12 inches away from the steam, breathe deeply through your nose for several minutes. *Caution:* Do not use peppermint internally if you have heartburn or esophageal reflux.

Peppermint

Licorice Root (*Glycyrrhiza glabra*)

Anti-inflammatory and antiallergy, licorice has actions that are similar to cortisone drugs. There are two kinds of licorice. One is used long-term to help heal ulcers and is labeled DGL licorice. For hay fever, you want whole licorice, not the DGL variety. *Typical dosage:* up to six 400- or 500-milligram capsules per day; or 20 to 30 drops of tincture up to 3 times per day. *Caution:* Do not use licorice for longer than six weeks. Do not use if you are pregnant or nursing, or have high blood pressure, diabetes, thyroid, kidney, liver, or heart disease. Also, if you are already taking corticosteroid allergy medications, consult a doctor before adding licorice to your treatment regimen.

Feverfew (*Tanacetum parthenium*)

Best known for preventing migraines, feverfew possesses anti-inflammatory properties that may relieve allergies. Although scientific studies have yet to confirm this, many herbalists view feverfew as an antiallergy herb. You can nibble one to two fresh leaves a day or make them into a tea, but the bitter taste may drive you to using a liquid extract or capsule. *Typical dosage:* up to three 400-to 500-milligram capsules per day; or 15 to 30 drops of tincture per day. *Caution:* About 10 percent of people report mouth ulcers, tongue inflammation, or lip swelling. Those allergic to other members of the daisy family may be allergic to feverfew. Do not use during pregnancy.

Garlic (*Allium sativum*)
This pungent bulb contains the anti-inflammatory substance quercetin, which can help calm the allergic response during hay fever season. Garlic is a potent antibacterial and antiviral agent, too, so it could help ward off sinusitis and make your mucous membranes less of a target for opportunistic cold and flu viruses. *Typical dosage:* up to three 500- to 600-milligram capsules per day (look for products that deliver a daily dose of 4,000 to 5,000 micrograms of allicin); or just eat one or more fresh, raw cloves per day. *Caution:* Consult your doctor before taking garlic if you have stomach inflammation, take warfarin or other blood thinners, or expect to have surgery soon.

Reishi (*Ganoderma lucidum*)
This Chinese remedy boasts several healthful effects, including an ability to reduce allergies. Reishi inhibits some of the body chemicals that trigger inflammation, including histamine. In China, it is used to treat asthma and other allergic disease. It's available in capsules, tablets, syrups, and teas. *Typical dosage:* up to five 420-milligram capsules per day; or up to three 1,000 milligram tablets up to 3 times per day.

THE MYTH OF THE STOIC SNEEZER

Hay fever isn't just an annoyance; doctors know that it increases your risk of other diseases. Lingering inflammation of the upper respiratory tract—one of hay fever's typical symptoms—can result in middle ear infections, sinus infections, allergic conjunctivitis (pinkeye), chronic cough, recurrent nosebleeds, and nasal polyps. One study even found a link in women between year-round hay fever and recurrent vaginal yeast infections. And other allergic conditions, such as asthma and eczema, often go hand in hand with hay fever. So toughing out your hay fever symptoms may not be a good option for your overall health.

Headaches

Not all headaches are created equal. Some produce a dull ache that is a nuisance but doesn't ruin your day. Others come with pain levels that bust the charts and send you to bed. Causes also vary.

Tension headaches, by far the most common kind of recurrent headache, arise from tight muscles in the shoulder, neck, and scalp. Often, these headaches come on during the course of the day and resolve after rest or a good sleep. Given sufficient stress, they can persist for several days.

Migraine headaches result from a narrowing of the arteries in and around the brain. When that happens, the insufficient blood flow sometimes produces what's called an aura (when the symptoms are only visual) or prodrome (when they include different types of sensory disturbances). This stage of the headache is marked by symptoms such as sensitivity to light, abdominal discomfort, sweating, moodiness, transient numbness or weakness on one side of the body, difficulty speaking, and visual disturbances, such as moving black dots, zigzag lines, and blurred vision. After this phase the brain arteries dilate, which causes pain—typically a throbbing pain on one side of the head. The pain may later become constant and involve the whole head. Usually the headache lasts two to three hours, but it can persist for a few days. Vomiting often breaks the headache. Sleepiness follows. Common triggers of migraines include stress, insufficient sleep, sleeping late, a less-than-optimal diet, menstrual periods, excessive noise, and bright lights.

Cluster headaches are severe, begin suddenly, and produce one-sided pain that localizes in the area around or behind the eye. Whereas a migraine makes a person want to lie in a dark, quiet room, cluster headaches produce restlessness. This type of headache is much less common than a migraine. Though the pain is intense, it usually goes away within 30 to 45 minutes. The term "cluster" refers to the occurrence of such headaches in episodes; for instance, one every afternoon for a month, followed by its disappearance for months or years before recurring.

Other less frequent causes of headache include head injury, sinus

SOME LIKE IT HOT

You can often find some relief from headache by using hot or cold applications. It's easy to tell whether a hot or cold compress makes your own headache worse or better. If heat seems to work, try wrapping a damp, hot towel around your neck and shoulders. This promotes circulation and helps relax tight muscles. You can also fill a clean athletic sock with a grain such as lentils, corn, or rice, knot the top, and microwave it for a minute or less. Test to see that it's not too hot; if it is, wait a minute or two or wrap it in another towel to buffer the heat. If cold is more soothing, apply a commercial cold pack or a bag of frozen vegetables to forehead, neck, or shoulders.

infections, other infections, temporomandibular joint disorder, hangover, depression, overuse of over-the-counter pain relievers, brain tumor, congenitally malformed blood vessels in the brain, bleeding into the brain, and high blood pressure.

DRUG TREATMENT

Analgesics
Aspirin, acetaminophen, ibuprofen, naproxen, ketoprofen. *Function:* ease headache pain. *Aspirin side effects:* heartburn, indigestion, stomach irritation, and mild nausea or vomiting. *Acetaminophen side effects:* chronic use or higher dosages may damage the liver and the kidneys. *Ibuprofen, naproxen, and ketoprofen side effects:* continuous use may irritate stomach lining; long-term high-dose use may damage the liver and the kidneys. *Note*: Using analgesics regularly and then quitting them abruptly can produce chronic headache with worse pain.

Prescription Analgesics
Isometheptene with acetaminophen and dichloralphenazone (Midrin), butalbital with aspirin and caffeine (Fiorinal). *Function:* ease more severe headache pain. *Midrin side effects:* drowsiness, dizziness. *Fiorinal side effects:* drowsiness, dizziness, nausea; risk of dependency.

Caffeine
Combination analgesics (Anacin, Excedrin Extra-Strength, others); with ergotamine (Cafergot). *Function:* constrict arteries to tame headache. *Side effects:* rapid heartbeat, hunger, anxiety, jitteriness; chronic, heavy use of caffeinated beverages can lead to headaches.

Triptans
Sumatriptan (Imitrex), zolmitriptan (Zomig), naratriptan (Amerge). *Function:* mimic the action of serotonin, a mood-controlling brain chemical thought to be involved in migraines; sometimes also used for cluster headaches. *Side effects:* burning, tingling, or redness at injection site; nausea and vomiting.

Beta Blockers
Propranolol (Inderal, Novopranol), metroprolol (Lopressor, Novo-Pindol), atenolol (Apo-Atenolol, Novometoprol), nadolol (Corgard, Syn-Nadolol). *Function:* prevent migraine or cluster headaches. *Side effects:* fatigue, nausea, depression, slow heart rate, low blood pressure, constricted airways, nightmares.

Calcium Channel Blockers
Nifedipine (Adalat, Apo-Nifed, Novo-Nifedin, Procardia), verapamil (Calan, Isoptin, Verelan). *Function:* prevent migraine headaches. *Side effects:* rapid heartbeat, depression, weight gain, constipation. Also, because these drugs dilate blood vessels, some people experience migraine-like headaches—the very condition the drugs are intended to relieve.

Tricyclic Antidepressants
Amitriptyline (Elavil) and nortriptyline (Aventyl, Pamelor). *Function:* prevent migraines and recurrent tension headaches. *Side effects:* headache, dry mouth, constipation or diarrhea, nausea, indigestion, weakness, fatigue, drowsiness, nervousness, anxiety, insomnia, tremor, excessive sweating.

Other Drugs
Ergotamine (Ergostat, Gynergen). *Function:* constrict blood vessels and mimic the action of serotonin to relieve migraines. *Side effects:* dizziness, nausea, diarrhea, vomiting; continuous use may cause worse headaches upon abrupt withdrawal.

HERBAL REMEDIES

Feverfew (*Tanacetum parthenium*)

Since the 1980s, three studies have shown feverfew's benefits for people with migraines. It seems to work for about two-thirds of the people who try it. Feverfew contains parthenolides, compounds that seem to inhibit the release of the mood-controlling brain chemical serotonin from blood cells called platelets. That's how researchers believe it prevents constriction of brain arteries. Many of today's feverfew products are standardized to a specific parthenolide content, but whether standardization is necessary isn't clear. For best results it's probably best to use the whole plant—the fresher the better. One laboratory study found that fresh leaf extracts blocked blood-vessel constriction, which is desirable in preventing migraines, whereas dried leaf extracts elicited contractions. Although you can eat the fresh leaves (one to four per day), they taste very bitter and produce mouth sores in some of those who eat them. Better to take feverfew as a tea or as capsules of the freeze-dried leaf. *Typical dosage:* up to three 300- to 400-milligram capsules per day; or up to 2 average-sized leaves per day; or 15 to 30 drops of tincture per day. *Caution:* Do not use during pregnancy.

Feverfew

Bay (*Laurus nobilis*)

This familiar culinary herb, like feverfew, contains parthenolides. James Duke, Ph.D., author of *The Green Pharmacy,* suggests using bay in combination with feverfew to prevent migraine. A typical dose is not well established, so you may want to check with your herbal practitioner.

Cayenne (*Capsicum annuum*)

Laboratory studies have shown that the capsaicin in cayenne blocks a chemical involved in the nerve transmission of pain.

Eating to Stop Headaches

Several studies have shown that many people who experience migraines have food allergies or a more subtle version of an allergy: food intolerance. Reducing or removing the amounts of these foods in the diet often reduces or eliminates the headaches. As a bonus, the patients who give up these foods often get rid of other allergy-linked problems, such as asthma and eczema. So which are the big allergy offenders? Topping the list are cow's milk, wheat, chocolate, eggs, citrus fruits, strawberries, cheese, tomatoes, rye, and the food additives tartrazine and benzoic acid.

Other foods and additives may cause headaches in sensitive people, not because they act as allergies, but because they contain substances that influence the diameter of blood vessels. Culprits may include chocolate, red wine, aged cheeses, caffeinated beverages, processed meats, the food additive monosodium glutamate (MSG), and aspartame (Nutrasweet). The best way to figure out if these foods and additives might be at the root of your own headaches is to take a look at how often you consume them and to try eliminating them one at a time. Standard allergy tests may pick up some, but not all, food allergies.

Cayenne is also rich in salicylates, natural aspirin-like compounds. One study found that repeated topical applications of capsaicin just inside the nose prevented the occurrence of cluster headaches, but the patients involved reported burning in their noses. Consult a qualified medical or herbal practitioner if you want to try this treatment. But you don't need a doctor's supervision to eat cayenne in your chili. At the first sign of any type of headache, you can eat pepper-spiked food (with plenty of water as a chaser) or swallow encapsulated cayenne. Another way to use cayenne is to massage a balm containing it into your temples. Just be sure to wash your hands well with soap afterward. *Typical dosage:* up to three 400- to 500-milligram capsules per day; or 5 to 10 drops of tincture per day. For topical creams, follow the manufacturer's recommendations.

OTHER WAYS TO CHASE AWAY HEADACHES

Acupressure and acupuncture can help relieve both tension and migraine headaches. In acupressure, the same points are stimulated with fingertips instead of with needles. In a study of more than 500 people with recurrent headaches, self-stimulation of acupressure points worked well enough to replace prescription headache drugs.

Two other strategies to try: relaxation training and biofeedback. Your doctor may be able to direct you to classes in both techniques.

Ginger (*Zingiber officinale*)

With its long history of use in relieving and preventing headaches and its good safety record, you'd think more people would know about this use of ginger. Laboratory studies show that it acts as an anti-inflammatory and decreases the tendency of platelets to clump together. Both attributes would help ease headaches, including migraines. Ginger also contains a substance called 6-shogaol, which seems to acts like the capsaicin in cayenne to decrease pain. Plus, it helps ease nausea, including the queasiness that comes with migraines. Its warming effect makes it useful when a migraine causes a person to feel chilled. Ginger combines well with turmeric, which is also anti-inflammatory and pain-relieving. *Typical dosage:* up to eight 500- to 600-milligram capsules per day; or 10 to 20 drops of tincture in water three times per day; or ½ to 1 teaspoon of the ground root per day.

Peppermint (*Mentha × piperita*)

When used internally or externally, peppermint's menthol reduces pain. Like ginger, it also settles the stomach. A triple-whammy approach is to brew a cup of peppermint tea and sip it while sitting in a bath spiked with 10 drops of essential oil of peppermint. Next, keeping the oil away from your eyes, massage your temples, forehead, and neck with about two drops of peppermint oil in a teaspoon of olive or almond oil. *Typical dosage:* 6 to 12 drops of oil in water up to three times per day; or 10 to 20 drops of tincture in water per day; or 1 cup of tea as often as needed (steep 1 to 2 tea-spoons of dried leaves in 1 cup of hot water for 15 minutes). *Caution:* Do not take peppermint if you have heartburn or esophageal reflux. Do not exceed recommended dosage of essential oil.

Willow (*Salix* spp.)
The bark of this family of trees contains salicylates, chemical close relatives to the acetylsalicylic acid in aspirin. *Typical dosage:* up to six 400-milligram capsules per day; or up to 3 cups of tea per day (steep ¼ to ½ teaspoon of powdered bark in 1 cup of hot water for 10 to 15 minutes).

Ginkgo (*Ginkgo biloba*)
This anti-inflammatory and antioxidant herb makes platelets less sticky and improves blood flow. All these properties would seem to reduce the risk of a migraine attack. Although studies have not looked at the effectiveness of ginkgo in preventing migraines, try-ing this nontoxic herb might be worth a shot. *Typical dosage:* 3 capsules of at least 40 milligrams standardized extract per day; or follow manufacturer's or practitioner's recommendations. *Caution:* Do not use with aspirin. In some people, ginkgo may inten-sify headaches.

Passionflower (*Passiflora incarnata*)
A gentle relaxant, passionflower helps unwind agitated minds and tight muscles during a tension headache. Herbalists often use this flower in combination with other traditional headache herbs. *Typical dosage:* 20 to 40 drops of tincture up to 4 times per day, or ⅓ cup of tea three times per day (steep ½ teaspoon of dried herb in 1 cup of hot water for 10 to 15 minutes).

Valerian (*Valeriana officinalis*)
More strongly sedating than passionflower, valerian is an herb to save for when you absolutely want to go to sleep despite a headache. *Typical dosage:* 300 to 400 milligrams of capsules stan-dardized to 0.5 percent essential oil per day; or 20 to 30 drops of tincture per day. *Caution:* Avoid during pregnancy.

HEART DISEASE

FORTY MILLION AMERICANS HAVE IT. Nearly one-third of the deaths in the United States can be blamed on it—and the statistics are just as bad for most of western Europe. But that doesn't mean we completely understand this major killer known as heart disease. So here's a brief tour of the terminology used to describe the things that can go wrong with the human heart.

Atherosclerosis is a condition in which fatty deposits called plaques accumulate in arteries, the blood vessels that carry oxygenated blood to the body's tissues. Think of plaques as biological shingles. As they gather into clusters and adhere to the interior of arteries, they narrow the diameter of the arteries to the point where the blood supply becomes inadequate and tissue damage occurs.

Plaques can stick to the walls of any artery. When they build up in coronary arteries, which carry oxygen to the heart, heart disease is the result. Symptoms of heart disease include angina (or chest pain), poor tolerance for exercise, weakness, dizziness, fatigue, and eventually heart attacks. But by the time these symptoms occur, heart disease is usually well advanced.

Atherosclerosis is a complex process. It appears to begin in childhood and progress with aging. Elevated blood cholesterol is an important contributing factor, but it is not the whole story. Two

DON'T SELF-TREAT HEART DISEASE

Heart disease is a very serious, potentially life-threatening illness. You *must* continue to see your family physician or cardiologist on a regular basis. If you are taking medications for heart disease, you should work with your doctor and possibly with an experienced herbalist to construct an individualized program, because many herbs interact with heart medications. *Never stop taking your prescription medications without consulting your doctor.*

main types of cholesterol exist in the bloodstream: LDL (low-density lipoprotein, or "bad" cholesterol) and HDL (high-density lipoprotein, or "good" cholesterol). The "bad" LDL tends to accumulate in damaged areas of arteries, while the "good" HDL tends to protect against this process.

Platelets also play an important role in heart disease. When platelets aggregate or clump together, they release compounds—including prostaglandins—that significantly contribute to plaque formation.

Though all this may seem complicated, it is important to understand why atherosclerosis happens. Then you can appreciate the ways that herbal and nutritional treatments can help to prevent and treat heart disease.

Based on what is known about heart disease, treatment should focus on:

◆ Decreasing total cholesterol and LDL while increasing HDL cholesterol

◆ Preventing and healing arterial injuries that lead to the accumulation of plaque

◆ Preventing platelet aggregation

◆ Shrinking plaques that are already present

◆ Dilating coronary arteries

◆ Strengthening the heart muscle in general, especially by boosting its efficiency in using energy and oxygen

If you have a strong family history of heart disease or have elevated cholesterol, it's never too early to start preventive strategies. Begin eating a heart-healthful diet, quit smoking, and add exercise to your daily routine—now, not tomorrow.

Drug treatment of heart disease is complex and depends on a variety of factors. They include whether high blood pressure, heart rhythm irregularities, or congestive heart failure are present and whether other disease, such as asthma, is present. Many patients require more than one drug.

Herbs that have an effect on the health of the circulatory system take time—weeks to months—to do their work. Be patient. Most important: Heart disease is not a condition to take lightly. Consult with your doctor about any symptoms of heart disease and be completely honest with him or her about herbs you plan to take. Do not

FIRST THINGS FIRST

Even though conventional medications and herbal remedies can help heal heart disease, the best treatment is
prevention: in other words, exercise and good diet. If you
have heart disease, your commitment to an exercise program and a good diet helps determine your ability to recover from it. Work with your doctor or other practitioner to
safely make these important lifestyle changes.

To prevent future heart disease, here are the steps to
take:

◆ **What should your cholesterol levels be?** Agencies
  and researchers are continually revising their guidelines. Check with your doctor for the most current ones.

◆ **Get up and sweat.** Regular exercise helps lower cholesterol and strengthens the heart. Any kind of aerobic
  exercise will work, but never exercise to the point of
  angina (chest pain) or exhaustion, which can damage
  your heart. If you are currently sedentary, start slowly,
  gradually increasing your pace and distance. Walking is
  an excellent exercise for this purpose.

◆ **Don't smoke and if you do, quit.** Even if you've been
  a lifelong smoker, it's never too late to realize the health
  benefits of quitting.

◆ **Open your heart.** This vital organ isn't merely a machine that pumps blood—the metaphor of the broken
  heart is not an empty one. Many scientific studies have
  implicated stress, loneliness, and isolation in the development of heart disease. If you are isolated, connect
  with others through your church, volunteer activities,
  classes, or other hobbies. If you are stressed, a variety
  of meditation and relaxation techniques can help ease
  the effects of stress on your body.

◆ **Eat better.** Western diets, with high animal fat and low
  vegetable fiber content, are predisposing factors in the
  development of heart disease. Many good books and
  classes are available on heart-healthy diets.

change your regimen of prescription or other pharmaceutical drugs without your doctor's supervision.

Drug Treatment

Nitrates
Nitroglycerin (under-the-tongue tablets or spray), isorbide dinitrate (Dilatrate-SR, Isordil, Sorbitrate), isorbide mononitrate (Imdur,

VITAMINS FOR HEART HEALTH

Diet is crucial to a healthy heart, but supplementation is the best kind of insurance, especially because switching to healthier foods is usually a long process for most people. Here are some supplements you may want to investigate if you have heart disease or are at risk for it.

◆ **L-carnitine.** This amino acid is involved with energy metabolism at the cellular level. It increases the efficiency of the heart muscle, reduces cholesterol metabolism, and prevents plaque formation. *Typical dosage:* 500 to 1,500 milligrams per day.

◆ **Coenzyme Q$_{10}$.** This vitamin-like antioxidant helps cells make energy and improves cholesterol levels. It decreases the frequency of angina and improves exercise tolerance. *Typical dosage:* 100 to 150 milligrams per day.

◆ **Niacin.** This B vitamin lowers cholesterol, but doses tend to be limited by the uncomfortable flushing that it can cause. Sustained-release or long-acting forms of niacin produce less flushing but may damage the liver. An appropriate alternative is a niacin precursor called inositol hexaniacinate, which does not cause flushing even at high doses; even better, it's harmless to the liver. Studies show this form of niacin to be as effective

Ismo, Monoket), nitroglycerin ointment (Nitrobid). *Function:* reduce angina by relaxing smooth muscles in the coronary blood vessels. *Side effects:* headache, slight decrease in blood pressure.

Beta blockers

Propranolol (Inderal), metroprolol (Lopressor), labetalol (Normodyne, Trandate), others. *Function:* decrease the heart's oxygen consumption by reducing blood pressure, heart rate, and the strength of contractions. *Side effects:* heart failure, too-low heart

as other forms, with no side effects reported. *Typical dosage:* 50 to 100 milligrams three times per day.

◆ **Vitamin E.** There are many kinds of vitamin E. The tocotrienol form may be especially helpful in lowering cholesterol. It actually inhibits cholesterol production, a feature that makes this form a good choice for people whose bodies make higher than normal amounts of LDL cholesterol, despite changes in diet. *Typical dosage:* 25 to 100 milligrams per day.

◆ **Vitamin B6.** Deficiency of this key B vitamin appears to be a major cause of heart disease. It can be taken as part of a good quality multivitamin or a B-complex combination. *Typical dosage:* 25 to 50 milligrams of B_6 per day.

◆ **Magnesium.** Many studies link magnesium deficiency with heart disease, sudden cardiac death, heart attacks, and dangerous irregular heart rhythms. This mineral may help decrease plaque formation, lower total cholesterol, raise "good" HDL cholesterol, and inhibit platelet aggregation. *Typical dosage:* 500 to 1,000 milligrams per day. *Caution:* If diarrhea occurs, reduce the dose.

◆ **Bromelain.** Made from proteolytic enzymes found in pineapple, this supplement has anti-inflammatory effects and inhibits platelet accumulation. It has been shown in clinical studies to break down plaques and ease angina. *Typical dosage:* 250 to 500 milligrams three times per day on an empty stomach. *Caution:* Occasionally, bromelain causes upset stomach.

rate, shortness of breath, decrease in HDL cholesterol, cognitive problems, problems with memory and concentration, depression, sexual dysfunction, altered sleep, fatigue.

Calcium Channel Blockers

Nifedipine (Adalat, Procardia), diltiazem (Cardizem, Dilacor, Tiazac), verapamil (Calan, Covera, Isoptin), others. *Function:* inhibit calcium transport into cells, leading to dilation of coronary vessels and reduced demands for oxygen by the heart. *Side effects:* flushing, low blood pressure, dizziness, swelling, headache, heart failure, heart rhythm irregularities.

Aspirin

Function: decrease risk of heart attacks by preventing platelets from sticking together. *Side effects:* heartburn, indigestion, stomach irritation, mild nausea or vomiting.

HERBAL REMEDIES

Garlic (*Allium sativa*) and Onion (*A. cepa*)

Both of these delicious, aromatic herbs contain substances that prevent platelets from sticking together, lower total cholesterol and triglycerides (a type of blood fat), and increase "good" HDL cholesterol. Garlic also promotes the breakdown of certain types of blood clots and lowers blood pressure. If you like these fragrant foods and want to include them in your diet rather than take a supplement, eat at least one clove of garlic or half a small onion a day. *Typical dosage:* capsules that provide at least 10 milligrams of allicin per day (your garlic capsules should specify how much allicin they contain). *Caution:* Some people cannot digest garlic or onions; the result is upset stomach, bloating, and gas. (If you experience a mild form of this side effect, try the culinary trick of adding lots of fresh parsley to a dish made with garlic or onions.)

Ginkgo (*Ginkgo biloba*)

Much scientific research has confirmed the traditional value of ginkgo in the treatment of heart disease. It's antioxidant, enhances heart efficiency, increases blood supply to the extremities, and has a tonic effect on blood vessels, gradually improving their health. It also prevents platelets from sticking together. Ginkgo may be particularly helpful if atherosclerosis has affected brain function or arteries in the arms or legs. It is common for people with coronary artery disease to have plaques in arteries throughout the body. *Typical dosage:* 40 to 80 milligrams of capsules standardized to 24 percent heterosides three times per day. *Caution:* Rare cases of gastrointestinal upset, headache, and dizziness have been reported by people who use ginkgo.

Hawthorn (*Crataegus* spp.)

We now know that hawthorn leaves, flowers, and berries dilate coronary arteries, thus increasing blood supply to the heart. Hawthorn benefits heart health in other ways as well. It improves metabolic processes in the heart, including oxygenation and energy production. It also decreases lactic acid, the waste product of exertion that causes muscle pain. Hawthorn also strengthens artery walls. It's antioxidant, antiinflammatory, and reduces cholesterol. *Typical dosage:* 1 cup of tea three times per day (simmer 1 teaspoon of dried berries or steep 1 teaspoon of leaves and flowers in 1 cup of hot water for 10 to 15 minutes); or ½ to 1 teaspoon of tincture three times per day; or 100 to 250 milligrams in capsules standardized to 20 percent proanthocyanidins three times per day.

Hawthorn

Ginger (*Zingiber officinale*)

This aromatic herb lowers cholesterol and prevents platelets from accumulating by decreasing the absorption of dietary cholesterol, and by stimulating its excretion in bile—one of the primary ways the body removes excess cholesterol. Ginger works best if eaten fresh and taken on an empty stomach. *Typical dosage:* up to a quarter-inch slice of an average-sized root per day; or 250 milligrams per day of freeze-dried fresh root in capsules. *Caution:* Ginger may cause upset stomach in some people, especially at higher doses.

Alfalfa (*Medicago sativa*)

The leaf from this grain decreases cholesterol levels and shrinks plaques that are already present. Often available in powdered form, it is to be taken according to package directions. *Typical dosage:* up to eight or nine 400- to 500-milligram capsules per day; or 15 to 30 drops of tincture four times per day.

Bilberry (*Vaccinium myrtillus*)

With a well-deserved reputation in the treatment of eye diseases, bilberry has significant potential benefits for cardiovascular disease as well. It is rich in anthocyanosides, which help it prevent the damage to the interior of blood vessels that allows narrowing to begin. Bilberry inhibits atherosclerosis, protects the heart during exertion, decreases inflammation, and strengthens artery walls—all of which means that bilberry does for blood vessels what spinach did for Popeye; it simply does so more slowly. *Typical dosage:* 80 to 160 milligrams in capsules standardized to 25 percent anthocyanidin content per day.

Yarrow (*Alchillea millefolium*)

Yarrow dilates arteries and helps to lower cholesterol. It is considered a blood vessel tonic, improving arterial health in general. *Typical dosage:* 1 to 3 cups of tea two or three times per day (steep 1 teaspoon of dried herb in 1 cup of water for 10 to 15 minutes); or ⅛ to ½ teaspoon of tincture two to three times per day. *Caution*: Do not use during pregnancy.

BERRY GOOD FOR THE HEART

Huckleberries and blueberries have chemical compounds similar to those of the more medicinal bilberry. They may have similar benefits for the heart, too, so you have a good excuse to include these delicious berries in your diet.

The pie crust that often accompanies them, however, is *not* part of a heart-healthful diet! Try eating these berries with low-fat ice milk, or by adding them to unsweetened, nonfat yogurt with a dash of maple syrup. Or add them to oatmeal, bran flakes, or a similarly fiber-rich cereal.

Motherwort (*Leonurus cardiaca*)

Another traditional heart tonic, motherwort is known to lower cholesterol, reduce platelet accumulation, and generally strengthen the heart. It also slows a too-rapid heart rate, especially when anxiety is a contributing factor, because it relaxes the nervous system in general. *Typical dosage:* 1 cup of tea two or three times per day (steep ½ to 1 teaspoon of herb in 1 cup of hot water for 10 to 15 minutes); or ¼ to 1 teaspoon of tincture two or three times per day.

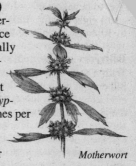

Motherwort

Siberian Ginseng (*Eleutherococcus senticosus*)

This herb works by acting on the adrenal glands, the primary stress-managing glands in the body. It tends to correct disease-producing processes in the body. In people with heart disease, it appears to lower cholesterol and reduce blood pressure. It is especially appropriate when chronic stress is part of the picture. *Typical dosage:* up to nine 400- to 500-milligram capsules per day; or 20 drops of tincture up to three times per day. *Caution:* At high doses, Siberian ginseng may cause insomnia, irritability, or anxiety. If these occur, reduce the dosage.

HEARTBURN

EVER WONDER HOW ANYONE COULD drink water standing on his head? You'd think the liquid would come right back out. But the human body being the engineering marvel that it is, it's able to keep the water moving in the right direction.

Wrapped around the gastrointestinal tract is a remarkable kind of smooth muscle that's designed to push solids and liquids in one direction—from the mouth to the anus. In addition, each section of the digestive tract is separated from the others by a thick ring of muscular tissue called a sphincter. The sphincters serve to keep food from moving backwards.

Although the gastrointestinal tract is really just one long tube, its individual sections have very different functions and very different inner linings. The stomach is lined with a thick layer of mucus designed to withstand exposure to potent acid. The esophagus, on the other hand, has a lining that's relatively thin and very sensitive to acid.

If the sphincter that separates the esophagus from the stomach relaxes too much, it can allow acid to splash back from the stomach into the esophagus. The symptoms resulting from this phenomenon can be quite painful—an intense burning or pressure that begins underneath the lower breastbone and radiates up to the throat or out into the chest. No wonder it is called heartburn.

Heartburn pain typically occurs within an hour or two after eating. (In contrast, the pain of stomach and duodenal ulcers tends to increase on an empty stomach and is often relieved by eating.) In advanced cases, heartburn is associated with a condition called hiatal hernia.

Normally, the muscles of the diaphragm help keep the esophagus tucked inside the chest cavity and the stomach inside the abdomen. These muscles act in concert with the lower esophageal sphincter. When the muscles of the diaphragm become lax and when there is sufficient pressure in the abdomen—such as after a large meal—all or part of the stomach can slide up into the chest. People with hiatal hernia can have reflux of partially digested food along with stomach acid and other fluids. The pain is often intense.

What makes the lower esophageal sphincter open inappropriately? One cause is mechanical: eating too much in one sitting, which can stretch out the sphincter. Thus, eating a large meal and lying down afterward is a definite no-no because it makes food more likely to flow in the wrong direction. This is especially true for obese people who already have constant external pressure on the stomach. Another cause is chemical: Certain foods and chemicals can make the muscles of the sphincter relax. The best examples are cigarette smoke, alcohol, high-fat foods, mints, chocolate, onions, and caffeine.

In addition to making lifestyle changes, using herbs can prove quite effective for heartburn. Along with avoiding troublesome foods and chemicals (listed above), stay away from fennel, lemon balm, peppermint, and spearmint—members of a group of herbs called carminatives, which relax the lower esophageal sphincter.

KEEPING STOMACH ACID WHERE IT BELONGS

In the case of heartburn and its cause, gastro-esophageal reflux, prevention is crucial. Studies show that the leakage of stomach acid into the lungs while a person sleeps is at fault in some cases of asthma. But that's not the worst news. Medical studies have shown that recurrent reflux over a period of months or years can lead to inflammation of the esophageal wall. It appears that people with such inflammation are at very high risk for developing esophageal cancer, which is extremely life-threatening and difficult to treat. It's all the more reason to take heartburn seriously.

Do:

◆ Stick to smaller, more frequent meals.

◆ Cut back on saturated fats—especially deep-fried foods—and alcohol, coffee, tea, white sugar, and unrefined carbohydrates.

◆ Try elevating the head of your bed six to nine inches. This slant may prevent acid reflux during sleep.

Don't:

◆ Eat a large meal just before bedtime.

◆ Lie down for a nap after eating.

◆ Eat spicy foods, onions, and acidic juices such as citrus or tomato.

◆ Take nonsteroidal anti-inflammatory drugs (aspirin, ibuprofen, or naproxen) unless you absolutely must, because these drugs can further irritate the esophageal lining.

DRUG TREATMENT

Antacids

Calcium carbonate tablets (Tums, many others), magnesium and aluminum hydroxide (Maalox, Mylanta, Gaviscon, others). *Func-*

tion: neutralize excess stomach acid for a short period of time. *Side effects:* possible rebound acid, meaning the stomach produces more acid when the treatment is discontinued.

Histamine-2 Receptor Antagonists

Cimetidine (Tagamet), ranitidine (Zantac), nizatidine (Axid), famotidine (Pepcid). *Function:* block the receptor for histamine in the stomach to reduce the secretion of acid. *Side effects with long-term use:* headache, muscle aches, rashes, mental disorientation.

Proton Pump Inhibitors

Lanosoprazole (Prevacid), omeprazole (Prilosec). *Function:* affect cells in the stomach wall to dramatically reduce production of acid. *Side effects:* because these drugs are usually prescribed for a few months' duration, long-term effects are unknown.

Promotility Agents

Cisapride (Propulsid), metoclopramide (Reglan). *Function:* improve tone of the lower esophageal sphincter and enhance downward contraction of smooth muscles in the esophagus and stomach. *Cisapride side effects:* diarrhea. *Metoclopramide side effects:* depression and anxiety.

HERBAL REMEDIES

Licorice Root (*Glycyrrhiza glabra*)

Studies have shown that licorice accelerates the healing of intestinal ulcers. It is anti-inflammatory and very soothing to mucous membranes. To use licorice for heartburn or reflux, choose a special kind called DGL (deglycyrrhizinated) licorice. It is just as effective as regular licorice without affecting the body's sodium-potassium balance. *Typical dosage:* for mild heartburn, drink 1 cup of tea after meals as needed (steep 1 to 2 teaspoons of dried, chopped root in 1 cup of hot water 10 to 15 minutes); for moderate to severe symptoms, use ⅛ to ¼ teaspoon of powdered root or liquid extract dissolved in ¼ cup of water after meals and at bedtime; or one to two tablets of DGL licorice, chewed thoroughly just after eating or as needed, up to 8 tablets per day. *Caution:* Do not use whole licorice for longer than six weeks. Do not use it at all if you have high blood pressure, diabetes, heart, thyroid, kidney, or liver disease, or if you're pregnant or nursing.

Aloe (*Aloe vera*)

Aloe gel contains very large sugar molecules called mucopolysaccharides. These special sugars have been shown to help heal burns, ulcers, and inflamed intestinal walls. Side effects are uncommon, but be sure to obtain a pure source of aloe pulp (not the rind, which can cause stomach cramps and diarrhea). Also, many commercial aloe juices contain citric acid, which can aggravate reflux. The best form of aloe for treating heartburn is a food grade freeze-dried powder. *Typical dosage:* ¼ to ½ teaspoon in ¼ cup of water just after meals or any time symptoms occur. Increase dose to 1 or more teaspoons if necessary.

Cabbage (*Brassica oleracea*)

Cabbage juice is not just a folk remedy—a medical study has shown that regular consumption can heal stomach ulcers. The active ingredient is an amino acid called L-glutamine, which appears to work by nourishing cells lining the esophagus and stomach so they repair themselves. Another advantage to cabbage, like its first cousin broccoli, is that it contains cancer-preventing agents called glucosmolates. *Typical dosage:* 4 to 8 ounces of fresh or bottled juice after meals. (If taking the juice gives you gas, instead take ½ to 1 teaspoon of L-glutamine, mixed in ¼ cup of water, just after eating.)

Calendula (*Calendula officinalis*)

A time-honored remedy for wounds, mouth sores, ulcers, and gastritis, calendula is so gentle it is often given to children for upset stomach. Its astringent and anti-inflammatory properties make it particularly useful for treating heartburn and reflux. *Typical dosage:* 1 to 2 cups of tea as needed (steep 1 to 2 teaspoons of dried flowers in 1 to 2 cups of hot water for 10 to 15 minutes); or 15 to 30 drops of tincture four times per day after meals.

Hemorrhoids

H EMORRHOIDS. They even sound awful. But more than half of Americans over the age of 50 have them and younger people can get them as well. These swollen and inflamed vein tissues in the rectal area are extremely common.

Typical symptoms of hemorrhoids are rectal pain, burning or itching, and bright red blood seen on toilet tissue, in the toilet bowl, or on the surface of the stool after defecation. Round swellings or protrusions in the anal area may also be present. But because all these symptoms can be caused by other, more serious conditions, it's important to get a doctor's diagnosis to know whether what you have is, in fact, hemorrhoids.

Why do hemorrhoids happen—and can anything be done to prevent them? Hemorrhoids are caused by genetic weakness of the veins in the rectal area, sitting or standing for long periods of time, and anything that causes increased pressure in the veins (pregnancy, heavy lifting, frequent straining during elimination). In Western countries, low-fiber diets with their resulting constipation are considered a major cause. The main reasons to seek medical attention

PUTTING MEDICINE WHERE IT HURTS

Herbs applied directly to hemorrhoids can ease symptoms, stop bleeding, and speed healing. Look for creams, salves, or suppositories that contain combinations of soothing, anti-inflammatory, and astringent herbs such as calendula, comfrey, chamomile, lavender, St.-John's-wort, and plantain. Distilled witch hazel is also an excellent astringent that shrinks swollen hemorrhoids and controls bleeding (do not take internally, though). And cypress essential oil may help shrink swollen veins and reduce bleeding.

RX FOR HEMORRHOIDS

This blend combines soothing herbs that foster wound healing with cooling, astringent witch hazel.

- 4 tablespoons distilled witch hazel
- ½ tablespoon comfrey tincture
- ½ tablespoon horse chestnut tincture
- 50 drops lavender essential oil
- 50 drops cypress essential oil (optional)

Combine all the ingredients in an airtight amber glass bottle with a tight lid and label. Store away from heat and light. To use, shake well and apply gently with a cotton ball twice a day and after each bowel movement. If internal hemorrhoids are present, insert the soaked cotton ball briefly into the rectal opening to allow the herbs to soak this area; be sure to keep a grip on the cotton ball so you don't lose it.

are intolerable pain, severe bleeding (which may be enough to cause anemia), or swelling severe enough to prevent normal defecation.

Although prescription cortisone and anesthetic products may reduce the pain and swelling of hemorrhoids, they can't address the causes. Herbs and other botanical medicines can help strengthen and tone blood vessels, decrease inflammation, and stop bleeding. They can also help the constipation that often accompanies hemorrhoids.

DRUG TREATMENT

Topical Anti-Inflammatories
Cortisone, anesthetics such as benzocaine or pramoxine (Analpram, Anusol, Cortifoam, Epifoam, Proctifoam). *Function:* reduce pain and swelling. *Side effects:* topical allergic reactions, thinning of the skin and mucous membranes.

Other Topical Drugs
Ointments and creams (Anusol, Tonolane, Preparation H). *Function:* reduce pain and swelling. *Side effects:* allergic reactions, rashes.

TAKING THE WATERS

A bath in warm water often provides temporary relief from hemorrhoids by soothing inflamed tissues and stimulating circulation. To make that bath more effective, add soothing herbs in the form of essential oils or tea to the water. Good candidates are calendula, comfrey, chamomile, lavender, and St.-John's-wort. Be careful, however; if you're adding essential oils, dilute them first. Add no more than 5 drops of essential oil to one fluid ounce of a neutral vegetable-based oil such as olive or almond.

HERBAL REMEDIES

Ginkgo (*Ginkgo biloba*)
Extracts of ginkgo leaf help strengthen the blood vessels. Ginkgo is also anti-inflammatory, just what you're looking for in conditions that include pain and itching among their symptoms. *Typical dosage:* 40 to 60 milligrams of capsules standardized to 24 percent flavone glycosides and 6 percent ginkgolides two or three times per day; or ¼ to 1 teaspoon of tincture two to three times per day.

Horse Chestnut (*Aesculus hippocastanum*)
A traditional treatment for strengthening and toning the veins, horse chestnut is anti-inflammatory and therefore decreases swelling. It is also astringent and tends to reduce bleeding. This herb can be used both internally and topically. *Typical dosage:* 1 cup of tea three times per day (simmer 1 teaspoon of dried seeds in 1 cup of water for 10 to 15 minutes); or ⅛ to 1 teaspoon of tincture three times per day. To use horse chestnut externally, allow the tea to cool. Soak a clean washcloth in the tea and wring out. Apply to swollen tissues as often as needed.

Horse chestnut

THE RID-OF-'ROIDS DIET

Foods rich in fiber and in proanthocyanidin and anthocyanidin, two compounds that improve the health of blood vessels, can help prevent future hemorrhoids and help current ones heal. Blackberries, blueberries, and cherries are among the foods that contain these ingredients. If constipation is a factor, you may want to consider a fiber supplement, such as psyllium seed husks (1 tablespoon per day) mixed with water or juice. If your diet is less than healthy, add a good multivitamin to ensure that you're getting all of the important blood-vessel-healing nutrients. Dairy products, meat, and fatty foods tend to be constipating, so it's a good idea to cut back on these products.

Butcher's Broom (*Ruscus aculeatus*)

This herb decreases inflammation and strengthens blood vessels. *Typical dosage:* 1 cup of tea three times per day (steep 1 to 2 teaspoons of dried leaf in 1 cup of hot water for 10 minutes); or ½ to 1 teaspoon of tincture three times per day on an empty stomach.

Witch Hazel (*Hamamelis virginiana*)

This strongly astringent herb stops bleeding and helps shrink swollen tissues. Apply commercial witch hazel preparations or distilled extract products three times per day and after each bowel movement. *Caution:* Never use these products internally.

Dandelion (*Taraxacum officinale*) and Yellow Dock (*Rumex crispus*)

These two herbs share some key characteristics. They're both considered weeds; you can eat the young greens of either; and the roots of both plants are mild, gentle laxatives. It's the roots you want for treating the constipation that sometimes comes with hemorrhoids. *Typical dosage:* 1 to 3 cups of tea per day (steep 2 teaspoons of dried, chopped root in 1 cup of water 15 minutes); or ½ to 3 teaspoons of tincture per day.

HERPES

HERPES HAS NO CURE, AND THERE'S no vaccination or immunity against it. Although symptoms disappear, the virus remains contagious and lies dormant in nerve cells, reactivating in response to stress, sunlight, or other causes. It's a secret you can usually hide: Up to 70 percent of those infected show no symptoms. On the other hand, if you're among the non-monogamous sexually active, there's no telling which potential partner might have given you herpes. Plus you certainly don't want to give it to anyone else.

Genital herpes is caused by a virus that's a member of the herpes family, herpes simplex type 2. The first sign of infection is usually tingling or itching of the genital area or anus, followed by painful sores, swollen lymph nodes, sore muscles, and headaches. The first outbreak, usually the most painful, can last up to two weeks. Later outbreaks usually last four or five days; blisters heal in one to three weeks.

Factors that can trigger herpes outbreaks in addition to stress and sun exposure include weakened immunity, diet, surgery, skin

TOPICAL HERPES TREATMENT

If the alcohol of this tincture stings too much, substitute glycerites or infused oils of the same herbs.

- ½ teaspoon St.-John's-wort tincture
- ½ teaspoon licorice root tincture
- 5 drops tea tree essential oil
- 3 drops myrrh essential oil

Combine all ingredients. Shake well, then apply directly to herpes lesions up to three times per day.

rashes, menstruation, hormonal fluctuations, and prolonged sexual activity. Genital herpes is diagnosed by smears or cell cultures.

Up to 70 percent of those infected with herpes show no symptoms. Unfortunately, while antiviral drugs may reduce the chances of infecting others, they can't eliminate that chance. And those who have genital herpes may be infectious to others at times when they're not aware of an outbreak.

Drug Treatment

Oral Antiviral Drugs
Acyclovir (Avirax, Zovirax), valacyclovir (Valtrex). *Function:* inhibit (but not eliminate) the herpes simplex virus to shorten the duration of outbreaks and reduce the risk of infecting others. *Side effects:* loss of appetite, nausea and vomiting, constipation or diarrhea, excessive sweating, dizziness, headache, confusion.

FOOD AND SUPPLEMENTS TO MANAGE HERPES

To minimize herpes outbreaks, limit foods containing the amino acid arginine. That means avoiding chocolate, walnuts, hazelnuts, Brazil nuts, peanuts, and peanut butter.

Another amino acid, lysine, may help prevent outbreaks. Get your lysine by eating plenty of turkey, chicken, fish, cottage cheese, ricotta cheese, and wheat germ. You can also take lysine in capsule form. *Typical dosage:* 3,000 milligrams of lysine per day for 3 months, then 1,000 milligrams per day to prevent outbreaks.

Meanwhile, take zinc at the first sign of an outbreak to limit its length and severity. *Typical dosage:* 30 to 60 milligrams during the outbreak and for several days after. You can also apply cream or ointment containing zinc sulfate to the sores.

Analgesics

Acetaminophen, aspirin, ibuprofen. *Function:* relieve pain. *Acetaminophen side effects:* chronic use or higher dosages may damage the liver or kidneys. *Aspirin side effects:* heartburn, mild nausea, vomiting. *Ibuprofen side effects:* dizziness, stomachache, nausea, headache, diarrhea.

Topical Anesthetics

Lidocaine (Viscous Xylocaine), benzocaine (Topicaine). *Function:* numb the lesion. *Side effects:* possible allergic reactions.

Herbal Remedies

Lemon Balm (*Melissa officinalis*)

This antiviral herb has recently shown its potential for accelerating the healing of herpes sores, especially when treatment is started early in the outbreak. Because it's also a mild sedative, lemon balm may help you sleep if the pain of an outbreak is keeping you awake. *Typical dosage:* 25 to 40 drops of tincture two times per day; or 3

HERPES-IMMUNE SYSTEM TINCTURE

Blending your own tinctures is easy to do; you simply purchase commercial tinctures and blend them in a dark glass bottle. You can blend larger amounts of the tinctures in this recipe; just keep the proportions the same.

½ teaspoon echinacea tincture
½ teaspoon St.-John's-wort tincture
½ teaspoon bupleurum tincture
½ teaspoon licorice tincture
½ teaspoon barberry tincture

Combine the tinctures. Take one dropperful of the mix four to six times per day as soon as you feel symptoms of an outbreak coming on and for as long as they continue.

THREE QUICK, EASY REMEDIES

Got tea bags on hand? How about aloe or vitamin E? Here are three quick, easy ways to quell the sting of a herpes lesion.

◆ **Apply a damp bag of black tea.** Steep it in hot water a few moments to allow the tiny pieces of leaves to unfurl; let it cool and place on the lesion.

◆ **Pop open a vitamin E capsule.** Apply the oil to lesions to ease the itch and promote healing.

◆ **Use pure aloe vera gel.** It's as good for any minor skin wound as it is for kitchen burns. Slice open a leaf, scoop out the fresh gel, and apply, or purchase a bottled pure aloe vera product.

cups of tea per day (steep 1¼ to 4 teaspoons of dried leaf in 1 cup of hot water for 10 to 15 minutes). In addition, you can apply a commercial lemon balm cream or ointment to the sores three or four times per day. Other effective herbs to look for in topical lemon balm products: aloe vera, calendula, chamomile, and plantain.

Echinacea (*Echinacea angustifolia, E. purpurea, E. pallida*)

This herb is useful in any condition involving the immune system. Begin taking echinacea as soon as you feel an outbreak beginning; continue for up to two weeks. *Typical dosage:* up to nine 300- to 400-milligram capsules per day; or 60 drops of tincture three times per day.

St.-John's-Wort (*Hypericum perforatum*)

A well-known virus fighter and wound healer, St.-John's-wort can be used in several ways to fight herpes. *Typical dosage:* 300 milligrams in capsules three times per day; or 15 to 40 drops of tincture three times per day; or 3 cups of tea per day (steep 1 teaspoon of dried herb in 1 cup of hot water for 10 minutes). To use externally, apply a compress made with the tea to the cold sores three times per day. You can also apply an infused oil or tincture of the flowering tops to active lesions. *Caution:* May cause increased reactions to sun exposure. Do not take St.-John's-wort internally if you are on an antidepressant drug.

Licorice (*Glycyrrhiza glabra*)

In studies, licorice inactivates the herpes simplex virus. It also has a potent anti-inflammatory effect. When an outbreak first occurs, you can take commercial products that contain licorice extract or apply a licorice compress or poultice several times per day. *Typical dosage:* 1 cup of tea per day (steep 1 to 2 teaspoons of dried, chopped root in 1 cup of hot water for 15 minutes); or up to six 400- or 500-milligram capsules per day; or 20 to 30 drops of tincture up to three times per day. *Caution:* Do not use licorice internally for longer than six weeks. Do not take it at all if you have heart disease, high blood pressure, liver disease, take diuretics or digitalis, or if you're pregnant.

HIGH BLOOD PRESSURE

Y OUR HEART IS AN ENGINEERING marvel: an elegant pump that receives oxygen-rich blood from the lungs and uses just the right amount of force to push it back through the arteries and out to the body's tissues.

When all goes well, there is just enough pressure inside the arteries to maintain a steady flow of blood. But such pressure can be affected by exercise, stress, diet, and hormones, as well as by blood loss from menstruation or severe injury. To keep the system working correctly in the face of constantly changing conditions, the heart makes continual adjustments. Its rate of beating speeds up or slows down, and the strength of its contractions increases and decreases. At the same time, arteries relax and dilate or contract and constrict, and the kidneys either retain salt and water (thus raising blood pressure) or release salt and water (allowing blood pressure to drop).

DOING THE BLOOD-PRESSURE NUMBERS

Blood pressure is measured in terms of how much the arteries contract (systolic pressure) and dilate (diastolic pressure). Although a reading of 140 (the upper, systolic number) over 90 (the lower, diastolic number) has been designated as the upper limit of normal for the American population, comparative studies of other populations suggest these figures may be too high. For example, the Tarahumara Indians of Mexico, who lead a very active lifestyle, often walking or running several miles daily up and down steep canyon walls, have an average blood pressure of 90 over 60 and a much lower rate of heart attacks and strokes than Americans do.

Instead of waiting until your blood pressure reaches someone else's arbitrary limit and then trying to lower it after the fact, a better strategy is to keep an eye on this barometer of health on a regular basis. Experts suggest beginning intervention on a number of fronts—diet, exercise, and natural remedies—when readings regularly exceed 120 over 80. Blood pressure should be checked once a year if normal, and four times a year if it is ever found to be elevated.

Given the intricacy of the system, it's no surprise that chronically elevated blood pressure, or hypertension, is one of the most common of all diseases, affecting more than 50 million Americans. It's even more common among African Americans than among people of other ethnic backgrounds, for reasons that remain unclear.

The trouble with high blood pressure is that it's symptomless. It can hang around for 10 to 20 years, damaging vital organs such as the brain, kidneys, and eyes, without giving you any clues that you have it.

Massive public health measures have been initiated to identify and treat people affected by high blood pressure. But figuring out whether you're one of them is not always easy. In some people, blood pressure readings can vary by 20 to 60 points in the course of a day. And many people notice that their blood pressure tends to increase in a doctor's office, a phenomenon called white-coat hypertension.

DRUG TREATMENT

Beta Blockers

Propranolol (Inderal), betaxolol (Kerlone), carvedilol (Coreg), atenolol (Tenormin), metoprolol (Lopressor, Toprol XL), labetolol (Trandate, Normodyne). *Function:* block chemical processes that lead to increased heart pressure and heart rate; often given after a heart attack. *Side effects:* tiredness, excessively slow heart rate, impaired sexual functioning; dramatic increases in blood pressure upon sudden discontinuation of treatment.

Alpha Blockers

Clonidine (Catapress), guanabenz (Wytensin), guanfacine (Tenex), prazosin (Minipress), doxazosin (Cardura), terazosin (Hytrin). *Function:* chemically block responses to stress that raise blood pressure and heart rate. *Side effects:* dry mouth, dizziness, fatigue, nausea, impaired sexual functioning; as with beta blockers, sudden discontinuation of treatment can result in dramatic increases in blood pressure.

Diuretics

Hydrochlorthiazide (HCTZ, HydroDiuril), hydrochlorthiazide with triamterene (Dyazide, Maxzide), hydrochlorthiazide with amiloride (Moduretic), indapamide (Lozol), metolazone (Zaroxolyn),

A SALTY DEBATE

It used to be a sure thing that you'd be told to pass up the salt if you had high blood pressure. More current research, however, has shown that reducing sodium helps lower blood pressure for less than half of those who try it.

On the other hand, most people do eat too much salt—a daily average of 2 to 3 teaspoons—and would benefit by cutting back to 1 teaspoon. A simple way to do this is to stop adding extra salt to food.

FIRST THINGS FIRST

Drugs to lower blood pressure are among the most frequent reasons a doctor gets out a prescription pad. Although these drugs are usually effective, their value is diminished by side effects such as fatigue and depression. They can also impair your ability to exercise or enjoy sex. And they're expensive. So if you've been newly diagnosed with high blood pressure, it's a natural to ask your doctor if you can avoid having to take such drugs by making some changes in your lifestyle.

Fortunately, because so many Americans suffer from high blood pressure, a great deal of research has been done on ways to fight the disorder. Stress management techniques that have been proven to help include meditation, biofeedback, and regular aerobic exercise. Losing weight and decreasing alcohol consumption may also have a big impact. Some people, especially those with Type II diabetes, find that restricting carbohydrates can dramatically lower their blood pressure.

furosemide (Lasix), and bumetanide (Bumex). *Function:* stimulate the kidneys to excrete more salt and water, lowering blood volume and blood pressure. *Side effects:* dangerously low levels of potassium and magnesium, elevations in uric acid (which can cause gout attacks), increases in blood cholesterol.

Calcium Channel Blockers
Amlodipine (Norvasc), diltiazem (Cardizem), verapamil (Calan, Isoptin, Verelan), nifedipine (Adalat, Procardia). *Function:* relax blood vessel walls to make them dilate, thus lowering blood pressure. *Side effects:* constipation, dizziness, nausea, fluid retention.

ACE (Angiotensin-converting enzyme) Inhibitors
Enalapril (Vasotec), captopril (Capoten), benazepril (Lotensin), lisinopril (Prinivil). *Function:* block an enzyme in the bloodstream that produces angiotensin II, a chemical that raises blood pressure by constricting blood vessels. *Side effects:* chronic cough, acute swelling in the face, lips, and throat.

Eight Ways to Fight High Blood Pressure

Here are eight more tips for lowering high blood pressure and reducing or preventing a dependence on blood pressure drugs.

◆ Eat fewer calories. Lowering your body weight if it's too high is one key way to lower your blood pressure.

◆ Avoid refined carbohydrates such as white flour and sugar, white potatoes (especially French fries), and sugar-sweetened soft drinks. All of these supply "empty" calories, meaning they're unusually bereft of nutrients and they lead to weight gain. They also fill you up so that you have no room left for healthful foods.

◆ Don't drink more than one 8-ounce glass of beer, or 4 ounces of wine, or 1 ounce of hard liquor per day. Higher amounts of alcohol are known blood pressure boosters.

◆ Eat high-fiber foods such as flaxseed meal and other whole grains and vegetables. In addition to boosting dietary fiber, these foods contain nutrients that lower blood pressure. And fiber makes you feel full, which helps you lose weight if you need to.

◆ Eat deep-sea fish that are rich in essential fatty acids, such as salmon, cod, mackerel, and tuna. The omega-3 fatty acids in fish tend to relax artery walls, reducing blood pressure. They also make blood thinner and less likely to clot.

◆ Emphasize foods high in magnesium, potassium, and calcium. On the list: nuts and seeds, green leafy vegetables, legumes, whole grains, tofu, bananas, oranges, apples, avocados, and melons.

◆ Stop smoking. Cigarette smoking raises your blood pressure by constricting arteries. It also damages heart muscle and other tissues by decreasing the amount of oxygen they get.

◆ Engage in regular aerobic exercise for 30 or 40 minutes three or four times a week. Such exercise has been shown to lower blood pressure and prevent heart attacks.

Angiotensin II Blockers

Candesartan (Atacand), irbesartan (Avapro), losartan (Cozaar), valsartan (Diovan). *Function:* block the effect of angiotensin rather than its production. *Side effects:* rare.

HERBAL REMEDIES

Hawthorn (*Crataegus* spp.)

The leaves, flowers, and berries of this tree have a well-deserved reputation as general tonics for the cardiovascular system. Hawthorn is perhaps the best-known botanical medicine used in the treatment of mild high blood pressure. A hawthorn extract is commonly used by herbalists for improving heart function and treating congestive heart failure, irregular heartbeats, and angina. It is a rich source of oligomeric proanthocyanidins (OPCs) and antioxidant bioflavonoids, both of which nourish the tissues of the heart and the blood vessels.

Hawthorn lowers blood pressure by relaxing and dilating artery walls. How the herb does this is only partly understood. It appears to possess similarities to ACE inhibitors, beta blockers, and calcium channel blockers. Since hawthorn can take weeks or even months to work, it should not be used by itself for significantly high blood pressure (above 160 over 100). But it is the ideal herb to use in the early stages of high blood pressure. *Typical dosage:* 150 to 1,500 milligrams of powdered standardized extract (one that contains 10 to 18 percent OPCs or 1.8 percent vitexin-4'-rhamnoside).

MINERAL "MAGIC"

One of the deadliest consequences of high blood pressure is stroke. But it is also the one with a proven dietary therapy. The DASH (Dietary Approaches to Stop Hypertension) study, performed at four medical centers and sponsored by the National Institutes of Health, showed that people who ate foods rich in potassium, magnesium, and fiber had a lower incidence of stroke.

Reishi (*Ganoderma lucidum*)

This mushroom is prized in Japan and China, where its rejuvenating qualities have been known for over 4,000 years. Scientific studies have confirmed its medicinal properties. Published studies in humans show that it lowers blood pressure and reduces "bad" LDL cholesterol and triglycerides, another type of blood fat. It also reduces the tendency of blood platelets to accumulate, thus making blood less likely to clot and provoke heart attacks and strokes. Since the raw mushroom is woody and inedible, the traditional method of preparing reishi is to make a tea by simmering it for a long time in water. Fortunately, it is also available in a powdered form. *Typical dosage:* 1,000 to 9,000 milligrams in capsules per day; or 50 to 75 milligrams in concentrated capsules three times per day.

Garlic (*Allium sativum*)

This common seasoning has been used as a medicine in many cultures for more than 3,000 years. It is known to lower blood pressure and cholesterol, treat infections, and prevent cancer. The surefire way to lower blood pressure with garlic is to eat one to three raw or lightly cooked cloves every day. If you can't handle the garlic breath that results, or you suffer from heartburn or an easily irritated stomach, garlic is available in other forms. *Typical dosage:* 1 to 3 standardized tablets (guaranteed to provide at least 4,000 micrograms of allicin each) per day.

Coleus (*Coleus forskohlii*)

An extract of this herb, forskolin, is used extensively in India to treat numerous conditions, including high blood pressure and asthma, though it is little known in the United States. Forskolin has been shown to increase the concentration of a chemical called cAMP, found in smooth muscles. Increased levels of cAMP relax those smooth muscles, thus dilating the walls of arteries. Forskolin also appears to help heart muscle work more efficiently. Since the root contains only small amounts of the active ingredient, it is important to use a concentrated extract. *Typical dosage:* 50 milligrams three or four times per day.

Dandelion (*Taraxacum officinale*)

The leaves of your favorite lawn weed are a popular home remedy for fluid retention. By gently increasing urine flow, dandelion leaf helps to lower blood pressure as well. In very high doses, the herb can have a diuretic effect. The advantages of using dandelion are twofold: It does not appear to cause potassium loss—a significant problem with some prescription diuretics—and at the right time of year, almost anyone can find fresh dandelion greens to throw into a salad or make into a juice or tea. (Avoid leaves that have been treated with chemicals.) *Typical dosage:* 2 to 6 cups of tea per day (simmer 1 to 2 teaspoons of dried leaves in one cup of water for 5 minutes); or 1 to 2 dropperfuls of tincture up to three times per day; or one 500-milligram capsule three or four times per day.

HIGH CHOLESTEROL

ELEVATED BLOOD CHOLESTEROL IS ONE of the most common medical conditions among Americans. This blood chemical plays a major role in heart attacks, strokes, and other life-threatening health problems. So keeping watch over your own levels of cholesterol and a similar group of chemicals called triglycerides is an important step in staying healthy.

Since you can't "feel" your own levels of blood fats—and because they can change slowly over time—you may have no idea that they're high. It's becoming increasingly common for older people to know their own cholesterol and triglyceride levels, but for other high-risk folks, it can be important to be tested regularly, starting as young as age 19.

What is cholesterol, anyway? It's no more than a special type of fat, one required by every cell in the body to function properly. Approximately 25 percent of your cholesterol supply comes from your diet; the other 75 percent is manufactured in your liver. When your body is working as it should, it burns dietary fat for energy and uses cholesterol to manufacture hormones (such as estrogen and cortisone) and nutrients (such as vitamin D). But when your body makes excessive cholesterol or triglycerides, or its systems for disposing of the excess are inefficient, these blood fats build up along with calcium deposits, clogging and hardening blood vessels.

You've probably heard low-density lipoprotein (LDL) referred to as "bad" cholesterol, and high-density lipoprotein (HDL) referred to as "good" cholesterol. That's an oversimplification, but it's essentially true. LDLs carry the type of cholesterol that can build up in the arteries; the cholesterol that HDL carries actually reduces heart-disease risk by removing fats from the bloodstream.

What researchers have discovered about cholesterol is that it's not the numbers, but the ratios of total cholesterol to HDL and of triglycerides to HDL that matter most. In both cases, the lower the better.

Nearly 30 million prescriptions per year are written for drugs that lower blood cholesterol and triglycerides. But while these drugs may reduce your risk of high blood fats giving you a heart attack or stroke, studies haven't proven that they'll increase your life span. Your best bet for lowering cholesterol is an approach that combines dietary and

THE VITAMIN THAT'S A DRUG

Since the 1950s, doctors have prescribed niacin, or vitamin B_3, for lowering cholesterol. But the dosages recommended—500 to 3,000 milligrams per day—make this use of the vitamin more like a drug. Niacin lowers not only total cholesterol but also LDL, triglycerides, and fibrinogen, a blood protein responsible for clot formation. It also raises HDL levels. Pure, crystalline niacin can cause a harmless but unpleasant flushing reaction. Taking an aspirin tablet before taking niacin, or using timed-release niacin, can prevent flushing. There have been reports of liver damage, however, with some forms of timed-released niacin. It should probably be avoided for this reason.

A new, better choice is inositol hexaniacinate, which is niacin bound to inositol, a B-complex-like vitamin. This substance has been used for years in Europe and appears to avoid niacin's side effects on the liver. All forms of niacin have side effects for some people, so consult your doctor to calculate a dosage.

DOING THE NUMBERS

What should your cholesterol levels be? Agencies and researchers are continually revising their recommendations. Here are the current guidelines.

◆ Total cholesterol: below 200 milligrams per deciliter

◆ LDL: below 130 milligrams per deciliter

◆ HDL: above 35 milligrams per deciliter

◆ Total cholesterol to HDL ratio: less than 5

◆ Triglycerides: below 100 milligrams per deciliter

◆ Ratio of triglycerides to HDL: controversial, but some experts recommend a ratio of less than 3

lifestyle changes with other natural remedies—plus cholesterol-lowering drugs if your doctor thinks it's critical to lower your cholesterol quickly.

DRUG TREATMENT

Bile Acid Sequestrants
Cholestyramine (Questran), colestipol (Colestid). *Function:* help the bowel excrete the body's excess cholesterol. *Side effects:* gas, bloating, constipation, impaired absorption of fat-soluble vitamins; may increase triglyceride levels.

Fibric Acid Derivatives
Gemfibrozil (Lopid), clofibrate (Atromid-S), fenofibrate (Tricor). *Function:* lower triglycerides by blocking their production in the liver and activating an enzyme in muscles that breaks them down into simple fats. *Side effects:* potential liver damage, gallstones, abdominal pain, nausea; possible increased risk for breakdown of muscle tissue and cancer.

HMG CoA Reductase Inhibitors
Referred to as statins (Mevacor, Pravachol). *Function:* compete with the key liver enzyme involved in the manufacture of choles-

terol. *Side effects:* liver damage, muscle aches, nausea, headaches, coënzyme Q_{10} deficiency, insomnia, fatigue, rashes.

Herbal Treatment

Guggul (from the myrrh tree, *Commiphora mukul*)
This sticky resin is used extensively in the ancient Indian system of medicine known as Ayurveda. An extract of this resin, called gugulipid, has been shown to lower LDL cholesterol and triglycerides while raising HDL cholesterol. It also appears to protect the heart from damage by unstable molecules called free radicals. Gugulipid is sold as an extract standardized to contain 5 to 10 percent of guggulsterone, the active ingredient. *Typical dosage:* 25 milligrams of guggulsterone three times per day with meals. You may have to take it for one to three months

FIRST THINGS FIRST

You've surely heard it before, but it remains as true as ever: The single most important natural way to lower a high cholesterol level is to change your diet. Reducing your intake of saturated animal fats can help. Cut back on high-fat red meats and avoid fried foods and lard. Replace saturated oils and fats with monosaturated ones, such as olive and avocado oil, and with polyunsaturated fats such as those found in raw nuts, seeds, flaxseed oil, and fish oils. This approach can lower LDL levels without significantly lowering HDL levels.

Increase your fiber intake by adding crispy vegetables and fibrous whole grains, especially oat and rice bran. Aim for a total fiber intake of 50 grams or more per day.

Try eating more soy, too. Soy protein and other soy foods have also been shown to reduce cholesterol when included regularly in the diet.

In addition, an exercise program consisting of both aerobic and weight resistance, performed at least three times per week, has been shown in medical studies to increase HDL levels while decreasing LDL levels.

THE DYNAMIC DUO

Combining garlic with fish oil (such as salmon or cod-liver extract) has been shown to increase the effectiveness of both products in lowering LDL cholesterol and triglycerides. A typical dosage of fish oil might be 1,000 to 3,000 milligrams per day.

for it to have an effect on cholesterol, but guggulsterone appears to have no significant side effects and it can be taken long-term.

Artichoke (*Cynara scolymus*)

The artichoke plant's leaves and roots contain a chemical called cynarin. This substance blocks the absorption of cholesterol in the intestines and inhibits its production in the liver. Cynarin also affects triglycerides; in one medical study, patients saw their triglycerides drop after six weeks of use. Similar to its cousin milk thistle, artichoke appears to assist the liver in breaking down toxic chemicals. Although eating artichoke leaves on a regular basis can definitely help lower cholesterol, to get a more consistent effect, use a powdered extract. *Typical dosage:* 500 to 3,000 milligrams per day, divided into three doses, taken before meals. *Caution:* Do not use if you have gallstones or gallbladder problems.

Garlic (*Allium sativum*)

This pungent bulb has been used medicinally in many cultures for more than 3,000 years. Its active ingredient is a compound called allicin; sometimes you'll see products standardized to a particular percentage of this chemical. Garlic inhibits at least two of the enzymes involved in the production of cholesterol by the liver, thus lowering cholesterol synthesis. *Typical dosage:* 1 to 3 raw or briefly cooked cloves per day; or in tablets or capsules, enough to total at least 4,000 micrograms of allicin potential daily.

Psyllium Seed (*Plantago ovata*)

The seed of the psyllium plant is rich in mucilage, the soluble fibers similar to those found in oat bran, flaxseed meal, and guar

gum. Although it is traditionally used to treat constipation, research shows that psyllium seed reduces
high cholesterol and triglyceride levels. Exactly
how it does this isn't known, but it appears to bind
with dietary cholesterol and fat to prevent their absorption. It also binds bile acids and prevents their reabsorption in the intestines, thus taking cholesterol
out of circulation. Psyllium needs to be consumed
quickly, because once you combine it with water, it
quickly thickens to the point of undrinkability. *Typical
dosage:* 2 to 4 teaspoons of powdered seed or 1 tablespoon of the ground seed husks dissolved in 1 cup of
water, once or twice per day. *Caution:* May cause gas,
bloating, or diarrhea; to avoid these side effects, start with half the
above dose and build up slowly.

Psyllium

Hives

HIVES ARE RAISED PATCHES OF SKIN somewhat circular in shape.
You might see only one, or a whole crop that breaks out and
lasts one to three days. They can be white, pink, or red, as small as
a dime or as large as a Frisbee. And they itch. Oh, how they itch!
They may also burn or sting.

Hives are basically an allergic skin reaction, during which certain cells release histamine and other inflammatory chemicals.
These chemicals make the small blood vessels in the area leak,
thereby producing localized swelling called a wheal. As the small
arteries dilate, the skin reddens. If your allergic reaction involves
other body systems, you might also appear flushed, wheeze, and
have swollen lips and eyelids.

Things that produce hives include certain medications, foods, insect bites, and exposure to cold. Less often, inhaling animal dander,
molds, and pollens can lead to hives as well as respiratory symptoms. Rarer still, parasitic infestations, other infectious illnesses,
and cancer can produce hives.

WHEN HIVES ARE AN EMERGENCY

Call for emergency medical transport if you experience wheezing or difficulty breathing along with swelling of your lips, tongue, and throat. If you suspect a new medication has produced the hives, call your doctor. No matter what the trigger, bear in mind that the next time you are exposed to that substance, you may have a much more severe reaction. To prevent this, you must identify and eliminate the cause of the reaction.

DRUG TREATMENT

Nonsedating Antihistamines

Cetirizine (Zyrtec), loratadine (Claritin), astemizole (Hismanal). *Function:* relieve itching without producing drowsiness. *Side effects:* dry mouth, nose, and throat. *Astemizole side effects:* may cause disturbances in heart rhythm.

Sedating Antihistamines

Diphenhydramine (Benadryl), chlorpheniramine (Chlor-Trimeton), brompheniramine (Dimetapp), clemastine (Tavist-1). *Function:* relieve itch and assist sleep. *Side effects:* drowsiness, dryness of mouth, nose, and throat.

Other Drugs

Hydroxyzine (Anxanil, Apo-Hydroxyzine, Atarax, Multipax, Novo-Hydroxyzin, Vistaril). *Function:* relieve allergic itching. *Side effects:* drowsiness, nausea, dryness of mouth, nose, and throat.

Epinephrine by injection. *Function:* restore normal breathing when allergic reaction has impeded it. *Side effects:* jitteriness, trembling, rapid heartbeat.

Topical corticosteroids such as hydrocortisone (Cortaid, Cortef), triamcinolone (Kenelog, Aristocort), dexamethasone (Decaderm, Decadron), desoximetasone (Tropicort), and others. *Function:* decrease inflammation. *Side effects:* uncommon when used short-term on a small area of skin.

HERBAL REMEDIES

Licorice (*Glycyrrhiza glabra*)

With its anti-inflammatory and antiallergy properties, licorice acts in a way that's similar to cortisol, the body's own anti-inflammatory hormone. Use whole licorice, not the DGL, or deglycyrrhizinated, form. *Typical dosage:* up to six 400- to 500-milligram capsules per day; or 20 to 30 drops of tincture three times per day; or 2 cups of tea per day (simmer 1 teaspoon of dried chopped root in 1 cup of water for 10 minutes). You can also cool the tea and apply it to the affected skin with a clean cloth three or four times a day. *Caution:* Limit internal use to six weeks. Do not use if you are pregnant or if you have high blood pressure, diabetes, or a disease of the thyroid, kidney, liver, or heart. If you are already taking corticosteroid allergy medications, consult a doctor before using licorice.

Chamomile (*Matricaria recutita*)

This effective anti-inflammatory herb also helps you sleep—a welcome attribute if the burning and itching of hives keeps you awake. *Typical dosage:* 3 to 4 cups of tea per day (steep 1 teaspoon of dried flowers in 1 cup of hot water for 10 minutes). You can also cool a cup in the refrigerator, moisten a clean cloth and apply it to your hives three to four times a day. Or brew about a gallon of tea and pour it into a lukewarm bath (hot water usually aggravates itching). *Caution:* If you're allergic to other daisy family plants, you might be allergic to chamomile. Apply the tea to a small patch of skin that doesn't have hives and wait 24 to 48 hours. If the chamomile produces inflammation, don't use it.

Yarrow (*Artemesia millefolium*)

This flower is in the same botanical tribe as chamomile and is also anti-inflammatory. *Typical dosage:* 3 to 4 cups of tea per day (steep 1 teaspoon of dried flowers in 1 cup of hot water for 10 minutes). You can use it externally in the same way as chamomile—but the same cautions apply. *Caution*: Do not use internally during pregnancy.

Yarrow

Burdock (*Arctium lappa*)

This plant is a traditional treatment for skin conditions, including hives. The roots, seeds, and leaves can all be used. *Typical dosage:* up to 3 cups of tea per day (steep 1 teaspoon of dried root in 1 cup of hot water for 10 to 15 minutes); or up to six 400- to 500-milligram capsules per day; or 20 to 30 drops of tincture three times per day.

Stinging Nettle (*Urtica dioica*)

Nettles may seem an odd choice to heal hives, because a serious case of them can result if you merely brush against the fresh plant. But taken internally, this plant somehow has an antiallergy effect. If stinging nettles grow near your home, wear thick gloves, long sleeves, and long pants. Pick a couple of handfuls, steam them, and eat as a vegetable. *Typical dosage:* 1 to 2 cups of tea per day (steep 1 teaspoon of dried leaves in 1 cup of hot water for 10 minutes); or up to six 400-milligram capsules per day.

Aloe (*Aloe vera*)

If you grow this plant, slice a leaf lengthwise, scoop out the inner gel, and apply as needed to your hives. It will reduce inflammation and feel cool and soothing on irritated skin. You can also use a commercial preparation of pure aloe vera gel, preferably one without artificial colorings or preservatives.

Ginger (*Zingiber officinale*)

This spice's strong anti-inflammatory powers come with a helping of heat, so you might not want to use it if your skin already feels hot. *Typical dosage:* up to 2 cups of tea per day (simmer 1 teaspoon of fresh grated root or ½ teaspoon of dried root in 1 cup of hot water for 10 minutes). You can also cool a batch to sponge onto your skin.

Hypothyroidism

Y OU DON'T KNOW IT'S THERE. You can't feel it working. But the functioning of the butterfly-shaped thyroid gland, located at the base of your neck, influences every organ system and every function of your body. So if your thyroid gland is not operating as it should, the effects on your body are widespread.

Hypothyroidism is a condition in which the thyroid gland does not produce enough thyroid hormones, which regulate the rate of metabolism in the cells of the body. The condition can range from very mild to severe, leading to coma or even death.

In infants and children, hypothyroidism causes severe mental and physical retardation. In adults, typical symptoms include low body temperature, sensitivity to cold, weight gain, dry skin, hair loss, constipation, lethargy, fatigue, depression, memory and con-

SUPPLEMENTS FOR THYROID HEALTH

The thyroid needs iodine to do its work. Dietary sources of iodine include salt-water fish, other seafoods, seaweeds, and iodized table salt. If you suspect you're deficient in iodine, include these foods in your diet or take 150 to 300 micrograms of iodine per day. Don't exceed this dose, because excess iodine may actually inhibit thyroid function.

The amino acid tyrosine is another building block of thyroid hormones; you may want to try taking 250 to 500 milligrams per day.

Although some foods can boost iodine levels, others may actually block the thyroid from using iodine. Foods to avoid include soybeans, peanuts, millet, pine nuts, turnips, cabbage, and mustard. Cooking, however, appears to inactivate the substances that cause this effect, so don't be afraid to eat cooked foods containing these ingredients.

centration problems, muscle weakness and stiffness, and decreased libido. In women, menstrual problems, infertility, miscarriages, and other problems with pregnancy can occur. In the long run, untreated hypothyroidism increases the risk of atherosclerosis and heart disease.

A number of factors may cause hypothyroidism. How it is treated depends on what causes it. So if you think you may have an underactive thyroid, see your doctor for a complete medical evaluation.

The most common cause of hypothyroidism is called idiopathic or sluggish thyroid. This means that the gland, for reasons that are not clear, is not quite doing its job. Other causes include autoimmune conditions (Hashimoto's thyroiditis), iodine deficiency, and, rarely, problems with the hypothalamus or pituitary gland.

If your gland's malfunction is caused by an autoimmune condition, you'll want to seek a treatment plan that addresses the autoimmune condition as well. Some herbs should not be used in such cases, so consult your doctor and/or a professional herbalist.

When mild or moderate hypothyroidism is caused by a sluggish thyroid, herbal and other natural remedies can help. You'll still need to see your doctor after a month or so of taking herbs because you'll want to learn whether the herbal remedy is working.

If you're taking thyroid drugs now, you may be able to switch to herbs, but do so slowly and carefully, with your doctor's help in monitoring the effects. If you have a child with an underactive thyroid, it's best to stick with the drugs, because the consequences of having an underactive thyroid in childhood can be severe and irreversible.

DRUG TREATMENT

Thyroid Supplements
Synthetic and natural thyroid supplements (Synthroid, Armour Thyroid). *Side effects:* none when dosage is correct (calculating the proper dosage can be difficult).

HERBAL REMEDIES

Bitters
This group of herbs has an overall stimulating effect on the body, including the digestive system and the hormone-producing en-

docrine system that the thyroid gland is a part of. In the clinical experience of many doctors, bitters are the most effective treatment for mild to moderate hypothyroidism. Bitters are named for their taste; their strong taste boosts the body's production of digestive fluids, so you get more nutrients from eating the same foods. The more bitter the taste, the better they work. You have to actually taste the bitterness, so swallowing capsules won't do the trick. Many commercial bitters tinctures are on the market; look for those that contain gentian. *Typical dosage:* ⅛ to ½ teaspoon of tincture three times per day before meals; or 1 cup of tea three times per day before meals.

Myrrh (*Commiphora myrrha*)

This tree resin stimulates the thyroid, although researchers haven't figured out how. Resins don't extract in hot water, though, so myrrh doesn't work in tea form. *Typical dosage:* ⅛ to ¼ teaspoon of tincture three times per day.

Bladderwrack (*Fucus vesiculosus*)

This iodine-rich seaweed is one of several seaweeds that can help balance and nourish the thyroid. *Typical dosage:* ⅛ to ½ teaspoon of tincture three times per day.

Bladderwrack

INDIGESTION

COMMERCIALS ENCOURAGE YOU TO go ahead and eat the whole thing—simply take an antacid afterward. But overindulging isn't the only reason you may find yourself wanting a stomach remedy.

Technically, indigestion means not being able to properly digest food. This covers everything from heartburn, sour stomach, acid overproduction, and stomach upset to pain, nausea and vomiting, heartburn with acid regurgitation, and gas that causes flatulence, burping, or bloating.

Often indigestion results from an overproduction of stomach acid. It can also result from a shortage of acid. Sometimes the culprit is the esophageal sphincter, the valve between the stomach and esophagus. If the sphincter fails to close properly, it allows partially digested food and acid to leave the stomach and come back up to the throat, causing heartburn. A sluggish digestive system may be at fault; so can bouts of stress and anxiety. And certain drugs can produce indigestion as a side effect.

One thing you can be sure of: If any weak links exist in your digestive system, overeating or eating problematic foods is bound to bring on indigestion.

If your bouts of indigestion are chronic, they could signal an underlying problem. So be sure to let your doctor know. Peptic ulcer, gallbladder disease, chronic appendicitis, stomach inflammation, and hiatal hernia are just some of the chronic gastrointestinal ailments that can have indigestion as a symptom.

Simple and occasional indigestion can be helped with herbs. Some herbs help dispel gas and ease overactive bowels; others can be used before eating to set the stage for better digestion. Some soothe irritated tissues in the digestive tract; another category eases the spasms or cramps that sometimes accompany indigestion. Some herbs for digestion have more than one of these benefits.

DRUG TREATMENT

Antacids
Simethicone (Gelusil), aluminum hydroxide (Maalox), magnesium hydroxide (Mylanta-DS), calcium carbonate (Tums). *Function:* neutralize excess acid and eliminate excess gas. *Side effects:* constipation or diarrhea, white or pale stools, stomach cramps.

Colloidal Bismuth Compounds
Bismuth subsalicylate (Pepto-Bismol). *Function:* bind to and coat the lining of the stomach to protect it from irritation by excess stomach acid. *Side effects:* may cause skin rash, weakness, joint pain, diarrhea, or stomach irritation when taken in large doses.

Histamine Antagonists

Ranitidine (Zantac), famotidine (Pepcid), cimetidine (Tagamet). *Function:* reduce the secretion of acid and digestive enzymes in the stomach. *Side effects:* confusion.

Antimuscarinic Agents or Cholinoreceptor Agonists

Anisotropine (Valpin), atropine, clidinium (Quarzan), isopropamide (Darbid), oxyphencyclimine (Daricon). *Function:* block nerve endings to prevent the secretion of acid in the stomach. *Side effects:* nervous system stimulation, increased or decreased heart rate, narrowed airways leading to shortness of breath.

Proton Pump Inhibitors

Omeprazole (Prilosec). *Function:* block the mechanism that pumps acid into the stomach. *Side effects:* growth of bacteria in the stomach.

Prokinetic Agents

Cisapride (Propulsid), metoclopramide (Reglan). *Function:* decrease the amount of time food spends in the stomach and intestines. *Cisapride side effects:* dizziness, vomiting, sore throat, chest pain, fatigue, back pain, depression, dehydration, diarrhea,

DRUGS THAT MAY CAUSE INDIGESTION

Many widely used drugs can cause digestive disturbances. Here are just a few.

◆ Antibiotics

◆ Aspirin, acetaminophen, and ibuprofen

◆ Corticosteroids

◆ Digoxin (a heart medication)

◆ Iron supplements

◆ Narcotic pain relievers

◆ Theophylline (an asthma medication)

SIMPLE STEPS FOR AVOIDING INDIGESTION

A few easy precautions can help reduce digestive upset.

◆ Give yourself time for meals—don't eat on the run.

◆ Decrease your consumption of fat and sugar, which can increase gas.

◆ Eat smaller portions.

◆ Chew food thoroughly.

◆ Eat whole foods that contain fiber, which move more easily through your intestines.

◆ Drink plenty of water, at least eight glasses per day, to help keep your intestinal contents moving.

abdominal pain, constipation, flatulence, runny nose. *Metoclopramide side effects:* fatigue, apathy, depression, rash.

Digestive Enzymes

Pancreatin (Creon). *Function:* promote digestion and relax the intestines. *Side effects:* drowsiness, headache, dizziness, blurred vision, nausea, vomiting, hot and dry skin, difficulty swallowing, constipation.

HERBAL REMEDIES

Chamomile (*Matricaria recutita*)

A time-honored, soothing digestive herb, chamomile helps dispel gas, soothe the stomach, and relax the muscles that move food through the intestines. Many people use chamomile as a sedative. It makes an excellent bedtime tonic for an upset stomach. Mix it with peppermint for a tasty, effective tea to treat indigestion. It may be more effective as a tincture than a tea since many of its components evaporate quickly. *Typical dosage:* 3 to 4 cups of tea per day (steep ½ to 1 teaspoon of dried flowers in 1 cup of hot water for 10 minutes); or 10 to 40 drops of tincture three times per day.

Peppermint (*Mentha × piperita*)

Any member of the mint family is good for indigestion, so if you don't care for the taste of peppermint, try lemon balm (*Melissa officinalis*). Mint acts as a muscle relaxant and can calm an overactive digestive tract. *Typical dosage:* 6 to 12 drops of essential oil in water three times per day; or 1 to 2 capsules three times per day after meals (if irritable bowel syndrome is a factor in your indigestion, use enteric-coated capsules); or up to 3 cups of tea per day (steep 1½ teaspoons of dried leaf in 1 cup of hot water for 10 minutes); or 10 to 20 drops of tincture in water after meals. *Caution:* Because peppermint relaxes the valve between the stomach and the esophagus, it can worsen heartburn. If this is one of your symptoms, don't use peppermint.

Marshmallow (*Althaea officinalis*)

The root of this herb soothes the digestive tract's mucous membranes. It's also a mild immune-system stimulant, good for those whose indigestion may have a viral or bacterial cause. Usually the root is used, but the leaves also contain some of the substance that soothes an upset stomach. *Typical dosage:* up to six 400- to 500-milligram capsules per day; or 1 cup of tea per day, divided into three doses (simmer 1 teaspoon of dried root in 1 cup of hot water for 15 minutes); or 20 to 40 drops of tincture up to five times per day.

Marshmallow

Angelica (*Angelica archangelica*)

The fruit, leaf, and root of this herb stimulate digestion, help dispel gas, and calm the nerves. Angelica is especially good when bloating or cramps are part of indigestion. You might see it included with other bitter herbs, such as dandelion, in commercial bitters preparations. *Typical dosage:* up to 3 cups of tea per day, taken 30 minutes before meals (steep 1 teaspoon of dried root in 1 cup of hot water for 10 minutes); or 10 to 40 drops of tincture up to three times per day. *Caution:* May cause sun sensitivity. Avoid during pregnancy and nursing.

OTHER WAYS TO CALM AN UPSET STOMACH

Try these approaches for stubborn cases of indigestion.

◆ **Take probiotics.** Often referred to as the "good bacteria," these are similar to the bacteria that normally inhabit your intestinal tract. Probiotics include bacteria of the genus *Lactobacillus* and *Bifidobacterium.* They are beneficial for a number of reasons. They reduce the chances for harmful bacteria to proliferate and cause diarrhea; they improve digestion; and they make B vitamins—especially niacin, vitamin B_6, and folic acid—much easier to absorb. Often, they can calm an irritated digestive tract.

There are two other ways to get their benefits. You can eat yogurt that contains live cultures (check the label to be sure that it does). Or you can eat more fruits, vegetables, and grains, all of which encourage the growth of probiotic bacteria.

◆ **Take digestive enzymes.** For indigestion caused by insufficient digestive enzymes, a few supplements may ease symptoms. Bromelain, from pineapple, and pancreatin, an extract of pancreatic enzymes, are two commonly used products. *Typical dosage for bromelain:* one or two capsules containing 2,400 milk-clotting units or gelatin-dissolving units per day, taken with food. *Typical dosage for pancreatin:* 350 to 1,000 milligrams of product labeled 10X USP three times per day.

Ginger (*Zingiber officinale*)

Ginger stimulates digestion and dispels gas. It also helps move food through the intestinal tract and reduce irritation. Studies show that ginger can prevent motion sickness. Typical dosage: up to eight 500- to 600-milligram capsules per day; or 1/2 to 1 teaspoon fresh ground root per day; or 10 to 20 drops of tincture in water three times per day.

Fennel (*Foeniculum vulgare*)

Fennel relieves gas and stimulates the digestive tract. If you expect to eat a vegetable that you have trouble digesting, such as cabbage, try adding fennel seeds to your recipe. *Typical dosage:* up to 2 teaspoons of raw seeds eaten after meals; or 1 cup of tea per day (simmer 2 to 3 teaspoons of crushed seeds in 1 cup of hot water for 10 to 15 minutes); or 30 to 60 drops of tincture in water up to four times per day.

INSECT BITES AND STINGS

INSECTS. YOU KNOW THEY HAVE FUNDAMENTAL, environmentally beneficial purposes, but sometimes you just can't imagine what those purposes might be. Particularly when a swarm of bugs buzzes around your head and feasts on your blood. Some insects bite, some sting. Biting insects include mosquitoes, chiggers, lice, bedbugs, fleas, and flies. None of the insects in this group are poisonous.

Stinging insects include fire ants, honeybees, hornets, and wasps. These bugs inject venom when they strike. If they sting you inside the mouth or throat, if you receive multiple stings, or if you develop a serious allergic reaction, seek immediate medical attention. A serious allergic reaction is one that results in severe local swelling, hives, nausea, vomiting, stomach cramps, wheezing or other breathing problems, difficulty swallowing, or swelling of the lips, face, eyes, or tongue.

Spiders, scorpions, and ticks belong to a separate class altogether: arachnids. Even though all spiders inject venom when they bite, most spider bites aren't serious. Two American spiders that can cause serious reactions are brown recluse spiders (tan with a dark violin-shaped mark on the back) and black widow spiders (usually black with a red hourglass shape on its underside). Bites from tarantulas (large and hairy) and scorpions (lobster-like with a stinger on a flexible tail) can also be serious. Reactions to such bites vary according to the species. Ticks burrow their heads into the skin to suck blood. Although most ticks are benign, some transmit illnesses such as Colorado tick fever, Rocky Mountain spotted fever, and Lyme disease.

BASIC BUG-BITE FIRST-AID

Washing an insect bite with soap and water usually prevents infection. If a honeybee was the offending critter and it left a stinger, gently flick or scrape the stinger out with a fingernail or credit card. Do not squeeze it between fingernails or tweezers, as this could release more venom. You can neutralize bee stings, which are acidic, with an alkaline substance such as baking soda.

For wasp stings, which are alkaline, apply vinegar or lemon juice. If a bite or sting burns, itches, or swells, apply a cold compress. Sometimes just rubbing an ice cube on the spot helps. You can also use certain herbs in compress form.

For a bite from a spider or tarantula, wash the bite with soap and lots of water. To reduce circulation of the venom, lie down. If possible, position the bitten body part below the level of your heart and apply a cold compress to the bite. Do not use a tourniquet. Seek medical attention if you have a serious reaction: severe pain or numbness around the bite, skin discoloration or rash, muscle rigidity, headache, dizziness, nausea, vomiting, an all-over sick feeling, or difficulty breathing.

If you discover a tick embedded in your skin, grasp it with fingers or tweezers as close to your skin as possible and pull steadily until the tick releases its grip. Avoid using undue force or you might separate the tick's body from its head. If parts of the head or mouth remain in the skin, they can cause infection later. After you dispose of the tick, wash the bite thoroughly with soap and water and apply an antiseptic ointment. Call your doctor if you can't remove the tick or remove only part of it, or if days later you develop an infection or ulcer around the bite, fever, flu-like symptoms, skin rash, or swollen lymph nodes.

Drug Treatments

Analgesics

Aspirin, acetaminophen, ibuprofen, naproxen (Alleve). *Function:* reduce pain; all but acetaminophen may also help reduce inflammation. *Aspirin side effects:* heartburn, indigestion, stomach irritation, mild nausea or vomiting. *Acetaminophen side effects:* doses higher than recommended can damage the liver and kidneys. *Ibuprofen and naproxen side effects:* dizziness, nausea, stomachache, headache.

Antihistamines

Diphenhydramine (Benadryl). *Function:* relieve itching and hives. *Side effects:* drowsiness, dryness of mouth, nose, and throat.

Corticosteroids

Hydrocortisone cream (Cortaid, many others). *Function:* prevent further inflammation from stings. *Side effects:* rare.

Oral prednisone (Deltasone). *Function:* Alleviate severe allergic reactions. *Side effects:* increased appetite, indigestion, nausea, headache, insomnia, dizziness, weight gain, fluid retention.

Tranquilizers

Diazepam (Valium), others. *Function:* act as a sedative and relax muscle spasms after a spider bite. *Side effects:* clumsiness, drowsiness, dizziness; when used with alcohol, increases sedation.

Muscle Relaxants

Methocarbamol (Robaxin), others. *Function:* relax muscle spasms after an insect bite. *Side effects:* clumsiness, drowsiness, dizziness; when used with alcohol, increases sedation.

Other Drugs

Calamine and calamine with topical anaesthetics (Dermarest). *Function:* dry oozing sores and relieve itching. *Side effects:* allergic reactions.

Herbal Remedies

Plantain (*Plantago major, P. lanceolata*)

Plantain contains a soothing, gooey substance called mucilage. Even better, this weed grows almost everywhere in the United

HERBAL INSECT REPELLENT

Aromatic herbs can deter insects. The secret is to apply them liberally and frequently. If you can't smell this concoction any longer, it's likely that the bugs can't either. That means it's time to reapply.

- **6 drops eucalyptus essential oil**
- **5 drops cedar essential oil**
- **4 drops lavender essential oil**
- **3 drops tea tree essential oil**
- **3 drops citronella essential oil**
- **3 drops lemongrass, lemon, or lemon thyme essential oil**
- **2 drops peppermint essential oil**
- **¼ cup almond or other vegetable oil**

Combine all ingredients, preferably in a brown glass jar. Label the jar. Apply to the skin as often as necessary. *Caution:* Do not take internally, get in your eyes, or get near the nose of an infant or toddler.

States. Mash the fresh leaves and apply to the insect bite or sting as needed.

Aloe (*Aloe vera*)
Soothing and antibacterial, aloe hastens healing. Simply slice a leaf, scoop out the gel, and apply to the bite or sting. Or buy a commercial aloe vera gel product and use it in the same way.

Witch Hazel (*Hamamelis virginiana*)
An extract of the bark of this tree is soothing and helps shrink swollen tissue. Just pick up the fluid concentrate at a drugstore and follow label instructions.

Calendula (*Calendula officinalis*)
Also known as pot or flat-leafed marigold, calendula is anti-inflammatory, mildly analgesic, antiseptic, and helps heal wounds. If you grow this plant, you can rub its fresh flowers directly on a bite

or sting. Or steep 1 teaspoon of dried petals in 1 cup of hot water for 5 minutes. Strain, cool, and apply with a clean cloth. Many commercial herbal salves contain calendula.

Lavender *(Lavandula angustifolia)*
The essential oil of this flowering herb is anti-inflammatory and can help ease the discomfort of bites and stings. It's also one of the very few essential oils you can apply undiluted to the skin; dab it directly on the injury.

Comfrey *(Symphytum officinale)*
Allantoin, a compound in comfrey, is antiseptic and accelerates wound healing. You can crush fresh or dried leaves or root, add enough water to moisten, and apply directly to a bite or sting. Or steep 1 heaping teaspoon of the dried plant in 1 cup of hot water for 10 minutes. Strain, cool, and apply to the insect bite with a clean cloth. Many commercial herbal salves contain comfrey. *Caution:* Do not take internally.

Tea *(Camellia sinensis)*
That's right, plain old antioxidant-rich tea helps shrink swollen tissues, including those caused by a bite. Just grab a tea bag, moisten it, and apply to the skin.

Tea Tree *(Melaleuca alternifolia)*
This antiseptic oil is good to have around when a bite or sting threatens to become infected. Simply apply undiluted tea tree oil to the bite or sting as needed. Tea tree oil also acts as a natural insect repellant, so you're less likely to get more bites.

Echinacea *(Echinacea angustifolia, E. purpurea)*
A tincture of this immune-boosting herb can be applied to a bite or sting to numb the pain. It also helps disinfect the site of the attack. Several tribes of Native Americans used echinacea internally against venomous bites. Chemical analyses of the herb now offer a possible reason why: There's an enzyme in venom called hyaluronidase that digests the "cement" holding our cells together. When this "cement" is gone, the venom can spread throughout the cells. Echinacea interferes with the action of hyaluronidase. If you get bitten by a snake or poisonous spider, you could take 2 dropperfuls of echinacea tincture every 15 minutes while you're on your way to the doctor or emergency room.

Kava-Kava (*Piper methysticum*)

This herb helps reduce anxiety and, in larger doses, eases pain and muscle spasms. If you receive a venomous spider bite that results in muscle spasms, you might want to try it. *Typical dosage:* up to 3 standardized capsules containing 180 to 210 milligrams of kavalactones. *Caution:* Don't drive or operate heavy machinery while taking kava.

Valerian (*Valeriana officinalis*)

While best known for relieving anxiety and insomnia, valerian can also ease muscle spasms. *Typical dosage:* up to 3 cups of tea per day, if you can tolerate the musty taste (simmer 2 teaspoons of dried root in 2 cups of hot water for 10 minutes); or 1 to 1½ teaspoons of tincture per day; or two 300- or 400-milligram capsules per day; or 150 to 300 milligrams per day of a standardized extract containing 0.8 percent valeric acid.

INSOMNIA

YOU TOSS, YOU TURN, YOU SIP warm milk, you count sheep, you pray to your deity of choice. And still, sleep won't come.

If you are sometimes plagued by insomnia, you are not alone. A survey conducted on behalf of the National Sleep Foundation found that one of every two Americans has trouble sleeping at some time and that 12 percent of the population experiences frequent insomnia.

The main cause of temporary insomnia is psychological stress and the worry and anxiety that arise from it. Other culprits include consuming caffeinated beverages or other stimulants before bedtime.

Insomnia is one condition that often is better treated with herbs than with drugs. Most herbs have far fewer side effects than pharmaceutical sleep aids. They're effective for sleeplessness from a wide variety of causes. Their effects range from very mild relaxants to effective sleep aids. They can be taken internally or used topically as bath teas or essential oils.

The sedative herbs discussed in this chapter appear in order from strongest to mildest.

Drug Treatment

Benzodiazepines

Temazepam (Restoril), triazolam (Halcion), diazepam (Valium), estazolam (ProSom), quazepam (Doral), flurazepam (Dalmane). *Function:* act on the central nervous system to reduce anxiety and induce sleep. *Side effects:* clumsiness, drowsiness, dizziness; may be habit-forming or cause temporary impairment of short-term memory.

SETTING THE STAGE FOR SLEEP

Almost all people with chronic insomnia need behavioral treatment, says Sonia Ancoli-Israel, Ph.D., director of the sleep disorders clinic at the Veteran's Administration Medical Center in San Diego and author of *All I Want Is a Good Night's Sleep.* Both herbs and drugs are temporary remedies. If you frequently have insomnia, you may need to revamp your nighttime routine. A report in the *Journal of the American Medical Association* found that adopting good sleep habits works better in the long run than taking sleeping pills.

Here are ways to practice good sleep habits.

◆ **Eliminate stimulants.** Cut out coffee, tea, caffeinated sodas, chocolate, and sugar-laden desserts, or at least don't consume them within six hours of bedtime. Two stimulant herbs to watch out for are guarana and ephedra.

◆ **Avoid alcohol and tobacco.** And definitely don't partake within a couple of hours of bedtime.

◆ **Check your medications.** Many drugs can interfere with sleep. Ask your doctor whether something you're taking may be giving you insomnia.

Antihistamines
Diphenhydramine (Benadryl Allergy, Nytol), doxylamine (Nytol Maximum Strength). *Function:* cause sedation. *Side effects:* grogginess, clumsiness, dry mouth, constipation, visual disturbances.

Other Drugs
Zolpidem (Ambien). *Function:* act on the central nervous system to induce sleep. *Side effects:* daytime drowsiness, lightheadedness, dizziness, clumsiness, headache, diarrhea, nausea.

- ◆ **Wind down with pleasant rituals.** Try yoga, a hot bath, sex, light reading, massage, or meditation.
- ◆ **Get regular exercise.** People who are sedentary often have trouble sleeping because their bodies simply aren't tired. Be aware, on the other hand, that strenuous workouts right before bedtime can disrupt sleep.
- ◆ **Nap with caution.** Naps not only make you feel groggy afterward but also can interfere with nighttime sleep. Try exercising instead. If you choose to snooze, do so before 3 P.M. and for only a half-hour.
- ◆ **Wait until you're truly sleepy.** Light sleepers who stay in the sack long hours are sometimes cured by spending less time in bed, which results in deeper, more efficient sleep.
- ◆ **Establish regular bedtimes.** Do so even if it reminds you of a parental voice saying "no more television!" Avoid sleeping late on weekends, which can lead to Sunday-night insomnia.
- ◆ **Set aside a worry time.** Rather than fretting in bed, designate a time earlier in the day to worry, plan, and make to-do lists—in a room that's not the bedroom.
- ◆ **If you can't sleep, get up.** Go do something soothing. Reading may help, but it's best to do it in another room.

Herbal Remedies

Valerian (*Valeriana officinalis*)

This is the best-studied herbal sleep aid. Like benzodiazepine drugs, valerian puts you to sleep but doesn't cause a morning hangover, interact with alcohol, or lead to addiction. Research shows that extracts of the root not only help you fall asleep faster but also improve sleep quality. *Typical dosage* (taken 30 to 45 minutes before bedtime): one 150- to 300-milligram capsule standardized to 0.8 percent valeric acid; or 300 to 400 milligrams in nonstandardized capsules; or ½ to 1 teaspoon of tincture in water. *Caution:* Valerian is not addictive, but if you're convinced you can't sleep without it, you could develop a psychological dependence. For a very small percentage of people, valerian produces a stimulating rather than a sedating effect. If this occurs, stop using it.

California Poppy (*Eschscholzia californica*)

The above-ground parts and roots of this wildflower show promise in the treatment of insomnia. Higher doses of California poppy are sedating; lower doses reduce anxiety. A commercial formula that combines California poppy and corydalis (*Corydalis yanhusuo*) is used in Europe to treat insomnia, agitation, and anxiety. *Typical dosage:* up to 4 cups of tea per day (steep 1 teaspoon of dried plant in 1 cup of hot water for 10 minutes); or 30 to 40 drops of tincture two to three times per day. *Caution:* Not recommended for use during pregnancy.

Lemon Balm (*Melissa officinalis*)

This common garden herb has many virtues, including an ability to ease insomnia. It also relieves fever, fights viral illness, calms the digestive tract, and eases headaches. So if your insomnia comes with any of these annoyances, lemon balm is a good choice. It also tastes good, so you can include it in a blend with other not-so-palatable insomnia herbs. *Typical dosage:* 1 to 2 cups of tea (steep 2 teaspoons of dried leaf in 1 cup of hot water for 10 minutes); or one to two 300- to 400-milligram capsules. Take before bedtime.

Passionflower (*Passiflora incarnata*)

Extracts of this herb have been shown in a study to decrease anxiety and induce sleep. Some herbalists find passionflower especially good for times when worry or an overactive mind interferes with sleep. *Typical dosage:* 1 cup of tea before bedtime (steep ½ teaspoon of dried herb in 1 cup of hot water for 10 minutes); or 20 to 40 drops of tincture in water before bedtime. *Caution:* Do not take passionflower with monoamine oxidase-inhibiting (MAO) antidepressants.

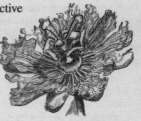

Passionflower

Kava-Kava (*Piper methysticum*)

When insomnia results from anxiety, this herb is particularly effective. Studies suggest that kava-kava promotes sleep by acting upon the brain's emotion centers and by relaxing muscles. Take kava-kava one hour before bedtime. *Typical dosage:* one or two 400- to 500-milligram capsules; or 20 to 30 drops of tincture in water; or a standardized extract containing 180 to 210 milligrams of kavalactones. *Caution:* Do not use kava-kava while pregnant or nursing, or in combination with alcohol or other sedatives.

Chamomile (*Matricaria recutita*)

A bright, daisylike flower, chamomile has an age-old reputation for calming nerves and gently aiding sleep. *Typical dosage:* 1 to 2

THE SWEET SMELL OF SLEEP

Marcel Lavabre, author of *Aromatherapy Workbook*, says that essential oils can coax sleep. His favorites are neroli (orange blossom), marjoram, spikenard, Roman chamomile, lavender, and ylang ylang. Lavabre recommends putting a couple of drops of undiluted neroli, marjoram, or lavender essential oils on your pillow, or adding 10 to 15 drops to a bath. Don't apply any of these oils to your skin, but you can blend a massage oil using 15 drops of essential oil and one ounce of almond or other vegetable oil. Rub the blended oils into your temples, forehead, and the back of your neck.

cups of tea before bedtime (steep 1 teaspoon of dried flowers in 1
cup of hot water for 10 minutes); or 10 to 40 drops of tincture in
water before bedtime. *Caution:* If you're allergic to other members
of the daisy family, such as ragweed, you might also be allergic to
chamomile.

Melatonin: Magic or Malarkey?

You may have heard about the supplement melatonin in
connection with insomnia. Melatonin is a hormone secreted at night by the pineal gland, a tiny gland deep inside the brain. It regulates several bodily processes,
including sleep. Production of this hormone usually begins to drop after the age of 40. Many senior citizens, but
not all, have decreased melatonin levels.

The results of studies using melatonin to treat insomnia
are inconsistent. Supplements of the hormone seem to
work best when they're used to reset the biological clocks
of people who perform shift work, who travel by jet across
time zones, who are blind, or who have become habitually
nocturnal. Although the optimal dosage of melatonin for insomnia has yet to be clearly defined, the typical recommendation is between 0.5 and 3 milligrams a half-hour to
an hour before bedtime. Because melatonin production requires the amino acid tryptophan, a safer bet may be to eat
plenty of tryptophan-rich foods such as turkey, fish, meat,
and beans.

Although no serious side effects have surfaced, most experts consider this hormone experimental. Authorities also
worry about product purity. Synthetic melatonin is safer
and probably more effective than a supplement derived
from animal sources. *Caution:* Avoid melatonin if you are
trying to get pregnant, are already pregnant, or have an
autoimmune disease. Children and adolescents should not
take it.

Skullcap (*Scutellaria lateriflora*)

Because it functions as both a nerve tonic and gentle sedative, skullcap is a time-honored remedy for anxiety and insomnia. *Typical dosage:* 1 cup of tea (steep 1 to 2 teaspoons of dried herb in 1 cup of hot water for 10 minutes); or 20 to 40 drops of tincture in water. Take at bedtime.

Catnip (*Nepeta cataria*)

Well-known to cat lovers, this herb has a gentle sedative effect on humans. It also expels intestinal gas, reduces fevers by inducing sweating, and is antispasmodic. So if your insomnia comes with these symptoms, catnip can be useful when blended with stronger sedative herbs. *Typical dosage:* 1 cup of tea before bedtime (steep 1 teaspoon of dried leaf in 1 cup of hot water for 10 minutes). *Caution:* Not for use during pregnancy.

INTERMITTENT CLAUDICATION

YOU KNOW YOU NEED EXERCISE so you decide to stroll the five blocks to the post office instead of driving. Halfway there, you get a crampy pain in your legs. You stop for a chat with a neighborhood gardener, and the pain goes away. But by the time you reach the mailbox, it's back—and it's worse.

What you are experiencing is called intermittent claudication. The term describes a particular type of pain that occurs in the legs when the arteries that feed blood to the lower extremities become partially blocked. What causes the blockage are atherosclerotic plaques—tiny deposits of cholesterol and related substances. These plaques build up slowly, gradually narrowing the passageways that move blood to the tissues. Eventually, the arteries become so narrow that the amount of oxygen-carrying blood getting through is insufficient to nourish the tissues, especially during exercise.

STOPPING THE SPASMS

In addition to using herbs that gradually improve artery health, people with intermittent claudication can benefit from herbs that relax smooth muscles to improve blood supply. The prime examples are motherwort (*Leonurus cardiaca*), cramp bark (*Viburnum opulus*), valerian (*Valeriana officinalis*), and skullcap (*Scutellaria lateriflora*). Because these herbs are also relaxants or sedatives, they're especially good if anxiety or stress is part of your symptoms. All can be taken in either tea or tincture form. *Typical dosage:* 1 to 3 cups of tea per day (steep 1 teaspoon of dried herb in 1 cup of hot water for 10 to 15 minutes); or ⅛ to 1 teaspoon tincture one to three times per day.

So what's a person with intermittent claudication to do? Clear those clogged pipes! But there's no Liquid Plum-R for blood vessels—at least nothing that works quickly.

If you are diagnosed with intermittent claudication, the quickest relief will come from expanding, or dilating, the involved arteries. You'll also need to shrink the plaques already present and heal damaged artery linings. To prevent future arterial narrowing, you'll want to prevent further damage to the inside walls of your arteries, reduce the clumping of a type of blood cell called platelets, and, finally, lower your blood cholesterol.

DRUG TREATMENT

Antiplatelet Agents
Aspirin, dipyridamole (Persantine). *Function:* reduce the progression of plaques (but do not relieve the symptoms of intermittent claudication). *Side effects:* gastrointestinal upset, gastrointestinal bleeding.

Other Drugs
Pentoxyfylline (Trental). *Function:* improve blood flow, provide modest relief of symptoms by making red blood cells more flexible, thinning blood, and altering platelet activity. *Side effects:* nausea, dizziness.

HERBAL REMEDIES

Ginkgo (*Ginkgo biloba*)
This is *the* herb for intermittent claudication. Ginkgo is an antioxidant, so it can help prevent arterial wall damage. It dilates blood vessels, has tonic effects on the blood vessels in areas that aren't getting enough oxygen, and helps prevent platelet accumulation. Multiple scientific studies have evaluated ginkgo in the treatment of intermittent claudication, comparing the herb with placebos (fake pills) and with various prescription drugs. Ginkgo actually worked better than the drugs.

The effect of ginkgo is cumulative: The longer it is used, the better it works. In one study, people with intermittent claudication took ginkgo for two years. By the study's end, they had increased their pain-free walking distance by an average of 300 percent. *Typical dosage:* 40

DON'T TREAT LEG PAINS YOURSELF

If you are taking medications for intermittent claudication, high or low blood pressure, or another condition of the heart or veins, you *must* consult your doctor before proceeding with herbal therapies—even if the drug you are taking is as common as aspirin. Certain drugs can have serious interactions with some herbs. Ginkgo, for example, has been known to induce spontaneous bleeding in those who take aspirin routinely. Work with an experienced herbalist to develop an individualized regimen based on your doctor's having checked for dangerous interactions.

In addition, gentle exercise is appropriate for people with intermittent claudication, but not beyond the point of pain. If you begin hurting, *stop*—you've reached the point where tissue damage begins.

Finally, intermittent claudication can be a sign of general circulatory or cardiovascular problems. A thorough medical exam is in order to detect any problems before they become serious.

to 80 milligrams of capsules standardized to 24 percent heterosides three times per day. *Caution:* Rare cases of gastrointestinal upset, headache, and dizziness have been reported by people who use ginkgo.

Garlic (*Allium sativum*) and Onion (*A. cepa*)

These tasty herbs contain substances that decrease platelet accumulation, prevent blood clots, and lower total cholesterol and triglycerides (a type of blood fat) while raising the so-called good

NUTRIENTS FOR HEALTHY LEGS

As with any disease involving the heart or blood vessels, it's important to refocus your diet on healthful low-fat, high-fiber foods. In addition, scientific studies have shown the following supplements to be useful.

◆ **Vitamin B₆.** Deficiency of this key B vitamin appears to be a major cause of heart disease. It can be taken as part of a good quality multivitamin or a B-complex combination. *Typical dosage:* 25 to 50 milligrams of B₆ per day.

◆ **Vitamin E.** One form of this vitamin inhibits the body's cholesterol production. *Typical dosage:* 25 to 100 milligrams of the tocotrienol form per day.

◆ **Magnesium.** It may help decrease plaque formation. *Typical dosage:* 500 to 1,000 milligrams per day. *Caution:* If diarrhea occurs, reduce the dose.

◆ **Niacin.** It lowers cholesterol. Take the niacin precursor inositol hexaniacinate; it doesn't produce niacin's usual side effects, such as flushing and liver damage. *Typical dosage:* 50 to 100 milligrams three times per day.

◆ **L-carnitine.** Among other benefits, this supplement prevents plaque formation. *Typical dosage:* 2,000 milligrams per day.

◆ **Bromelain.** Made from enzymes found in pineapple, bromelain inhibits platelet accumulation and has been proven in studies to break down plaques. *Typical dosage:* 250 to 500 milligrams three times per day.

cholesterol, HDL. If you like these pungent alliums and want to simply include them in your diet rather than take a supplement, eat at least one clove of garlic or half a small onion a day. *Typical dosage of garlic:* capsules providing at least 4,000 micrograms of allicin potential per day. *Caution:* Some people cannot digest garlic or onions; upset stomach and gas result.

Hawthorn (*Crataegus* spp.)

This herb is a valuable health-booster for the entire cardiovascular system. Rich in flavonoids and proanthocyanadins, hawthorn has antioxidant and anti-inflammatory effects, reduces cholesterol, and stabilizes and strengthens collagen, the substance that holds cells together. This means that it will prevent the development of plaques *and* decrease the size of plaques already present. And hawthorn has virtually no side effects. Products usually use either the leaves and flowers or the berries; both are useful, but the berries are strongest. *Typical dosage:* 1 cup of tea three times per day (simmer 1 teaspoon of dried berries in 1 cup of water for 10 minutes, or steep the same amount of leaves and flowers); or ½ to 1 teaspoon of tincture three times per day; or 100 to 250 milligrams of capsules standardized to 20 percent proanthocyanadins three times per day.

Ginger (*Zingiber officinale*)

This delicious spice has antioxidant and anti-inflammatory effects, helps lower cholesterol, and prevents platelet accumulation. This means that ginger, like hawthorn, helps shrink the stuff that's clogging your arteries while preventing new stuff from forming. If a new healthy diet has you craving sweets, try grating or thinly slicing fresh ginger root and mixing it with a little honey. *Typical dosage:* up to a ¼-inch slice of an average-sized root per day; or if fresh root is not available, 250 to 500 milligrams in capsules (preferably freeze-dried) three times per day. *Caution:* Ginger may cause upset stomach in some people, especially at higher doses.

Prickly Ash (*Zanthoxylum americanum*)

The bark of this member of the rue family is a traditional circulatory stimulant, thought to increase blood vessel tone throughout the body. *Typical dosage:* 1 cup of tea up to three times per day (simmer 1 teaspoon of dried bark in 1 cup of water for 10 to 15 minutes); or ⅛ teaspoon of tincture three times per day.

INTESTINAL PARASITES

PARASITES COME IN TWO MAIN VARIETIES: single-celled protozoa such as giardia and amoebas, and worms such as tapeworms and hookworms. Whatever the type, they can cause intestinal distress, fatigue, hunger, cramps, nausea, flatulence, diarrhea, and other problems.

Usually people pick up parasites by consuming contaminated food or water. Some parasites are present in water and soil and enter the body by penetrating bare skin.

Take an infestation of parasites seriously because they can spread easily. A doctor's diagnosis is important. If you have nausea, fever, and diarrhea that persists for three or more days, or if such symptoms become severe, consult your doctor. Be sure you tell your doctor if you are pregnant or plan to become pregnant. Many drugs for parasite infections, as well as many of the herbs recommended for them, have side effects for pregnant women.

Several herbs and foods have traditionally been used to treat parasites. They have fewer side effects than the drugs usually used, but they also take longer to work. In addition, little information is available about the dosage needed. If you plan to use herbs to treat parasites, do so under the guidance of a qualified health practitioner. Return for follow-up appointments to make sure you've gotten rid of the parasites. And if you're pregnant, don't take herbs unless you've first consulted a qualified health practitioner.

DRUG TREATMENT

Antiparasitic Drugs

Metronidazole (Flagyl). *Function:* treat infestations of giardia or amoebas. *Side effects:* headache, loss of appetite, vomiting, diarrhea, stomachache, metallic taste in the mouth, dizziness; abdominal distress, nausea, vomiting, flushing, or headache when combined with alcohol.

Furazolidone (Furoxone). *Function:* treat infestations of giardia. *Side effects:* occasional nausea, vomiting, headache; flushing, shortness of breath, slight temperature elevation when combined with alcohol.

Anti-Worm Drugs

Mebendazole (Vermox). *Function:* treat infestations of many parasites, including amoebas, pinworms, hookworms, roundworms, and *Trichinella spiralis. Side effects:* occasional diarrhea, abdominal discomfort.

Albendazole (Albenza). *Function:* treat infestations of a range of parasites. *Side effects:* occasional diarrhea, abdominal discomfort.

Thiabendazole (Mintezol). *Function:* treat infestations of the worm *Strongyloides stercoralis. Side effects:* headache, vomiting, dizziness, weakness, fuzzy thinking.

Ivermectin (Stromeotol). *Function:* treat infestation of the worm *Strongyloides stercoralis. Side effects:* headache, fever, joint and bone pain, tender lymph nodes, itchy skin.

Niclosamide (Niclocide). *Function:* treat tapeworms. *Side effects:* nausea, vomiting, abdominal discomfort, decreased appetite, diarrhea, drowsiness, dizziness, headache, itchy skin rash.

Praziquantel (Biltricide). *Function:* treat tapeworm. *Side effects:* mild headache, dizziness, abdominal discomfort, nausea.

Pyrantel (Antiminth). *Function:* treat pinworm and roundworm. *Side effects:* decreased appetite, vomiting, diarrhea, abdominal cramps, headache, dizziness, drowsiness, insomnia.

Pyrvinium (Vanquin). *Function:* treat a variety of worm infestations. *Side effects:* nausea, vomiting, cramping, diarrhea.

HERBAL REMEDIES

Oregon Graperoot (*Mahonia aquifolium, Berberis aquifolium*)

This herb contains berberine, which acts against the parasites *Entamoeba histolytica* and *Giardia lamblia.* One study in children showed that berberine was better at ridding them of giardia than the drug Flagyl or a placebo (fake pill). Other berberine-containing herbs include goldenseal (*Hydrastis canadensis*), gold thread (*Coptis chinensis*), and barberry (*Berberis vulgaris*). *Typical dosage:* 1½ to 3 teaspoons of tincture per day; or up to six 250- to 500-milligram capsules per day. *Caution:* Do not use during pregnancy.

Garlic (*Allium sativum*)

This bulb is a veritable pharmacy all by itself. A traditional treatment for several types of parasites, garlic's power to kill roundworm, pin-

The Citrus Cure

Grapefruit seed extract can be helpful in fighting both bacterial and parasitic infestations. It is made from the seed, pulp, and inner rind of grapefruit. Test-tube studies show that it inhibits the growth of giardia and amoebas. Dosage varies widely; follow the manufacturer's instructions.

worm, tapeworm, and hookworm has been confirmed by scientific studies. *Typical dosage:* 2 or 3 raw cloves of garlic per day; or three 500- to 600-milligram capsules of powdered garlic per day (look for products that supply a daily dose of 4,000 to 5,000 micrograms of the active ingredient allicin). *Caution:* Do not use if you have stomach irritation, if you will soon have surgery, or if you take the blood thinner warfarin. If you're on insulin, check with your doctor, as garlic can lower blood-sugar levels.

Ginger (*Zingiber officinale*)

This common seasoning works against several parasites, including the anisakis worm, which occurs in raw fish—a good reason for serving pickled ginger with sushi. *Typical dosage:* up to eight 500- to 600-milligram capsules per day; or ½ to 1 teaspoon ground root per day; or 10 to 20 drops of tincture in water three times per day. (Studies have not yet established optimum dosages for expelling worms; this dosage is only a guideline.) *Caution:* Do not take ginger continuously if you have gallbladder disease or are on blood-thinning medication.

Epazote (*Chenopodium ambrosioides*)

This herb contains a chemical called ascaridole, which is chemically related to the artemisinin found in Chinese wormwood. So it's no surprise that this plant inhibits parasites, including worms. *Typical dosage:* 3 cups of tea per day (steep ½ teaspoon of dried herb in 1 cup of hot water for 10 to 15 minutes). *Caution:* When taken internally, the essential oil of this plant is extremely toxic and has caused fatalities. Some people are highly allergic to this plant.

Quassia Bark (*Picrasma excelsa*)

This bark has a reputation among North American herbalists for treating giardia. Montana herbalist Sunny Mavor, coauthor of *Kids, Herbs, and Health,* heard a report of a man who resolved his giardia symptoms with 30 drops of quassia bark tincture three times per day for three weeks. Although this dose was effective, it irritated his stomach and made him nauseated. *Typical dosage:* up to 30 drops of tincture, three times per day.

Raw Pumpkin Seeds (*Cucurbita pepo*)

These seeds have antiparasitic action, though how they work isn't clear. They do contain zinc; when this mineral is in short supply, as it often is among the elderly, the stomach's production of hydrochloric acid drops. And insufficient stomach acidity often occurs in patients with parasites. Pumpkin seeds may work best in conjunction with conventional drugs or to prevent recurrences. *Typical dosage:* not well-defined for this use, but generally, several handfuls of raw pumpkin seeds every day for several weeks.

Long Pepper (*Piper longum*)

Also called Indian long pepper, this plant is a botanical cousin to black pepper. In India, the fruits are a traditional remedy against intestinal distress. A study on humans with giardia found that an Ayurvedic remedy prepared from long pepper and another Indian herb called palash (*Butea monosperma*) resulted in the complete disappearance of the parasite in 23 out of 25 patients. To use this herb, contact a qualified practitioner, because the dosage is not well-established.

Irritable Bowel Syndrome

Second only to bad colds, irritable bowel syndrome (IBS) is a common reason that people miss work. It is also one of the primary reasons that people visit doctor's offices.

IBS affects up to 35 million Americans, more than half of whom are women between the ages of 20 and 40. But its usual symptoms—constipation or diarrhea, along with severe bloating and gas—can be caused by a variety of other ailments or conditions. Be sure of your diagnosis before you begin exploring your treatment options.

Conventional drug treatments for IBS include laxatives, antispasmodics, and tranquilizers. In the past, when these didn't help, doctors often attributed a patient's symptoms to psychological factors. Although stress can certainly play a role in most digestive disorders, it's unlikely to be the sole cause of the problem. Today when you see a practitioner, you'll find him more willing to look for abnormalities

Is It Allergy-Related?

One source estimates that up to two-thirds of people with irritable bowel syndrome have one or more food allergies. But determining which foods cause allergies can be difficult and time-consuming. The most common offenders include dairy products and gluten-rich grains such as wheat; however, your own irritable bowel symptoms might be a reaction to almost anything. One of the easiest ways to help pinpoint your own possible culprits is to keep a detailed food diary, recording foods eaten and symptoms. If you notice that certain foods consistently make you feel bad, try eliminating them from your diet—one at a time—and see if your symptoms improve.

such as food allergies or intolerances and for digestive problems caused by insufficient pancreatic enzyme or stomach acid production.

It's also worth looking into your digestive system's ecology. Parasites from tainted food and water can cause the same symptoms as

TIPS FOR A HEALTHY BOWEL

Just as a garden that needs constant weeding and pruning, your intestines need regular attention and maintenance. This is especially true for people with irritable bowel syndrome. Part of that maintenance involves good eating habits, including the following strategies.

◆ **Take it easy.** Try to make mealtime as calm and stress-free as possible. Eating more slowly and taking time to chew food thoroughly is a great way to improve digestion.

◆ **Find the fiber.** Get enough of this key component from fruits, vegetables, and some grains. Fiber can help both constipation and diarrhea by regulating peristalsis, the involuntary muscle contractions that move food.

◆ **Pass up the gas-causers.** Avoid gas-forming foods such as beans, cabbage, or carbonated beverages. If you can't avoid them entirely, consume these foods in small quantities only.

◆ **Trim the sugar.** Because carbohydrates can ferment in the intestines and produce gas, many people find that cutting out refined sugars, or even all carbohydrates, can reduce or even eliminate symptoms.

◆ **Accept no substitutes.** Be aware that sorbitol and xylitol—indigestible carbohydrates used as artificial sweeteners—can aggravate irritable bowel symptoms.

◆ **Avoid irritants.** Fatty foods and coffee, regular or decaffeinated, can induce intestinal spasms, resulting in cramps or diarrhea. Try alternatives to your usual java fix and drive past the burger joints.

irritable bowel syndrome; antibiotic use can lead to the overgrowth of yeasts and other unhealthy bacteria. These microscopic organisms produce toxins that irritate the bowel wall, making it more sensitive and disrupting peristalsis, the normal flow of food through the digestive system.

DRUG TREATMENT

Antispasmodics

Hyoscyamine (Levsin), dicyclomine (Bentyl), hyoscyamine/atropine/scopolamine/phenobarbital (Donnatal), chlordiazepoxide/clinidium bromide (Librax). *Function:* relax the bowel wall and ease cramps. Librax and Donnatal also contain a sedative. *Side effects:* dry mouth, difficulty urinating, constipation, dizziness, blurry vision, nervousness, insomnia.

Antidiarrheal Agents

Loperamide (Imodium A-D), diphenoxylate/atropine (Lomotil). *Function:* affect the bowel wall to stop erratic or excessive digestive contractions. *Side effects:* allergic reactions, abdominal distension, constipation, drowsiness, dry mouth.

BOWEL-BOOSTING SUPPLEMENTS

One of the single most helpful supplements for irritable bowel syndrome is *Lactobacillus acidophilus.* This beneficial bacterium has been shown to suppress the overgrowth of unhealthy bacteria, yeasts, and parasites. *L. acidophilus* is commercially available as a powder or capsule. For best results, obtain a product that guarantees at least 2.5 billion live organisms per gram and take 1,000 to 4,000 milligrams per day.

Another very useful supplement is digestive enzymes, which assist in the thorough breakdown of foods. Several sources are available, including pancreatic extracts (from cows), papain (from papaya), bromelain (from pineapple stem), and cultured molds (such as *Aspergillus* species).

Laxatives

Lactulose syrup, magnesium citrate, phenolphthalein (Ex-Lax), bisacodyl (Dulcolax), magnesium hydroxide (Phillips' Milk of Magnesia). *Function:* activate muscles in the bowel wall to induce bowel movements. *Side effects:* diarrhea, bloating (from lactulose), cramping, dependence on laxative for proper bowel function.

Surfactants

Simethicone (Di-Gel, Gas-X). *Function:* theoretically to reduce and disperse trapped gas bubbles, but may not be effective. *Side effects:* unknown.

HERBAL REMEDIES

Peppermint (*Mentha × piperita*)

Pain-relieving, anti-inflammatory, and antimicrobial, peppermint has a long history of use for intestinal problems including indigestion, cramping, and bloating. It also fights yeast organisms. Mints are members of the group of herbs called carminatives, which relax the muscles of the lower esophagus and allow the release of gas trapped in the stomach.

The typical dosage is one to four capsules taken with meals, although dosage varies from one product to another. Follow the manufacturer's directions. All of these enzymes are safe to use for extended periods of time.

In Asia, rice bran oil is used extensively for cooking and salad dressing but is also recognized for its medicinal properties. Doctors in Japan use it as a treatment for numerous medical conditions, including irritable bowel syndrome and gastritis. It is rich in a substance called gamma oryzanol, which has been shown to normalize acid production in the stomach and to decrease inflammation of the intestinal lining, thus soothing the entire intestinal tract. Rice bran oil is widely available in gourmet and health food stores; it is also available as a dietary supplement. The typical dosage is 1 to 2 tablespoons of oil per day, mixed into foods; or one 100- to 200-milligram capsule of gamma oryzanol three times per day with food.

Although mint tea is useful for stomach upsets, peppermint essential oil is better for IBS. Several studies have confirmed that this oil acts directly on the smooth muscles lining the intestinal walls to decrease erratic contractions and alleviate spasms. For peppermint oil to reach the colon, however, it must be taken as an enteric-coated capsule, which shields the oil from the digestive enzymes of the stomach. *Typical dosage:* 1 to 2 capsules containing 0.2 milliliter of the oil two or three times per day as needed; or dilute a few drops of the oil in 1 fluid ounce of vegetable oil and rub directly on the site of discomfort such as the lower abdomen. *Caution:* Do not use peppermint internally if you have heartburn or esophageal reflux.

Psyllium (*Plantago ovata*)

The seed husks from this plant have a long history of use by herbalists and medical doctors alike for the treatment of constipation and recurrent diarrhea. Psyllium is rich in fibers similar to those found in oat bran, flaxseed meal, and guar gum. These fibers form a soft bulky material that gently regulates peristalsis. *Typical dosage:* up to 1 tablespoon of seed husks or 2 teaspoons of powdered seed stirred into 8 ounces of water, once per day (drink 30 minutes to 1 hour after eating or taking other drugs). Don't let the mixture set once mixed; the blend thickens quickly and becomes difficult to drink.

Chamomile (*Matricaria recutita*)

This popular, versatile herb acts as a sedative, relieves gas, calms intestinal spasms, and fights inflammation. It soothes the gastrointestinal tract and helps fight both constipation and diarrhea. *Typical dosage:* 3 to 4 cups of tea per day (steep ½ to 1 teaspoon of dried flowers in 1 cup of hot water for 10 minutes); or 10 to 40 drops of tincture three times per day; or up to six 300 or 400 milligram capsules per day in divided doses—all taken between meals. *Caution*: Avoid if you have heartburn or are allergic to other plants in the aster family, which includes ragweed.

Chamomile

KIDNEY STONES

MENTION THE WORDS *KIDNEY STONES* to anyone who knows anything about them and you're likely to get shudders and winces. This is a condition that literally makes grown men—and women—cry.

Up to 10 percent of American men and 5 percent of American women have a kidney stone at least once in their lifetime. These painful little pebbles are responsible for as many as one out of every 1,000 hospital admissions.

Most kidney stones are composed of calcium; a smaller number consist of uric acid or a substance called struvite. Stones form in the kidneys when an imbalance occurs among the amounts of water, calcium oxalate, uric acid, and phosphate that are normally present in the urine. Kidney stones can also form when the pH of the urine is abnormal or when the kidney's normal protective mechanisms are overwhelmed.

Other factors that may contribute to the formation of kidney stones include the following:

◆ Dehydration

◆ Sluggish or obstructed urine flow

◆ Systemic diseases such as gout, Cushing's disease, and hyperparathyroidism

◆ Hereditary metabolism problems

◆ Undergoing chemotherapy for cancer or receiving methoxyflourane anesthesia

◆ Using specific drugs, such as thyroid medications, vitamin D supplements, or aluminum salts (primarily antacids)

Whatever their cause, when kidney stones form, they are hard and crystallized. Thus, whenever such a stone is moving through the narrow urinary passageway, it causes excruciating pain in the side, usually below the ribs. The pain sometimes radiates into the lower abdomen or even the leg.

The pain from kidney stones is among the most severe caused by any disease. No one with this condition can be in doubt that something is terribly wrong. Sometimes the pain is accompanied by nausea, vomiting, inability to eat, and fever and chills.

In some cases a stone can completely block the flow of urine from the kidney. This can lead to infection and even to permanent kidney damage if not corrected. Usually blood is present in the urine during passage of a stone, even though it might not be enough to see with the naked eye.

Kidney stones always require prompt medical evaluation to rule out obstruction and secondary infection and to assess the cause of stone formation. Your doctor may recommend pain medication, surgery, or a procedure that uses sound waves to pulverize the stone.

Holistic and herbal approaches to kidney stones are appropriate to alleviate mild pain when there's no obstruction or infection involved and to help people prone to developing kidney stones avoid recurrences. Anyone having at least two episodes of stone formation should consider preventive treatment.

During an acute episode of kidney stone pain, strong painkillers are usually necessary. But if pain is mild and manageable, try using strong antispasmodic herbs to relax the ureter (the tube that connects each kidney to the bladder). Demulcent herbs form a protective coating on the urinary passages to minimize damage from the moving stone. Occasionally, such herbs are enough to ease pain and even allow the stone to pass out of the body.

Some herbs that may help fight recurring kidney stones contain compounds called anthraquinones, which bind with calcium in the urinary tract and prevent it from crystallizing into a stone. These herbs can have a laxative effect. If they give you loose stools or diarrhea, reduce your dose.

DRUG TREATMENT

There are no specific drugs to treat or prevent kidney stones, except in some very rare metabolic conditions. Depending on the type of stone you have, your doctor will likely recommend various dietary restrictions and an increase in your fluid intake.

HERBAL REMEDIES

Valerian (*Valeriana officinalis*)

This antispasmodic and strongly sedative herb may help the ureter relax enough to allow a small stone to pass. *Typical dosage:* 1 cup of tea every hour until the pain subsides (steep 1 to 2 teaspoons of dried herb in 1 cup of hot water for 10 to 15 minutes); or 1 teaspoon of tincture every hour until the pain subsides. This is a fairly high dose of valerian, so take it only for a day or so; discontinue if no results are seen by that time. *Caution:* Do not use during pregnancy.

Valerian

Skullcap (*Scutellaria lateriflora*)

Commonly used as a sedative, skullcap is also antispasmodic. *Typical dosage:* 1 cup of tea four times per day, or every hour until the pain eases (steep 1 to 2 teaspoons of dried herb in 1 cup of hot water for 10 to 15 minutes); or ¼ to 1 teaspoon of tincture four times per day or every hour until pain eases. If you see no results, try gradually increasing the dose.

Wild Yam (*Dioscorea villosa*)

This herb has long been used as an antispasmodic, but it's not a sedative. So if you need to stay awake, it may be a good alternative to valerian or skullcap. *Typical dosage:* up to two 400-milligram capsules per day; or ¼ to 1 teaspoon of tincture up to five times per day.

Khella (*Ammi visnaga*)

If some clinical studies and centuries of traditional use are any indication, this Middle Eastern herb may be helpful for kidney stones. It helps relax the muscles of the ureter and urinary tubules. Unfortunately, it is hard to find. *Typical dosage:* 250 to 300 milligrams of extract standardized to 12 percent khellin per day, in divided doses.

Marshmallow (*Althaea officinalis*)

This long-venerated demulcent may help soothe irritated urinary tissues. *Typical dosage:* up to six 400- to 500-milligram capsules

KIDNEY-FRIENDLY FOODS

The typical American or western European diet, with its high amounts of fat and sugar, appears to be a significant reason for the upswing in kidney stones. Stones are much less common in "developing" countries, where meals are higher in fiber and lower in animal protein. As a group, vegetarians have fewer kidney stones—but so do meat eaters who also eat lots of vegetables, fruit, and fiber. Obese people and those with diabetes are at increased risk of stone formation.

So, what's for dinner? Lots of leafy green vegetables. They're rich in vitamin K, which your body needs to build a urinary substance that normally prevents the formation of stones.

Magnesium and vitamin B_6 also reduce stone formation; include foods rich in these nutrients or take a daily supplement, 50 to 100 milligrams of each per day. In general, people with kidney stones shouldn't take calcium supplements. But if you need the extra calcium, take the citrate form, which is less likely to contribute to stones.

At meals, set a tall, cool glass of water by your plate—and a pitcher from which to refill it. Dehydration can set the

per day; or 1 cup of tea divided into three portions per day (steep 1 to 2 teaspoons of dried root in 1 cup of hot water for 10 to 15 minutes); or 20 to 40 drops of tincture up to five times per day. *Caution:* Marshmallow root may reduce the action of other drugs taken at the same time. If you're on any other medications, consult your doctor.

Slippery Elm (*Ulmus rubra*)

This useful bark contains high amounts of mucilage, the soothing, slippery substance that eases irritation and helps body tissues heal. *Typical dosage:* up to twelve 370-milligram capsules per day; or 2 to 3 cups of tea per day (steep ½ teaspoon of powdered bark in 1 cup of hot water for 10 to 15 minutes); or 10 to 30 drops of tincture up to five times per day. *Caution:* Slippery elm may reduce the actions of other drugs taken at the same time. If you're taking any other medications, consult your doctor.

stage for stone formation in susceptible people. You should drink six to eight 8-ounce glasses of water every day, especially after working up a sweat.

Two final tips: First, avoid antacids because they can increase your risk of stone formation. Second, if you smoke, quit. Cigarette smoking may contribute to kidney stones because it increases urine levels of cadmium, a heavy metal.

Foods Rich in Magnesium

- ◆ Dark green vegetables
- ◆ Nuts
- ◆ Seeds
- ◆ Legumes (peas, peanuts, some beans)
- ◆ Soy products
- ◆ Whole grains
- ◆ Avocados
- ◆ Dried apricots

Foods Rich in Vitamin B₆

- ◆ Brewer's yeast
- ◆ Egg yolks
- ◆ Fish
- ◆ Whole grains
- ◆ Legumes
- ◆ Sweet potatoes
- ◆ Cauliflower
- ◆ Avocados

Corn Silk (*Zea mays*)

Yes, it's those same strings you work so hard to get *out* of an ear of corn. Not only does a tea made from the fresh silk soothe and relax the urinary tubes, but it is also believed to have a beneficial effect on the kidneys themselves, reducing stone formation. *Typical dosage:* 4 to 6 cups of tea per day (steep 1 to 2 teaspoons of chopped dried herb, or a small handful of fresh herb, in 1 cup of hot water for 5 minutes); or ¼ to 1 teaspoon of tincture four or five times per day.

Aloe (*Aloe vera*)

This familiar burn remedy also contains anthraquinones, the compounds that help prevent kidney stones. *Typical dosage:* 1 teaspoon after meals, or follow practitioner's or manufacturer's directions. If you experience a laxative effect, reduce your dose.

Yellow Dock (*Rumex crispus*)

This traditional blood purifier also contains anthraquinones. While it's highly thought of in many herbal traditions, there hasn't been much research done on it. *Typical dosage:* up to four 500-milligram capsules per day; or 20 to 40 drops of tincture up to two times per day. *Caution:* If you experience diarrhea, decrease the dose. Avoid yellow dock during pregnancy.

LIBIDO PROBLEMS

DECREASED DESIRE FOR SEX IS OFTEN a side effect of an illness, an injury, or a drug. For instance, circulatory problems, diabetes, and high blood pressure can all cause a decrease in libido. These disorders should be treated by a doctor, but you may wish to consult a marriage counselor or other type of expert if you have trouble regaining your enjoyment of the things that bring you pleasure. Psychological issues such as stress, anxiety, guilt, and depression can be addressed through therapy.

Many drugs can decrease libido. If you experience this common side effect, see your doctor about trying other drugs or natural alternatives to them. If you're taking a prescription drug regularly, don't discontinue it or add herbs to your regimen without your doctor's advice.

One physiological cause of decreased libido is reduced hormone levels, specifically of the sex hormone testosterone. Both men and women can experience this phenomenon. It can be medically treated.

Erectile dysfunction, another cause of sexual problems in men, is not necessarily related to loss of desire—though it can certainly affect libido. Men who experience such dysfunction should see a doctor to diagnose any medical problems first. Any drug or herb that addresses this problem is bound to get considerable attention. (Before you fork over a lot of money for the next "herbal Viagra," for example, be sure to do your research on whether that remedy works and is safe for you to take.)

FEEDING YOUR DESIRE

Food can be the music of love—but there's also no accounting for tastes. Here are a few nutritional libido-boosters to investigate.

◆ **Oysters.** Scientists scoffed at oysters' sexual reputation until nutritionists discovered that the mollusks are exceptionally rich in the essential trace mineral zinc, which is related to male sexual health. Men with zinc-deficient diets are at high risk for infertility, prostate problems, and poor libido. University of Rochester researchers have restored sperm counts in infertile men using zinc supplements. Whole grains and fresh fruits and vegetables also contain zinc, but processed foods are often low in the mineral.

◆ **Caffeine.** If your sweetheart's thoughts turn to dreamland just as yours turn to dalliance, a cup of coffee with a chocolate bar on the side just might keep him or her awake long enough to make the most of the evening. But caffeine does more than simply keep the sandman at bay. One study found that regular coffee drinkers are considerably more sexually active than persons who don't drink coffee.

◆ **Chocolate.** Finally, an excuse to indulge! Chocolate contains not only caffeine but also high levels of phenylethylamine (PEA). Sexual medicine specialist Theresa Crenshaw, M.D., author of *The Alchemy of Love and Lust* and coauthor with James Goldberg, Ph.D., of *Sexual Pharmacology,* calls PEA the molecule of love. It's a natural form of stimulant and a natural antidepressant, according to Dr. Crenshaw. Both love and lust increase blood levels of PEA; but these levels plummet after a heartbreak.

Some experts say the PEA in chocolate gets metabolized so quickly that it couldn't have much effect. Perhaps. Nonetheless, giving chocolates is a longstanding, worldwide courtship ritual. Maybe it's the silky texture and creamy taste. Then again, maybe it's the PEA.

◆ **Oat bran.** Oat bran can provide an indirect sexual boost because of its effect on blood flow. It's now common knowledge that eating oat bran helps reduce artery-clogging cholesterol. Clear arteries to the genitals mean that more blood is available to produce erection in men and vaginal lubrication in women.

BEWARE THE TURNOFFS

If you want to rev up your sex life, first make sure that you don't shut it down. A surprisingly large number of everyday items don't mix with amorous intentions.

◆ **Alcohol.** In *Macbeth,* Shakespeare wrote that the substance used worldwide to coax reluctant lovers into bed "provokes the desire, but takes away the performance." Truer words were never penned. If people of average weight drink more than two beers, cocktails, or glasses of wine in an hour, the alcohol becomes a powerful central nervous system depressant. It interferes with erection in men and impairs sexual responsiveness in women.

◆ **Smoking.** One herb is bad news for sex: tobacco. Smoking narrows the blood vessels, impairing blood flow to the penis and causing an increased risk of erection impairment. In women, the same mechanism limits blood flow into the vaginal wall, decreasing vaginal lubrication.

◆ **Antidepressants.** A popular family of antidepressants, the selective serotonin reuptake inhibitors (SSRIs), which includes Prozac, Paxil, and Zoloft, elevate mood—but at a price. They carry a considerable risk of sexual side effects including loss of desire and difficulty reaching orgasm in both sexes, erection impairment in men, and lubrication problems in women. According to Jamie Grimes, M.D., chief of outpatient psychiatry at the Walter Reed Army Medical Center in Washington, D.C., they cause sex problems in more than half of those who use them. Other classes of antidepressants have similar sex-impairing side effects, except Wellbutrin.

Finally, some people find that as they age, their desire for sex wanes. But the belief that such decreases in libido are normal or unavoidable is only a myth. And there are natural ways to support your body's continued health and your own enjoyment. For those who simply want to know how to enhance an already satisfying sex life, there are some herbal remedies worth a try.

If you take an antidepressant, what can you do to preserve sexual function? Ask your physician about switching to Wellbutrin or trying a lower dose. St.-John's-wort, an herbal antidepressant, has no known sexual side effects.

◆ **Other legal drugs.** Many prescription and over-the-counter medications can cause sexual impairment—even the antihistamines that people take for allergies and cold symptoms. If the label says the drug may cause drowsiness, it can impair sexual desire or performance. Ask your doctor and pharmacist about the possibility of sexual side effects every time you get a prescription.

◆ **High-fat, high-cholesterol diet.** A study by researchers at the University of South Carolina School of Medicine in Columbia found that the higher a man's cholesterol, the more likely he is to suffer erection impairment.

Researchers tested the cholesterol levels of 3,250 men ages 25 to 83, then asked them to complete questionnaires that explored sexual issues. Compared with the men whose total cholesterol was below 180 milligrams per deciliter of blood, those with levels above 240 were almost twice as likely to report erection problems.

Cholesterol levels relate directly to consumption of dietary fat and cholesterol, found primarily in meats and dairy products. Ironically, many Americans consider meat a "virility food." In fact, it's the opposite. Men who want to enjoy sex without erection problems should forgo the steak and eat salads instead.

While some products marketed as natural aphrodisiacs are ineffective and even dangerous, newer research shows that sometimes herbalists of yore were on to something. A number of herbs or other natural products have physical effects that may qualify them as aphrodisiacs. And if you define *aphrodisiac* as anything that adds extra zing to lovemaking, then the possibilities are as boundless as the erotic imagination.

Drug Treatment

Hormone Replacement Therapy

Oral testosterone (Testex, Metandren), testosterone patch (Testoderm). *Function:* boost low testosterone levels to restore libido in men. *Side effects:* possible behavioral changes; patch can cause redness and itching.

Testosterone with estrogen (Estratest). *Function:* restore normal levels of testosterone in women. *Side effects:* acne, masculinizing effects such as slight growth of facial hair.

Other Drugs

Sildenafil (Viagra). *Function:* increase the amount of blood in the penis to cause stronger erections. *Side effects:* headache, stomach pain, nasal congestion, color blindness, significant drug interactions.

Herbal Remedies

Ginseng (*Panax ginseng*)

The Chinese and Koreans insist that ginseng strengthens exhausted sperm and impotent genitals. American scientists remain skeptical, but they acknowledge that several Asian animal studies show that ginseng stimulates sexual activity. While it is traditionally thought of as a man's remedy, some herbalists use it for women. Ginseng doesn't produce a quick fix and must be used regularly for several months before its effect becomes noticeable. *Typical dosage:* up to 2 cups of tea per day (steep ½ teaspoon of powdered root in 1 cup of hot water for 10 minutes); or follow manufacturer's instructions for packaged products. *Caution:* Consult your doctor before using ginseng if you have high blood pressure. Do not use during pregnancy.

Saw Palmetto (*Serenoa repens*)

Early American folk healers recommended the fruit of this small palm tree, which is native to the southeastern United States, as a diuretic and treatment for benign prostate enlargement, a common problem among men over age 50. Through the years, they extended saw palmetto's use to invigorating the genitals and enlarging women's breasts. Scientific research shows that saw palmetto won't boost anyone's libido or bra size, but it is a mild diuretic. About a dozen studies have shown that saw palmetto extract is about as effective in treating benign prostate enlargement as the drug Proscar. *Typical dosage:* up to three 585-milligram capsules of nonstandardized product per day; or 20 to 30 drops of tincture up to four times per day.

Wild Yam (*Dioscorea villosa*)

This tuber's sexual reputation springs from its use as a treatment for gynecological ailments. Wild yam is a potent source of diosgenin, a chemical that resembles female sex hormones and was used in the manufacture of the first oral contraceptives before scientists figured out how to make the required hormones in the laboratory. There is no credible evidence that wild yam arouses women sexually, but salves made from it can make intercourse more comfortable for women over 40 and are a fine substitute for estrogen creams used as vaginal lubricants. *Typical dosage:* use as needed.

Wild yam

Oats (*Avena sativa*)

Many ranchers swear that horses fed wild oats become friskier and more libidinous. When humans behave that way, we say they're "sowing their wild oats." The research is scant, but many herbalists recommend wild oats, often in combination with ginseng and yohimbe, in tea blends that supposedly possess aphrodisiacal effects. *Typical dosage:* up to 2 cups of tea per day (steep 1 tablespoon of dried tops in 1 cup of hot water for 10 to 15 minutes); or 25 drops of tincture three times per day.

Ginkgo (*Ginkgo biloba*)

Ginkgo, which has no traditional reputation as an aphrodisiac, is the newest arrival among sex-promoting herbs. During the past decade, a great deal of research has shown that it improves blood flow through the brain. Today, ginkgo is widely used in Europe to treat strokes and cerebral insufficiency, or poor circulation in the brain. Ginkgo also boosts blood flow into the penis. *Typical*

Sweat Is Sexy

Want more sexual heat? Then work up a sweat. One indisputable aphrodisiac is exercise. James White, Ph.D., professor emeritus of physical education at the University of California at San Diego, recruited 95 healthy but sedentary men with an average age of 47 to follow one of two exercise programs. One involved low-intensity, 60-minute walks four times a week, the other an hour of aerobics for the same amount of time. After nine months, both groups reported increased sexual desire and pleasure, but the aerobics group reported the greatest increase.

Exercise leads to fitness. And fitness, says Louanne Cole, Ph.D., a California sex therapist, boosts self-esteem. "You feel healthier and more attractive and you project that, so you look more alluring to prospective lovers," she explains.

The same could be said for weight loss—shedding a few pounds often boosts interest in sex. A psychologist at the Duke University Diet and Fitness Center in Durham, N.C., noticed that people who lost weight at the center often remarked that they felt more sexual. She surveyed 70 male program participants ages 18 to 65 before and after a weight loss of 8 to 30 pounds. After losing weight, they all reported more sexual desire. Excess weight makes most people feel less desirable and more anxious about being seen naked, she says. In other words, fat causes stress and stress interferes with desire. Carrying extra weight also requires a good deal of energy. Dropping pounds frees that energy for other uses.

dosage: 3 capsules per day, each containing at least 40 milligrams of standardized extract.

Damiana (*Turnera diffusa* var. *aphrodisiaca*)

Whereas many traditional aphrodisiacs have shown at least some stimulating effects, nothing even remotely libidinous has ever been discovered about damiana, despite the *aphrodisiaca* in its scientific name. This herb is safe, however, so it won't hurt you or your partner. And if you really believe it's an aphrodisiac, the placebo effect may turn it into one for you. *Typical dosage:* up to six 400-milligram capsules per day; or up to 3 cups of tea per day (steep 1 teaspoon of dried herb in 1 cup of hot water for 10 to 15 minutes); or 20 to 60 drops of tincture in water three times per day.

LIVER DISEASE

Y OU DON'T SEE IT, YOU DON'T FEEL IT, and you might even be unsure of its location, but all day long your liver is working for you. It's far more important to your overall health than you probably realize, unless you're already having problems with it.

We think of the liver as an organ of detoxification, but this is merely one of its more important functions. The liver also filters the blood, removing harmful bacteria and chemicals; breaks down excess hormones; and helps maintain water and body-fluid salt balances. The liver assists in the digestion and metabolism of fats, carbohydrates, and proteins, the storage and production of some vitamins and minerals, and the manufacture of a wide variety of proteins and immune substances. The liver makes glycogen out of sugar and then stores it. Glycogen can be converted into glucose, or blood sugar, when the body needs it. Because of its production of bile, the liver contributes not only to elimination of drugs and toxins but also to the absorption of fats and the fat-soluble vitamins.

But what's truly amazing about the liver is how quickly and efficiently it works. Every minute, over a liter of blood passes through it.

Much is known about the complex chemical events that occur when the liver does its work. The first phase involves the chemical alteration of certain substances into nontoxic forms. The second phase makes these compounds water soluble, enabling the body to excrete them via the kidneys.

Specific nutrients are required for each phase. When the body is subjected to higher-than-normal levels of contaminants, its entire supply of necessary nutrients could be depleted. When a deficiency of any one of the nutrients occurs, the chemical processes might slow or even stop.

During phase 1, the detoxification phase, your liver needs riboflavin, niacin, magnesium, iron, molybdenum, and essential fatty acids. When phase 1 is very active, the body needs extra vitamin A, C, and E. Phase 2 requires zinc, copper, molybdenum, thiamine, pantothenic acid, vitamin B_6, folic acid, a host of amino acids, and sulfur. You can see by this list the importance of a nutritious, varied diet that supplies a wide range of vitamins and minerals.

Many different factors and conditions affect liver function and lead to liver disease. These include viruses, metabolic disorders, hereditary conditions, cancers, exposure to toxins such as alcohol, and more. But someone not affected by these conditions might nevertheless develop subclinical liver disease, meaning that the disease isn't pronounced enough to show itself in symptoms but still negatively affects overall health.

The primary cause of this subclinical condition is the profound effect pollutants have on the environment. No matter how careful you are, there's almost no escaping unhealthy chemical exposure. Your liver can easily be overwhelmed or subtly damaged.

One common subclinical liver problem is cholestasis, sometimes called sluggish or congested liver. It's caused by an impaired flow of bile. The liver produces bile, stores it in the gallbladder and then, when fat is present in the digestive tract, releases it into the duodenum—the first section of the small intestine. A sluggish bile flow causes problems in digesting fats and detoxifying certain substances. Common symptoms of cholestasis include gas, bloating, constipation, fatigue, increased allergies, chemical sensitivities, and premenstrual syndrome.

If you have a liver disease, you'll want to take herbs to support the liver. But among the organ's wonderful attributes is its good response to preventive therapy. So certain herbs can also help people who must take drugs that are potentially toxic to the liver. Such herbs can also provide relief to those with hormonal imbalances, headaches, chronic skin conditions, fatigue, digestive complaints, allergies, and chemical sensitivities.

DRUG TREATMENT

With a few exceptions, no specific Western drugs exist for most non-hepatitis types of liver disease. Most doctors don't even recognize subclinical liver disease or cholestasis as a problem; it's rare that prevention of such ailments is addressed. The only common recommendation is that liver toxins such as alcohol should be avoided when low-grade liver disease is present.

HERBAL REMEDIES

Milk Thistle (*Silybum marianum*)

This herb is the quintessential liver protector and healer. A great deal of scientific research has verified how well it heals. This amazing herb protects liver cells from damaging molecules called free radicals, inhibits production of leukotrienes—inflammatory compounds responsible for some types of liver damage—and boosts the production of glutathione, one of the liver's hardworking chemicals, by 35 percent. Milk thistle alters liver cell membranes, making it more difficult for the toxins flowing past them to break in. It stimulates the flow of bile, which helps the digestive system do *its* work. Finally, this herb helps increase liver cell regeneration when damage has occurred. All this without side effects other than occasional loose stools. *Typical dosage:* 70 to 210 milligrams of capsules containing milk thistle's active ingredient, silymarin, three times per day; or ¼ to 1 teaspoon of milk thistle tincture three times per day.

Milk thistle

Dandelion Root (*Taraxacum officinale*)

Don't rid your yard of this weed; it's an excellent traditional liver remedy. The bitter constituents in the root enhance liver function by increasing production of bile and improving gallbladder function. Dandelion also contains choline, a form of B vitamin that's involved in normal liver function. Dandelion root is rich in vitamins and minerals, improves digestion, and may even lower cholesterol. *Typical dosage:* 1 cup of tea three times per day (simmer 1 teaspoon of dried, chopped root in 1 cup of water for 10 minutes).

Turmeric (*Curcuma longa*)

This aromatic yellow herb gives Indian curry dishes their unique flavor and color. In addition to its many other medicinal benefits,

A LIVER-LOVING LIFESTYLE

What else can you do to maintain a healthy liver? Here are a few sure strategies.

◆ **Eat well.** Vegetables of the *Brassica* family—the familiar broccoli, cabbage, and cauliflower plus the less familiar Brussels sprouts—all help spur the liver to do its detoxification work. Caraway and dill seeds have this effect, too, so try sprinkling them freely on a big bowl of steamed brassicas.

◆ **Work up a healthy sweat.** Physical activity increases the first phase of the liver's detoxification cycle by almost 60 percent—but only when you exercise regularly. It takes about a month of regular workouts for the effects to show up.

◆ **Avoid toxins when you can.** While you can't stop breathing, you can eat organically grown foods and avoid toxic chemicals in household cleaning products and lawn and garden supplies. Don't smoke, keep your alcohol consumption to a minimum, and never use drugs you don't absolutely need. Common over-the-counter drugs such as acetaminophen and ibuprofen can cause liver damage when used long-term; if you take these drugs routinely and drink, the effect is even worse. Finally, become an activist in your community to stop the spread of air, water, and soil pollution. You might make a difference in not just your own liver's health, but the overall health of those around you.

turmeric's antioxidant properties protect the liver from numerous toxic chemicals. It can nearly double bile output and increase the solubility of bile, thus preventing and treating gallstones. Finally, turmeric has been shown to reduce cancer-causing agents in the urine of smokers, lowering the level of these toxins in the body. *Typical dosage:* for general, preventive support of the liver, cook with turmeric about three times a week; or take 250 to 500 milligrams in capsules two to three times per day with meals; or ⅛ to ½ teaspoon of turmeric tincture or glycerite (glycerin extract) three times per day. Taking turmeric along with the same amount of bromelain, an enzyme found in pineapple, may increase absorption. *Caution:* Some people experience gastrointestinal irritation when using turmeric. The spice may increase hot flashes in menopausal women.

Licorice (*Glycyrrhiza glabra*)

This root has many medicinal benefits, inhibiting injury to the liver with an antioxidant compound called glycyrrhetic acid. Its antiviral effects make it especially helpful when viral hepatitis is the cause of liver damage. *Typical dosage:* ⅛ to 1 teaspoon of tincture up to three times per day; or 1 to 3 cups of tea per day (simmer 1 heaping teaspoon of dried, chopped root in 1 cup of water for 15 minutes). Be sure not to purchase DGL, or deglycyrrhizinated licorice; this form is used to treat ulcers and doesn't contain the necessary liver-healing compounds. *Caution:* Do not use for longer than six weeks unless under the supervision of a qualified practitioner. Do not use if you have heart disease or high blood pressure, if you are pregnant, or if you are taking digitalis-based heart medications.

Bupleurum (*Bupleurum chinensis*)

This traditional Chinese herb protects against liver damage. It also stimulates parts of the immune system. Studies on bupleurum have focused mainly on the treatment of viral hepatitis, where it has been proven to be beneficial. *Typical dosage:* ⅛ to 1 teaspoon of tincture three times per day; or 1 cup of tea three times per day (simmer 1 teaspoon of dried sliced root in 1 cup of water for 10 to 15 minutes).

Schisandra (*Schisandra chinensis*)

The berries of this plant protect the liver from damage by a variety of substances, probably via its antioxidant effects. It is also a mild adaptogen, meaning that it gradually improves overall health—a big help when chronic stress is part of your life. *Typical dosage:* up to six 580-milligram capsules per day; or 1 cup of tea three times per day (simmer ⅓ to 1½ teaspoons of dried fruit in 1 cup of water for 10 to 15 minutes); or ⅛ to 1 teaspoon of tincture or glycerite up to three times per day.

LYME DISEASE

WHEN IT COMES TO LISTS OF favorite creatures, nobody rates ticks very high. You'll never see them listed in glossy brochures that crow about the wildlife that graces a particular natural area or national forest.

But you can be sure that wherever warm-blooded animals thrive, ticks are likely to prosper as well. And depending on your location, some of these ticks are likely to be *Ixodes scapularis,* the deer tick. Deer ticks spread Lyme disease when a specific bacterium infects them. The tick bites you, the bacteria enter your bloodstream, and you're exposed to a chronic disease that can take years to become full-blown. Lyme disease causes a multitude of symptoms, including neurological problems, cardiac problems, and arthritis. It's enough to make an avid hiker stay home and watch the Outdoor Channel instead.

Lyme disease is one of those illnesses to which it is easy to underreact *and* overreact. It's difficult to diagnose because the symptoms are not only vague, but also similar to those of other diseases, especially the flu. Moreover, there are no definitive laboratory tests for Lyme disease. The disorder progresses in three seemingly unrelated stages. The first appears as a bull's-eye rash three days to four weeks after the tick bite. The rash may be accompanied by headache, fever, chills, and a feeling of tiredness. One key to diagnosis is noticing both the rash and the flu-like symptoms at the same time.

The second stage, which begins weeks to months later, brings pain in the joints and muscles, along with meningitis, irregular heartbeat, or inflammation of the sac surrounding the heart. When this stage occurs, the victim may have forgotten the first stage.

Finally, months or even years later, the third stage begins. It's characterized by more severe problems affecting the skin, nervous system, and joints.

As frightening as all this is, Lyme disease is usually over-diagnosed. Full treatment is often given to any patient suspected of having Lyme disease because the full-blown symptoms are so serious. Although this is an effective means of prevention, it results in

BITING BACK WITH NUTRIENTS

The following supplements may help you recover from an encounter with Lyme disease, actual or probable. And if it turns out to be a false alarm, the supplements are also good for overall health.

- **Essential fatty acids.** Plant sources include evening primrose oil, black currant seed oil, borage oil, and flaxseed oil. These oils can benefit many symptoms associated with Lyme disease, including fatigue, arthritis, heart disease, and neurological problems. *Typical dosage:* 1,400 to 3,000 milligrams per day of evening primrose oil, black currant seed oil, or borage oil. The less expensive option is 2 tablespoons per day of flaxseed oil.

- **Coenzyme Q$_{10}$.** Also called ubiquinone, this enzyme is an antioxidant and immune stimulant. It may improve stamina and general well-being. *Typical dosage:* 60 to 200 milligrams per day, divided into two doses if you are not a vegetarian. (Because coenzyme Q$_{10}$ is present in high amounts in vegetables, vegetarians already get enough.)

- **B-complex vitamins.** These vitamins are necessary for efficient nerve and immune function. Vegetarians in particular may want to take a B-complex supplement to treat the neurological symptoms of Lyme disease. *Typical dosage:* one to two 50-milligram B-complex capsules per day. Make sure they include 50 milligrams of thiamine, riboflavin, niacin, B$_6$, and pantothenic acid, plus 50 micrograms of B$_{12}$ and biotin and 100 micrograms of folic acid.

- **Magnesium.** This mineral is an important component of many cellular functions, including energy production. *Typical dosage:* 400 milligrams per day.

THWARTING TICKS AND LYME DISEASE

If you don't get bitten, you don't get Lyme disease. Here are some simple ways to keep ticks away.

◆ **Wear appropriate clothing when you go outdoors.** Roll socks over the cuffs of long pants; tuck in your shirt, and button the cuffs of long-sleeved shirts. This keep ticks from having access to the skin. And even if you hate chemical repellents, you can spray the clothing that covers your ankles and calves.

◆ **Do a tick check once you're indoors.** After returning home, trade tick checks with a partner. Generally, ticks must feed for 24 to 48 hours to pass on the infection, so you are safe if you find the little bloodsuckers right away.

◆ **Pluck them properly.** To remove a tick from your skin, use a tweezers to grab its head, not its body, and pull steadily.

the overuse of antibiotics. It may also mean doctors are missing other serious health problems because they're prepared to see only Lyme disease.

If you suspect you have Lyme disease, be safe and see a practitioner experienced in diagnosing and appropriately treating this condition.

There are no researched herbal treatments for Lyme disease. But James A. Duke, Ph.D., botanical medicine proponent and author of *The Green Pharmacy,* suggests using herbs that boost the immune system along with antibiotics, or taking just the herbs if you're not certain the bite was from a deer tick.

If you do take antibiotics, you will certainly need to replenish the beneficial bacteria that help your body digest food and fight off less harmful "bugs." So if your doctor prescribes antibiotics, eat yogurt containing active cultures or take a probiotic supplement containing *Lactobacillus acidophilus* and/or *Bifidobacterium bifidum.* Take as directed on the label.

Drug Treatment

Drug treatment for Lyme disease consists of high doses of antibiotics, usually tetracycline or penicillin. Sometimes such antibiotics are used—although with much controversy—to prevent the development of Lyme disease when a person knows she has been bitten by a deer tick. Most doctors are concerned that antibiotic-resistant strains of the bacteria that cause Lyme disease may develop because of the overuse of these antibiotics.

Penicillin side effects include decreases in some types of white blood cells. In children, they can include kidney inflammation, bleeding, rashes, and changes in blood pH. Tetracycline side effects may include deformities in growing bones, localized allergic reactions, nausea and vomiting, diarrhea, liver and kidney damage, bleeding, increased sun sensitivity in fair-skinned people, dizziness, and vertigo.

Herbal Remedies

Licorice (*Glycyrrhiza glabra*)

According to Dr. Duke, licorice contains the most antibacterial isoflavonoid compounds of any herb. He recommends it highly for bacterial conditions such as Lyme disease. *Typical dosage:* 5,000 to 6,000 milligrams of the dried, powdered root in capsules per day; or 1 to 2 cups of tea per day (simmer 1 teaspoon of dried, chopped root in 1 cup of hot water for 30 minutes). *Caution:* Do not use for more than six weeks unless under the supervision of a qualified practitioner. Not for use by those with heart disease, liver disease, or high blood pressure, or by women who are pregnant.

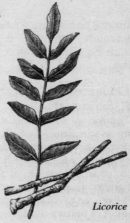

Licorice

Garlic (*Allium sativum*)

This bulb yields odoriferous oils, most notably allicin, that offer proven antibiotic activity against a wide range of bacteria and

THE NOT-QUITE VACCINE

At the time of this writing, a vaccine against Lyme disease had just been approved by the U.S. Food and Drug Administration—but the committee's approval was guarded. Many unanswered questions remain about the vaccine. Its long-term effectiveness and side effects are unknown, as are its safety and effectiveness for children.

Of most concern to some experts is the danger that vaccinated people will become complacent in their efforts to avoid tick bites. This puts those people at greater risk of other tick-borne diseases, including ehrlichiosis, babesiosis, Rocky Mountain spotted fever, and tularemia—all of which are serious or life-threatening.

The new vaccines also require three injections over the span of a year to reach a 92 percent effectiveness rate. It's likely that research into different and better vaccines will continue.

fungi. The oils have not been tested specifically against the bacteria causing Lyme disease, however. *Typical dosage:* Dr. Duke suggests capsules equivalent to 1,200 milligrams of fresh garlic per day.

Echinacea (*Echinacea angustifolia, E. pallida, E. purpurea*)

The root of this purple wildflower is the most well-known immune-stimulating herb. It can be taken along with garlic. Most herbalists recommend starting echinacea at the first sign of any symptoms and taking it frequently until symptoms have subsided, for up to eight weeks at a time. *Typical dosage:* 400 to 800 milligrams in capsules per day (when Dr. Duke suspected he had Lyme disease, he took capsules to equal 2,700 milligrams per day); or 60 drops of tincture three times per day.

MACULAR DEGENERATION

EVEN IF YOU HAVEN'T THE VAGUEST idea what macular degeneration is, it probably doesn't sound good. And it isn't: This eye condition, which involves the deterioration of the center of the retina, is the leading cause of progressive blindness in people age 65 and older.

Macular degeneration can be caused by exposure to light or chemicals as well as by normal metabolic processes. Another culprit is free radicals, those rogue compounds that steal electrons from healthy cells. Free radicals oxidize fatty acids in cell membranes and in enzyme systems. Within the retina of the eye, such cell damage can disturb energy production and the chemical balance of the eye's fluids.

Antioxidants in your body can counteract this process, but they can't do it fast enough when free radical levels are high or when your diet is deficient in antioxidants. That's why poor diet is a risk factor for macular degeneration.

Other factors include family history of the disorder, aging, high blood pressure, and heart disease narrowing the arteries.

Macular degeneration can be diagnosed in its earliest stages, a good reason to see your eye doctor annually even if you have no symptoms. People who already have macular degeneration should keep regular appointments with an eye doctor to monitor their response to treatment.

DRUG TREATMENT

Conventional Western ophthalmologists often suggest taking antioxidants as a treatment for macular degeneration. Several antioxidant brands, such as Ocutive, I-caps, and OcuGuard, are specifically formulated for the condition. Clinical studies have confirmed that best results are obtained when using combinations of selenium, vitamins C and E, and beta-carotene.

When macular degeneration is detected early, its progress may

KEEPING YOUR SIGHT CLEAR

Lifestyle changes not only can help treat macular degeneration but also can prevent it. If you have the disorder or have a family history of it, here are some tips.

◆ **Protect your eyes.** Avoid excess exposure to the sun; wear good-quality protective sunglasses to shield your eyes from the sun's ultraviolet radiation.

◆ **Stop smoking.** In addition to the other health problems they cause, cigarettes increase free radicals, one of the causes of macular degeneration.

◆ **Avoid other chemical exposures.** They're also a source of free radicals.

◆ **Boost antioxidants in your diet.** Eat more carrots, squash, and other orange and yellow vegetables, as well as dark, leafy greens and flavor-rich berries such as blueberries, huckleberries, blackberries, and cherries. Citrus fruits are high in vitamin C, the best-known antioxidant; beans and peas provide antioxidant amino acids.

be slowed by laser surgery, which preserves your sight for a longer period of time. Laser surgery is also used for a rare variety of the disease called exudative macular degeneration, in which a part of the retina discharges a pus-like substance.

HERBAL REMEDIES

Bilberry (*Vaccinium myrtillus*)
This anthocyanoside-rich herb has strong antioxidant effects. *Typical dosage:* one 80- to 160-milligram extract capsule standardized to 25 percent anthocyanidin three times per day. *Caution:* In rare cases bilberry may cause gastrointestinal upset, dizziness, or headaches.

Bilberry

Ginkgo (*Ginkgo biloba*)
Another powerful antioxidant, ginkgo has been shown to improve vision in people with macular degeneration. *Typical dosage:* one 40- to 60-milligram capsule standardized to 24 percent flavone glycosides three times per day. *Caution:* Ginkgo may cause gastrointestinal upset, dizziness, or headaches.

Memory Loss

MISPLACED YOUR KEYS LATELY? Or dialed a phone number and forgotten whom you were calling? Temporary lapses in memory are a common phenomenon. Unfortunately, they occur with greater frequency as you get older.

The ability to retain new information is one of the first mental functions that declines with aging. The odd consequence is that older people can sometimes remember an event that happened 10 years ago better than what they did 10 minutes ago.

The conversion of experience into memory is a complex biochemical process, of which scientists have only a limited understanding. In the same way that a computer has a working memory that is discarded if it is not saved onto a hard drive, your brain sorts through a lot of information that it does not retain unless you have a reason to preserve it. Vivid experiences that are rich in images, sounds, touch, or emotions tell the brain that something significant is happening—something worth remembering. So you are much more likely to recall information associated with these kinds of sensations than you are a telephone number.

Good memory requires the ability to not just store information but also retrieve that information on demand. Consequently, when your attention is distracted by something, you have a harder time learning new things and retaining them. Part of the "normal" age-related decline in memory results from the cumulative demands on attention that build over a lifetime.

Another aspect of age-related memory loss has to do with a deficiency of the brain's chemical messengers, called neurotransmitters. Although this deficiency may be years in the making, its symptoms rarely surface before you reach your early to mid-fifties. One chem-

KEEPING A HEALTHY MEMORY

The best way to help your brain work better is to keep your body healthy. The methods are probably nothing new to you, but the reasons these strategies affect brain function may be.

◆ **Get up and sweat.** A lifelong program of regular physical activity is essential. Aerobic exercise boosts circulation and sends more oxygen-enriched blood to the brain. The simple act of walking is a workout for the brain as well as the body. Exercise also helps decrease high blood pressure, which has been associated with mental deterioration.

◆ **Think about it.** A healthy attitude combined with ongoing mental stimulation is just as important for maintaining the skills of memory and concentration. Studies show that people who seek new intellectual challenges throughout their lives are more likely to stay mentally alert and active as they get older. Other research indicates that chronic stress interferes with concentration and damages brain cells. Meditation and other stress reduction techniques can be a valuable antidote.

ical appears to be intimately involved in the conversion of working memory into permanent memory: acetylcholine. Many of the drugs and nutritional supplements used to help improve memory do so by increasing levels of acetylcholine in the brain.

It is important to distinguish intermittent forgetfulness from permanent or progressive loss of memory. Everyone is familiar with the "absent-minded professor" character who is so preoccupied with a project that he forgets to put on his socks in the morning. This kind of forgetfulness may be amusing, annoying, or embarrassing, but it's not a cause for medical concern. But if memory loss involves information critical to your ability to function, this can indicate a medical problem. If you forget how to get back home from the grocery store or can't remember the name of your partner, consult a doctor for a thorough evaluation.

Progressive memory loss is part of a condition that neurologists

- **Colorize your diet.** By eating foods that are rich in carotenes and flavonoids—that's right, those colorful fruits and vegetables—you can help protect blood vessels and brain tissue. On the other hand, high amounts of saturated fats and trans-fatty acids (found in margarine and commercial baked goods) have been found to increase the risk of Alzheimer's disease. The polyunsaturated fats found in cold-water fish such as salmon, mackerel, halibut, and tuna are very beneficial to brain tissue and may protect against mental decline.

- **Boost your Es and Cs.** Two specific supplements have been found to be especially important to brain function. A daily dose of 400 IU of vitamin E appears to protect brain cells. In even higher amounts (1,000 to 2,000 IU per day), it has been shown to slow the progression of Alzheimer's disease. Vitamin C, in doses of 2,000 to 6,000 milligrams daily, may have similar effects.

- **Learn to love lecithin.** An extract of soybeans, lecithin is the source of several chemicals that help maintain healthy levels of neurotransmitters in the brain. Taken in doses of up to 10 grams daily, lecithin is an excellent preventive for age-related memory disorders.

and other brain specialists call dementia, a diagnosis that means a widespread disruption in the brain's ability to function properly. Along with loss of memory come impairments in concentration, judgment, reasoning, and comprehension that are severe enough to interfere with normal daily activities.

When dementia occurs in adults younger than 50, it may be related to any number of factors, including viral infection, syphilis, alcoholism, vitamin B_{12} deficiency, brain tumor, hemorrhage, blood clots, thyroid disorders, manic depression, or severe depression. In the elderly, the most common reasons for dementia are Alzheimer's disease and strokes associated with hardening of the arteries.

Because it is difficult to diagnose and treat, Alzheimer's disease is probably the most dreaded cause of memory loss. It affects up to two million Americans—nearly half of those who live to age 85. Despite extensive research, its cause remains unknown. What is known is that it involves the irreversible and widespread loss of brain cells, which can lead to death within eight to ten years. Alzheimer's may represent the end stage of a long process of brain-cell deterioration. About 15 percent of people with age-associated memory impairment progress to Alzheimer's disease every year.

DRUG TREATMENT

Acetylcholinesterase Inhibitors
Tacrine (THA, Cognex), donepezil (Aricept). *Function:* provide mild improvement in mental function for Alzheimer's patients. *Side effects:* nausea, vomiting, sweating, watery eyes, increased salivation, diarrhea.

MAO-B Inhibitors
Selegiline/deprenyl (Eldepryl). *Function:* prevent the destruction of certain neurotransmitters in the brain and increase their levels. *Side effects:* drowsiness, dizziness, sexual dysfunction, insomnia, drug interactions.

Other Drugs
Ergoloid mesylate (Hydergine). *Function:* improve overall memory and other brain functions. *Side effects:* mild nausea.

HERBAL REMEDIES

Ginkgo (*Ginkgo biloba*)
The leaves of this tree have been used for over 2,500 years as a Traditional Chinese Medicine for mental and respiratory disorders. About 30 years ago, a highly concentrated extract (50 pounds of leaf to make 1 pound of extract) was developed in Germany. Since that time, more than 50 studies have shown ginkgo's effectiveness in treating dementia from strokes and early-stage Alzheimer's disease. Its effectiveness is comparable to that of the drug tacrine. Ginkgo is also used to prevent and treat age-related memory loss and chronic tinnitus (ringing in the ears). *Typical dosage:* 120 to 140 milligrams daily of an extract standardized to 24 percent flavonoid glycosides and 6 percent terpene lactones. *Caution:* Do not combine with blood-thinning medications such as warfarin (Coumadin) or aspirin, or with high doses of vitamin E.

Bacopa (*Bacopa monniera*)

This plant, commonly called water hyssop, is the source of an extract used in India for centuries. It has specific benefits for the brain, and specialists in Ayurvedic medicine commonly use it to treat mental illness and epilepsy. Bacopa appears to strengthen memory and improve concentration by enhancing the conductivity of nerve tissue. It also has mild sedative and antianxiety properties. Bacopa is most often found in commercial formulas used for memory symptoms. As with all manufactured herbal products, read the label carefully and follow the manufacturer's directions on dosage.

Club Moss (*Huperzia serrata*)

An ingredient in the Traditional Chinese Medicine remedy Qian Ceng Ta, club moss has been used for centuries to treat fever and inflammation. More recently, Qian Ceng Ta was found to contain a substance called huperzine A (HupA). This substance acts similarly to the drugs tacrine and donepezil, but it appears to be more potent and cause fewer side effects. In recent years it has been used in China to treat more than 100,000 patients with dementia. Huperzine A also appears to shield brain cells from injury and it may be useful in treating strokes and epilepsy. Huperzine A is sold over the counter in health food stores. Although it is used primarily to treat the early stages of Alzheimer's, many people are taking it to improve memory and enhance mental alertness. *Typical dosage:* 50 to 100 micrograms in capsules twice daily.

Siberian Ginseng (*Eleutherococcus senticosus*)

This revered tonic from Eastern Russia was used as a folk medicine to help people endure harsh winters. The scientist who first studied Siberian ginseng coined the term "adaptogen" to describe the herb's ability to normalize the functions of many body systems. The effects were confirmed in several large medical studies performed in the former Soviet Union. In addition to improving overall health, Siberian ginseng restores memory, increases stamina, stabilizes blood sugar, and boosts the immune system. *Typical dosage:* 100 to 200 milligrams of standardized extract one to three times per day; or 30 drops of tincture one to three times per day.

Siberian ginseng

MENOPAUSE

SOME WOMEN SPEAK OF MENOPAUSE with an ominous tone of dread as a time of hot flashes, uncontrollable moods, and dwindling desires. Other women embrace The Change with a relentlessly upbeat attitude, heralding it as a glamorous, even fascinating time of life to be greeted wearing running shoes and a sexy smile.

VITAMINS AND SUPPLEMENTS FOR MENOPAUSE

Mounting evidence suggests that getting enough of certain vitamins and other nutrients can make menopause a breeze.

◆ **Vitamin E.** Tests dramatically support its use for hot flashes and other symptoms of menopause. In some tests, vitamin E worked better than barbiturates to calm anxiety, cool hot flashes, protect against heart disease, and ease vaginal dryness. *Typical dosage:* 200 to 800 IU per day.

◆ **Vitamin C with bioflavonoids.** Clinical studies of women in menopause found that half experienced relief from discomfort by using vitamin C with the bioflavonoid hesperidin. Leg cramps, bruising, and hot flashes significantly decreased. *Typical dosage:* 500 to 5,000 milligrams per day.

◆ **Calcium/magnesium.** This dynamic duo of minerals helps prevent osteoporosis and ease mental stress and anxiety. In fact, adding supplemental calcium to the diet as early as age 20 can increase bone density, which puts you ahead in the race against bone loss after menopause. Use absorbable forms such as calcium citrate, gluconate, or carbonate. *Typical dosage:* 1,000 to 1,500 milligrams of calcium per day in a 2:1 ratio with magnesium. So if you take 1,000 milligrams of calcium, take 500 milligrams of magnesium, too.

Regardless of how you feel about menopause, if you're female, you will go through it. But you'll have plenty of company: In the next two decades, more than 40 million American women will experience menopause. If you're one of these women, chances are that at least 25 years of your life will be post-menopausal. Now there's a reason for positive thinking: 25 years of being period-free.

Menopause occurs when the ovaries' production of the hormones estrogen and progesterone greatly decreases. This dwindling hormone supply can occur suddenly or it can take several months. Although it can cause a variety of physical and emotional symptoms,

- ◆ **B-complex vitamins.** These nutrients help to reduce water retention, combat fatigue, and prevent nervous and mental disorders. In fact, vitamin B_6 injections have been used to reduce hot flashes and treat mood disorders. Take a good daily B-complex supplement that provides at least 25 to 50 milligrams of vitamin B_6, 50 to 100 micrograms of B_{12}, and 400 to 1,000 micrograms of folic acid.

- ◆ **Selenium.** This mineral helps to maintain normal hormone function; some research suggests it may also brighten moods and help fend off heart disease. *Typical dosage:* 200 micrograms per day.

- ◆ **Acidophilus:** These beneficial bacteria work to prevent vaginitis, yeast infections, and cystitis, problems that can crop up more frequently after menopause. *Typical dosage:* 2 to 6 capsules daily; or 1 teaspoon of liquid one to three times daily.

- ◆ **Evening primrose oil.** This oil contributes to estrogen production and works as a sedative and a diuretic. It has also helped some women control hot flashes. Using flaxseed oil with evening primrose oil can help you maintain a healthy cardiovascular system. *Typical dosage:* 800 to 1,200 milligrams standardized to 20 percent gamma-linolenic acid, or GLA, per day. To help your heart, supplement your evening primrose oil with 1 to 2 tablespoons of flaxseed oil per day.

Danger Signs and Symptoms

Bleeding between periods or prolonged or excessive menstrual bleeding may indicate the presence of a uterine tumor. Bleeding after menopause is not normal; if this happens, contact your doctor for an evaluation.

there are some things it does *not* do: It does not redistribute fat, contribute to a loss of muscle tone, or cause wrinkles to appear. If you're experiencing these phenomena, blame other causes.

The first phase of menopause is sometimes called perimenopause. It is characterized by the fluctuation of estrogen levels, which can begin as early as age 35 in some women. Common symptoms of perimenopause include erratic periods, both in terms of length and amount of flow, breast tenderness, headaches, food cravings, irritability, forgetfulness, and mood swings.

Some women describe perimenopause as nothing more than a bad case of PMS, or premenstrual syndrome. So if you've always experienced PMS, you're probably wondering how to tell when those trials end and the trials of perimenopause begin.

Whatever symptoms you may have, the important thing is to anticipate menopause as a natural event and prepare for it. Exercise and proper nutrition can ease a woman's passage through the menopausal years, diminishing many symptoms to the point where drugs are unnecessary.

Hormone replacement therapy (HRT) is the most common drug treatment prescribed for symptoms of menopause. But it's also the subject of some controversy. Estrogen is thought to help slow osteoporosis and reduce a woman's risk for heart attack and heart disease, two of the leading killers of postmenopausal women. But some data challenge the notion that estrogen protects the heart.

What's more, HRT is not without its risks, including the possible development of ovarian, uterine, and breast cancer. It has even been linked to autoimmune disorders such as lupus. A safer technique might be to boost the intake of natural estrogen-like compounds called phytoestrogens in your diet.

In addition to HRT, tranquilizers, antidepressants, and sleeping pills are sometimes prescribed for specific menopausal symptoms. But these drugs have their own attendant side effects.

Several herbs can act as hormonal precursors—that is, they help the body build estrogen molecules when the hormone is running low. Other herbs help ease or even eliminate hot flashes, the anxiety and depression that may accompany menopause, and other symptoms associated with hormone fluctuation and dysfunction.

DRUG TREATMENT

Hormone Replacement Drugs

Estradiol (DepGynogen). *Function:* add estrogen when the body stops producing it to alleviate hot flashes, decrease bone loss, and

WORKING UP A SWEAT TO COOL HOT FLASHES

It's no joke: Clinical studies have found that women who engage in regular physical activity are half as likely to experience menopausal hot flashes as women who don't. Exercise is also one of the most important weapons against the increased risk of osteoporosis and heart disease that women are exposed to after menopause. And working up a sweat marshals endorphins, the body's own mood-menders and painkillers.

Most experts recommend an aerobic, weight-bearing workout three to five times per week for 35 to 45 minutes. There are lots of exercise options out there: cycling, brisk walking, tai chi, in-line skating. But if it's not weight-bearing, it doesn't strengthen bones (so swimming, while it does burn calories and boost aerobic capacity, isn't as helpful). Whether your exercise is social or solo, start slowly and check with your doctor or other health practitioner before taking up a new routine. Injuries, even minor ones, can derail good habits before they're ingrained.

protect the heart. *Side effects:* nausea, bloating, weight gain, breast tenderness.

Conjugated estrogens (Premarin). *Function:* alleviate symptoms associated with menopause. *Side effects:* nausea, bloating, weight gain, breast tenderness, increased chance of blood clots.

Other Drugs

Raloxifene (Evista). *Function:* guard against bone loss without increasing risk of breast and uterine cancer. *Side effects:* hot flashes, nausea, bloating, weight gain, breast tenderness.

Testosterone (Estratest). *Function:* sometimes given to decrease menopausal symptoms. *Side effects:* nausea, breakthrough bleeding, swelling, increased hair growth on body and face.

HERBAL REMEDIES

Black Cohosh (*Cimicifuga racemosa*)

This herb has proven to be such an effective remedy for menopausal and premenstrual complaints that it has received official recognition in Britain and Germany. Studies have confirmed that black cohosh root can mimic estrogen in the body. It also possesses antispasmodic and diuretic properties. It is useful for hot flashes, vaginal dryness, and even the depression sometimes associated with menopause. *Typical dosage:* one to three 500-milligram capsules standardized to 2 percent triterpene glycosides per day; or 10 to 25 drops of tincture up to every four hours. *Caution:* Do not exceed recommended dosage. Do not use if you are pregnant or nursing.

Black cohosh

Dang Gui (*Angelica sinensis*)

A staple of Traditional Chinese Medicine, this herb helps relieve a number of unpleasant symptoms associated with menopause. No other herb in Chinese medicine is as widely used for treating gynecological ailments. Dang gui acts as a phytoestrogen—in other words, it has similar, but milder, effects on the body than actual estrogen. Dang gui is traditionally believed to have pain-relieving properties, but this is probably due, in part, to its ability to calm spasms. It also boosts elimination and supports the cardiovascular system, valuable actions for women in menopause. *Typical dosage:* up to six 500- to 600-milligram capsules per day; or 5 to 20 drops of tincture up to three times per day. *Caution:* This herb should not be used by pregnant or nursing women or during a bout with the flu. It has made some people more sun-sensitive.

NUTRITION FOR A SMOOTHER PASSAGE

Smart eating, begun in the years that precede menopause, may help to decrease unwanted symptoms.

Vegetables from the cruciferous family—broccoli, Brussels sprouts, cabbage, cauliflower, kale, kohlrabi, rutabagas, and turnips—may help the body make substances called indoles. And indoles may help protect women from the dangerous effects of excess estrogen, among them breast cancer. Plus they're all good sources of vitamins and fiber. If you eat them without cheese sauce, they're all low-fat.

Here are more foods to seek out.

◆ Whole grains
◆ Garlic
◆ Sesame seeds
◆ Whole-grain pastas
◆ Sunflower seeds
◆ Flaxseed oil
◆ Almonds
◆ Dates
◆ Fresh vegetables
◆ Pomegranates
◆ Fresh fruits

Here are foods and substances to avoid.

◆ Rich dairy products
◆ Caffeine
◆ Sugar
◆ Alcohol
◆ Fried foods
◆ Cigarettes
◆ Red meats
◆ Nicotine

Vitex (*Vitex agnus-castus*)
Compounds in the berries of this plant act on the pituitary gland to stabilize hormone fluctuations. Good clinical evidence bears out the use of vitex in the treatment of menopausal symptoms. *Typical dosage:* 200 milligrams of product standardized to 0.5 percent ag-

THE POWER OF ISOFLAVONES

One reason Asian women tend to sail through menopause with few symptoms and lower incidences of hormone-related cancers is that they eat large amounts of soy products, such as tofu, tempeh, and miso. Most soybean products contain isoflavones, whose chemical structure closely resembles that of estrogen. More than a thousand clinical studies indicate that soy compounds act as weak estrogens in the body—filling in for "real" estrogen when there isn't enough, but blocking the body's own hormone when there's too much.

Phytoestrogens can also protect the heart against post-menopausal heart disease just as well as hormone replacement therapy; help protect against bone-mineral loss, the leading cause of osteoporosis; and help protect against breast and uterine cancer and post-menopausal psychological symptoms. Although no dietary guidelines have been established for soy, studies show that even small amounts of soy products, eaten twice a day, can improve women's health during menopause.

If you want to get isoflavones, but you just hate soybeans no matter how cleverly they're disguised, try incorporating other beans into your diet. Most legumes—including adzuki, black, fava, great Northern, kidney, lima, and mung beans, red and yellow lentils, and black-eyed peas—either come close to or surpass soybeans' level of genistein, one of the key isoflavones. In addition, they're low-fat, high-fiber protein, perfect heart-healthy foods.

And it's not cheating to get your isoflavones from a capsule, but you won't reap the side benefits of bringing a low-fat, high-fiber food to your table. *Typical dosage of supplemental isoflavone:* 6 to 20 milligrams of genistein, or total isoflavone consumption of 40 to 80 milligrams daily.

nuside, one to three times daily. *Caution*: Do not use during pregnancy or attempts to become pregnant.

Red Raspberry (*Rubus idaeus*)

Long used for various discomforts during pregnancy and childbirth, red raspberry also strengthens the uterus, stops hemorrhages, decreases excess menstrual flow, and increases deficient flow. It also relieves painful menstruation by relaxing the smooth muscles. *Typical dosage:* 1 to 2 cups of tea per day (steep 1 teaspoon of dried leaves in 1 cup of hot water for 10 to 15 minutes). *Caution*: Consult a qualified practitioner to use red raspberry during pregnancy.

Licorice Root (*Glycyrrhiza glabra*)

You'll find this root as an ingredient in about a third of all Chinese herbal formulas and in a majority of the formulas prescribed for female reproductive problems. Licorice works to control water retention, breast tenderness, and carbohydrate cravings. It also adjusts and boosts estrogen metabolism, helping to decrease the symptoms associated with hormone fluctuation. Licorice is believed to enhance the action of other herbs when taken in a formula. *Typical dosage:* up to six 400- to 500-milligram capsules per day; or 20 to 30 drops of tincture up to three times per day. *Caution:* Avoid licorice if you're pregnant or nursing, have high blood pressure, heart rhythm irregularities, or kidney disease, or if you are taking digitalis-based drugs, unless supervised by a physician. Taking licorice for extended periods of time can raise blood pressure. Taking potassium supplements with licorice is advised. Deglycyrrhizinated or DGL licorice avoids the side effects of this herb.

Saw Palmetto (*Serenoa repens*)

This shrub yields berries that were used for hundreds of years by Native Americans. Today saw palmetto has been scientifically and clinically proven effective for both prostate conditions in men and hormonal conditions in women. *Typical dosage:* 320 milligrams of capsules standardized to 85 to 95 percent fatty acids, per day.

St.-John's-Wort (*Hypericum perforatum*)

This well-known mood lifter and antiviral herb helps boost brain function and fight the anxiety and depression sometimes associated with menopause. It works by increasing blood supply to brain tissue and naturally raising serotonin, a mood-controlling brain chemical. It can help to control mood swings. *Typical dosage:* 300 milligrams of capsules standardized to 0.3 percent hypericum three times per day. *Caution:* May cause increased sun sensitivity. Don't take St.-John's-wort in combination with prescription antidepressants or with L-dopa, a drug for Parkinson's disease, unless advised to do so by your physician.

Menstrual Problems

EVERY WOMAN EXPERIENCES MENSTRUATION differently. For some, it's painless and predictable; for others, it's misery. Some women lose very little blood; others lose enough to bring on anemia, fatigue, and dizziness.

Most menstrual difficulties are caused by real physical conditions, not by one's imagination or mental illness, as had been believed at one time. Endometriosis, uterine infection, fibroid cysts, scar tissue, or a troublesome IUD may be involved. Anatomical problems, such as a tilted uterus, are occasionally at fault. Stress and emotional upsets, especially when intense and prolonged, can also affect menstrual symptoms.

As if the pain and inconvenience of a difficult period weren't enough, some women also experience premenstrual syndrome, widely known as PMS. This group of symptoms begins three to seven days before menstruation and ranges from mere discomfort and fatigue to debilitating cramps and depression. Various medical texts identify up to 150 symptoms.

About a third of all women have visited their doctors to discuss symptoms of PMS. To make matters worse, the immune system's ability to respond also drops just before the monthly cycle. This may lead to increased susceptibility to colds, flu, allergies, herpes outbreaks, and flare-ups of rheumatoid arthritis.

A few women develop other, less common menstrual difficulties. Those who haven't begun menstruating despite passing through puberty, or who begin menstruating but stop, have amenorrhea. Those who experience scanty menstrual flow or who skip periods for reasons other than pregnancy have oligomenorrhea. In addition, some women have irregular periods—which can make planning a pregnancy difficult. Others bleed on schedule, but so heavily that they experience light-headedness, exhaustion, and anemia.

Because many of these menstrual difficulties can be brought on by another physical condition—endometriosis, pelvic inflammatory disease, or nutritional imbalances, to name only a few—it's important to consult a doctor about any dramatic changes in what's customary for you or about factors related to your period that make life difficult. Work with your doctor or other health practitioner to examine all your treatment options, including changes in your diet, nutritional supplementation, and other natural remedies. There are times when drugs can work wonders, but

CRAMP-RELIEVING TEA

This tea helps ease one of the most common menstrual symptoms.

- 1 **teaspoon dried cramp bark**
- ½ **teaspoon dried motherwort herb**
- ½ **teaspoon dried chamomile flowers**
- ½ **teaspoon dried wild yam root**
- ½ **teaspoon dried California poppy, whole plant or root**
- ½ **teaspoon dried valerian root**
- ½ **teaspoon dried skullcap herb**
  Licorice or stevia, to taste
- 4 **cups water**

Combine the herbs and water in a pan. Bring to a boil, then lower the heat and simmer for 5 minutes. Remove from the heat, cover, and steep for 20 minutes. Strain and discard the herbs. Drink 1 cup as often as needed.

be sure you understand their side effects and repercussions for your hormones, fertility, and health.

DRUG TREATMENT

Analgesics

Aspirin, acetaminophen, ibuprofen. *Function:* reduce pain and suppress prostaglandins, the hormones that cause the uterine lining to thicken. *Aspirin side effects:* possible stomach and gastrointestinal bleeding. *Ibuprofen side effects:* can damage the liver in large doses. *Acetaminophen side effects:* can damage the liver if recommended dosage is exceeded or you generally consume three or more alcoholic beverages per day.

Gonadotropin Inhibitors

Danocrine (Danazol, others). *Function:* suppress some hormones during the middle of the menstrual cycle to relieve heavy periods. *Side effects:* weight gain, swelling, acne, hot flashes, increased hair growth and other male secondary sex characteristics.

TOO-HEAVY PERIODS TINCTURE

Blend this tincture and keep it on hand for times when your menstrual flow is uncomfortably heavy.

- 1 teaspoon shepherd's purse tincture
- 1 teaspoon yarrow tincture
- ½ teaspoon red raspberry leaf tincture
- ½ teaspoon vitex tincture

Combine all of the ingredients in a dark glass jar with a tight seal. Take three dropperfuls every 15 to 30 minutes for very heavy bleeding or two dropperfuls every hour for moderately heavy bleeding. (Try to purchase shepherd's purse tincture made from the fresh herb; it loses some of its strength when dried.)

Antidepressants
Selective serotonin reuptake inhibitors (Prozac, Zoloft, Paxil). *Function:* slow the uptake and breakdown of the mood-controlling brain chemical, serotonin, thereby diminishing mood swings. *Side effects:* headache, nausea, insomnia, nervousness.

Tranquilizers
Benzodiazepines (Xanax, Valium, Ativan). *Function:* reduce anxiety and promote sleep. *Side effects:* headache, nausea, tinnitus, insomnia, nervousness; can be habit-forming.

Other Drugs
Buspirone (BuSpar). *Function:* relieve anxiety and difficulty concentrating. *Side effects:* headache, dizziness, nausea.

Bromocriptine mesylate (Parlodel). *Function:* act on the pituitary gland to suppress excessive levels of the hormone prolactin and produce regular menstruation. *Side effects:* nausea, vomiting, dizziness, decreased blood pressure, appetite loss.

HERBAL REMEDIES

Vitex (*Vitex agnus-castus*)
An extract of the berries of this tree can ease fluid retention, mood swings, food cravings, premenstrual acne, constipation, and outbreaks of herpes. Scientists think that vitex works by regulating the pituitary gland, which sends signals to other glands, instructing them how much of each hormone to make. *Typical dosage:* 2 to 3 dropperfuls of tincture in water two times per day between meals; or three capsules two times per day. *Caution:* Do not use if you are taking oral contraceptives, because vitex may lessen their effectiveness. Do not use during pregnancy.

Black Cohosh (*Actaea racemosa*)
Sometimes recommended during menopause, black cohosh has the ability to relieve pain, cramps, and uterine swelling; it is often blended with vitex in commercial formulas for menstrual difficulties. It must be taken over a period of time to be effective. *Typical dosage:* 3 to 4 dropperfuls of the tincture two times per day. *Caution:* For some women, this herb brings on heavy menstrual bleeding.

Cramp Bark (*Viburnum opulus*) and Black Haw (*V. prunifolium*)

Each of these safe, time-tested remedies works to relax the uterine muscle. Cramp bark has long been used as an antispasmodic. If your cramps come with scanty bleeding, anxiety, and lower back pain, try black haw. Combine either herb with valerian or kava-kava to increase its effects. *Typical dosage:* 3 to 5 dropperfuls of tincture three to five times per day; or 2 to 3 cups of tea per day (simmer 1 to 2 teaspoons of dried bark in 1 cup of water for 10 minutes). If you want to relieve the anxiety as well as the cramps, try also taking kava-kava in a dosage of six 400- to 500-milligram capsules in three divided doses per day or 15 to 30 drops of tincture three times per day. If you prefer valerian, take six 425-milligram capsules of the powdered root in three divided doses per day; or 30 to 90 drops of valerian root tincture three times per day.

Cramp bark

Ginkgo (*Ginkgo biloba*)

Because ginkgo leaf extracts improve brain function and circulation, they may help alleviate any mental fuzziness you feel during your period. Improved circulation also means improved removal of fluids, so ginkgo can help relieve breast tenderness. Ginkgo must be used for six to eight weeks before it has an effect. *Typical dosage:* 3 capsules containing at least 40 milligrams of extract standardized to flavone glycosides or ginkgolides per day.

Feverfew (*Tanacetum parthenium*)

Feverfew diminishes migraines and the nausea that comes with them. A compound called parthenolide seems to be responsible for its healing effects. *Typical dosage:* up to three 300- to 400-milligram capsules per day; or two average-sized fresh leaves per day; or 15 to 30 drops of tincture per day. *Caution:* Avoid during pregnancy or attempts to become pregnant.

EASY CURES FOR MENSTRUAL DIFFICULTIES

Here are some easy, non-invasive ways to ease menstrual woes.

◆ **Get some sunlight.** Some studies suggest that sunlight may help regulate the menstrual cycle. Plus, sunlight produces vitamin D in the body.

◆ **Stay away from fried foods.** Potato and corn chips, crackers, baked goods, and anything that contains hydrogenated oils, including margarine, may increase menstrual discomfort.

◆ **Check your eating and exercise habits.** If excessive exercise, low body fat, or malnutrition is the likely cause of missed periods, increase your caloric intake and decrease the exercise.

◆ **Reduce your sugar intake.** To satisfy your sweet tooth, turn to fresh whole fruit in season, carob, nuts, and dried fruit.

◆ **Eat several small meals per day.** This strategy supports the immune system and reduces food cravings and emotional swings.

◆ **Avoid caffeine.** Reduce your intake of coffee, chocolate, and tea before and during menstruation.

◆ **Adjust your nutrition.** Before your period, increase whole grains in your diet to help stabilize moodiness. Then, once your period starts, eat fewer whole grains. When it ends, consume more protein.

◆ **Try ginger tea.** Ginger tea can relieve nausea and abdominal discomfort (grate 1 to 3 teaspoons of fresh ginger root; add to 1 cup of hot water and steep for 10 to 15 minutes; strain). Drink 1 to 3 cups per day.

◆ **Get regular aerobic exercise.** Exercise releases endorphins, the body's natural pain relievers. Many women with menstrual pain or premenstrual symptoms also benefit from yoga or meditation.

PMS TEA

This calming tea helps ease premenstrual symptoms.

- 1 **teaspoon vitex berries**
- 1 **teaspoon wild yam root**
- ½ **teaspoon burdock root**
- ½ **teaspoon dandelion root**
- ½ **teaspoon feverfew leaf**
- 1 **teaspoon orange peel, licorice root, or stevia (optional)**
- 4 **cups water**

Combine the herbs and water. Bring to a boil, then turn off the heat and let steep for at least 20 minutes. Strain out the herbs. Drink at least 2 cups daily as needed.

California Poppy (*Eschscholzia californica*)
This herb calms mild anxiety and promotes relaxation and refreshing sleep. *Typical dosage:* drink 1 cup of tea at night to promote restful sleep (steep 1 to 2 teaspoonfuls of dried herb in 1 cup of freshly boiled water for 10 minutes); or take 35 to 40 drops of the tincture at night. *Caution*: Avoid during pregnancy or attempts to become pregnant.

Hops (*Humulus lupulus*)
The strobiles, or flowers, of the hops plant promote sleep, calm heart palpitations, and help women who have low estrogen levels. *Typical dosage:* 1 cup of tea before bedtime (steep 1 heaping teaspoon of whole dried hops in 1 cup of hot water for 10 to 15 minutes); or 10 to 40 drops of tincture three times per day. *Caution:* Women who have had estrogen-driven breast cancer may wish to avoid this herb.

St.-John's-Wort (*Hypericum perforatum*)
The compounds in this bright yellow flower work over time to relieve mild to moderate depression, including that caused by monthly hormonal fluctuations. *Typical dosage:* 7 dropperfuls of tincture per day, divided into two doses; or 300 milligrams of capsules standardized to 0.3 percent hypericin, three times per day.

Kava-Kava (*Piper methysticum*)

This calming herb eases anxiety almost instantly. It also has pain-relieving effects comparable to aspirin. Because of this, you might want to begin taking kava-kava a few days before your period to ease PMS, then continue taking it for the first few days of menstruation to alleviate cramps. *Typical dosage:* 3 to 4 dropperfuls of tincture two to three times per day. *Caution*: Do not use during pregnancy or attempts to become pregnant.

Valerian (*Valeriana officinalis*)

With its reliable overall relaxing effect, this herb can relieve the nervousness, tension, and sleeplessness that often accompany cramps. If you want to merely take the edge off your nerves, use a lower dose; if you want to conquer insomnia, use more. *Typical dosage:* 1 to 2 dropperfuls of tincture per day; or one to five 500-milligram capsules per day.

PERIOD-REGULATING EXTRACT

This formula helps regulate hormones and improve mood. Use it to normalize periods and ease premenstrual syndrome.

- 1¼ teaspoons vitex tincture
- ¾ teaspoon black cohosh tincture
- ½ teaspoon motherwort tincture
- 1 teaspoon boldo or burdock root tincture
- 1 teaspoon St.-John's-wort tincture
- ½ teaspoon California poppy tincture

  Tincture of stevia or licorice root to sweeten (optional)

Blend the tinctures together. Take 1 teaspoon morning and evening, at least 30 minutes before or 30 minutes after meals. Take for at least four months.

Yarrow (*Achillea millefolium*)

Yarrow has long been used to treat menstrual pain, heavy periods, and excessive bleeding before menopause. In Germany, it's approved as a treatment for menstrual cramps. *Typical dosage:* 20 to 40 drops of tincture two to three times per day; or 1 to 3 cups of tea per day (steep 1 teaspoon of dried flowers in 1 cup of hot water for 10 minutes). *Caution*: Do not take during pregnancy or attempts to become pregnant.

Red Raspberry (*Rubus idaeus*)

The leaves of this berry-producing vine are an important remedy for most conditions involving the uterus. They can help relieve pain and excessive bleeding. *Typical dosage:* 1 to 2 cups of tea up to three times per day (steep 1 teaspoon of dried leaves in 1 cup of hot water for 10 to 15 minutes). *Caution:* Consult a qualified practitioner to use red raspberry during pregnancy.

Dang Gui (*Angelica sinensis*)

This herb is known in Traditional Chinese Medicine as a blood builder, meaning it can help boost the circulatory system and overall metabolism. It may be helpful to women seeking to regain their natural menstrual cycles. It is particularly effective when combined with an herbal hormone regulator such as vitex, described earlier. *Typical dosage:* 1 to 2 dropperfuls of tincture two times per day; or 1 cup of tea two or three times per day (simmer 2 teaspoons of dried root in 1 cup of hot water for 10 minutes). *Caution:* Do not take during pregnancy or attempts to become pregnant.

Morning Sickness

Pregnant? Flip a coin. Heads, you don't have morning sickness, tails, you do.

The odds are 50–50 that you'll experience nausea or vomiting early in your pregnancy. And despite the name, you can have morning sickness at any time of the day or night.

Although doctors don't know what causes morning sickness, some believe it might be related to the profound hormonal and metabolic changes that occur in a woman's body during the first trimester of pregnancy.

Low blood sugar, nutritional deficiencies, sluggish liver function, and hydrochloric acid deficiency are other possible contributors. Psychological factors may play a role as well.

Just because herbs are natural does not mean they are safe, especially during pregnancy. As a general rule, do not take any herb without consulting your obstetrician.

In particular, avoid any bitter-tasting herbs in early pregnancy, as they can cause uterine contractions and possibly induce miscarriage. Also avoid stronger medicinal herbs in general.

Gentle, pleasant-tasting, tonic herbs are the safest ones to use during pregnancy. Taking them in tea form means you boost your fluid intake as well. The herbs listed below are also rich in vitamins and minerals. Experiment with various combinations to find the ones that most appeal to you.

When nausea is severe, don't force yourself to drink something that tastes or smells unpleasant to you. And don't blame yourself if your preferences seem to change without warning or logic.

The herbs below can be taken hot or cold. Add honey or lemon juice if that sounds appealing.

Drug Treatment

Currently, most obstetricians avoid prescribing drugs for morning sickness, because any drug taken by the mother gets passed along to the developing fetus. Some women have severe enough vomiting to require treatment with intravenous fluids to prevent dehydration and correct body-fluid balances.

Herbal Remedies

Ginger (*Zingiber officinale*)

Researchers don't know how ginger calms nausea and stops vomiting, but they know that it does. It's a superior remedy for motion sickness as well as morning sickness. It may act on vomiting centers in the brain. Ginger also calms stomach spasms and reduces gas. *Typical dosage:* 1 to 3 cups of tea per day (simmer

More Tips for Easing Morning Sickness

Small changes can make a big difference in the frequency and severity of morning sickness. These ideas can help.

◆ **Eat small, frequent meals and snacks.** Make them wholesome foods, with plenty of protein and complex carbohydrates that help maintain stable blood sugar. Try whole-grain crackers with nut butters, hard-boiled egg slices on rye bread, or yogurt with fruit and some wheat germ.

◆ **Keep an eye on your fluid intake.** Dehydration can make nausea worse. If you are severely nauseated, sip fluids frequently or suck on ice chips. You can also freeze herbal teas in an ice tray.

◆ **Beef up your B$_6$ intake.** Vitamin B$_6$ deficiency is common during pregnancy. It could even be causing your nausea. Eat plenty of foods rich in B$_6$, such as nuts, legumes, wheat germ, whole grains, dark green vegetables, meat, and fish. Or take 50 milligrams of a B$_6$ supplement twice per day.

◆ **Check out hydrochloric acid.** It's necessary for normal digestion and helps the body absorb some vitamins. Deficiency is common in the early stages of pregnancy. You might consider a supplement if you get bloated or nauseated after meals, especially those that are high in protein. Such products, called Betaine H-Cl supplements, are available in most health food stores. They should be taken with meals, never on an empty stomach. Follow the manufacturer's or your doctor's instructions on dosage. If you experience abdominal discomfort, burning, or heartburn, discontinue use immediately.

(Later in pregnancy, heartburn is sometimes a problem—a sign of your body producing too *much* hydrochloric acid. So supplements of this acid are exactly the *wrong* thing to take at this stage.)

◆ **Assess your emotions.** Severe or longer-lasting morning sickness may indicate a need for psychological support to address any conflicts or negative feelings you may be having about being pregnant. In such cases, hypnotherapy might be an option to pursue.

OTHER HERBS TO TRY

Other safe herbs to try for morning sickness, or to look for in commercial teas, include fennel seed (especially good for gas and bloating), cinnamon, and lemon balm, and don't forget the demulcent, or soothing, herbs such as slippery elm, flaxseed, and oats.

1 to 2 teaspoons of fresh chopped ginger in 1 cup of water for 10 minutes); or one 250-milligram capsule two to four times per day. *Caution:* Do not use if you have gallstones.

Chamomile (*Matricaria recutitia*)

Gentle and soothing to both the digestive tract and the nervous system, chamomile makes a lovely tea. It is especially helpful if you are feeling a little stressed out in addition to your nausea. *Typical dosage:* 1 to 3 cups of tea sipped frequently throughout the day (steep 1 to 2 teaspoons of dried flowers or one tablespoon of fresh flowers in 1 cup of hot water for 10 minutes).

Peppermint (*Mentha × piperita*)

This aromatic herb soothes the entire digestive tract and is especially helpful if you feel gassy or bloated. *Typical dosage:* 1 to 3 cups of tea, sipped frequently throughout the day (steep 2 teaspoons of dried leaves or 1 tablespoon of fresh in 1 cup of hot water for 5 minutes). *Caution:* Avoid peppermint if you have heartburn or esophageal reflux; peppermint may worsen these conditions.

MOTION SICKNESS

I T'S ANOTHER GORGEOUS SUNDAY AFTERNOON—perfect for a long drive in the country. Too bad you have to settle for a walk around the block. Your feet seem to be the only mode of transportation that doesn't make you queasy.

If you experience motion sickness, it doesn't really matter what's providing the motion. A car, bus, boat, airplane, merry-go-round, even a swing can bring on dizziness and nausea.

Motion sickness is the result of your eyes perceiving one type of movement while your brain is processing another. The phenomenon can affect anyone—even people who seldom experience it.

DRUG TREATMENT

Over-the-Counter Antihistamines
Dimenhydrinate (Dramamine). *Function:* relieves motion sickness symptoms by reducing input from the inner ear to the central nervous system. *Side effects:* drowsiness and dry mouth.

Prescription Antihistamines
Hydroxyzine, meclizine (Antivert, Meni-D). *Function:* reduce symptoms by minimizing the body's histamine response. *Side effects:* drowsiness, dry mouth.

Other Drugs
Phenergan (Promethazine). *Function:* alleviate motion sickness via its antihistamine, sedative, and antinausea actions. *Side effects:* blurred vision, drowsiness, increased susceptibility to seizures, abnormal muscular contractions in the face and neck.

Prochlorperazine (Compazine). *Function:* reduce anxiety and nausea; sedate. *Side effects:* blurred vision, lowered blood pressure, drowsiness, increased susceptibility to seizures, abnormal muscular contractions in the face and neck.

Scopolamine (Transderm Scop). *Function:* act on the central nervous system to reduce nausea. *Side effects:* drowsiness, dry mouth, blurred vision, increased urinary symptoms in men with

Savvy Traveling

In addition to herbal treatments, here are a few more things you can do to minimize your chances of experiencing motion sickness.

◆ Avoid alcohol, both before and during a trip.

◆ If you are traveling by boat, stay in the middle of the boat and on the upper deck, if there is one.

◆ If you're small in stature, sit on a cushion so you can see straight ahead and focus on distant points.

◆ Don't sit in a seat that faces backwards.

◆ Wear headphones and listen to soothing music.

◆ Don't take nutritional supplements on an empty stomach; they can cause nausea. Some prescription drugs also need to be taken with food; check the label carefully.

◆ Avoid reading or other activities that cause you to put your head down. Likewise, don't move your head around to converse.

◆ Try an acupressure wristband, available in marine and travel stores. These devices use a trigger point in the wrist to calm nausea.

◆ Avoid heavy meals with a high fat content, but don't travel on an empty stomach, either.

◆ When booking a flight, reserve the low-fat, vegetarian, low-sodium, kosher, or diabetic meal. Or skip the airline food and bring your own saltines, melba toast, candied ginger, or bananas. The goal is to avoid stomach-upsetting fats, but still have something to eat that's easy on the digestion.

◆ Keep your area well-ventilated; overly warm or stuffy conditions aggravate nausea.

Calm Mind, Calm Stomach

Because motion sickness ebbs and flows, it can play havoc with your nerves. Alternately feeling relief as the nausea fades and anxiety as it returns may be the worst part of motion sickness. Classic antianxiety herbs can be helpful in such cases. Try passionflower, kava-kava, or valerian if anxiety plays a major role in your travel woes.

prostate enlargement, increased eye pressure in certain kinds of glaucoma.

Herbal Remedies

Ginger (*Zingiber officinale*)

This root acts as a strong gas-expeller that also settles the stomach. No automobile glove box or medicine chest should be without it. One British study found ginger root more effective than either Dramamine or a placebo (fake pill) in fighting motion sickness. In another study, ginger reduced nausea and vomiting after major surgery. Be aware that ginger may be more effective when taken at least four hours before your car or boat ride. *Typical dosage:* up to eight 500- to 600-milligram capsules per day; or 10 to 20 drops of tincture in water three times per day; or ½ to 1 teaspoon of the fresh ground root per day. Crystallized ginger or candied chunks of the root can also be eaten.

Peppermint (*Mentha × piperita*)

One of the oldest and most-used remedies for any kind of stomach upset, peppermint helps prevent vomiting and quiets stomach spasms. The tincture can be taken along on trips and drunk in a little bit of water. Or simply try a strong peppermint candy such as Altoids. *Typical dosage:* 10 to 20 drops of tincture in water after meals or before trips; or 1 cup of tea as needed (steep 2 to 4 teaspoons of dried, cut, and sifted leaf in 1½ to 3 cups of hot water for 15 minutes). *Caution:* Avoid undiluted peppermint essential oil; it can be irritating. Use peppermint with caution if pregnant or nursing.

Fennel (*Foeniculum vulgare*)

The seeds of this plant have been valued for hundreds of years as gentle digestive aids and antispasmodics. They can be especially helpful if that winding mountain road leads home from a favorite restaurant. *Typical dosage:* up to 20 of the raw seeds chewed well, as needed; or up to three 400- to 500-milligram capsules per day; or 1 cup of tea per day (simmer 2 to 3 teaspoons of crushed seed in 1 cup of hot water for 10 to 15 minutes); or 30 to 60 drops of tincture in water up to four times per day.

Fennel

MULTIPLE SCLEROSIS

ONE IN EVERY 1,000 AMERICANS is affected by multiple sclerosis (MS). But being diagnosed with the condition doesn't necessarily mean inevitable, increasing debility. On the other hand MS troubles doctors as well as those who have it, because its progress is unpredictable and no cure exists. There's not even a lot that conventional drugs can do.

Multiple sclerosis involves a tissue called myelin that covers nerve fibers in the spinal cord and brain. Myelin permits the rapid transmission of electrical nerve impulses. In a person with MS, the protective myelin sheaths begin to deteriorate, slowing down nerve impulses in the process. Eventually, scar tissue forms around the damaged nerves, causing a hardening or sclerosis.

MS usually strikes people between the ages of 20 and 40. It affects twice as many women as men. Although its cause remains unknown, researchers suspect a link to little-known viruses. MS is five times more common in temperate climates than in tropical climates but altogether rare in Japan, leading medical theorists to suspect that sun exposure, genetics, and diet also play roles. High consumption of animal fats and low consumption of essential fatty acids has been linked to MS.

The symptoms of MS include fatigue, stiffness, loss of muscle strength or feeling in the arms or legs, poor coordination, and loss of balance. The disease can also produce tremors, a constant tingling sensation, facial pain, blurred or reduced vision, and mood swings. Many people who are diagnosed with MS experience only minimal symptoms.

Unfortunately, medical science has little to offer people with MS. No drugs will stop or prevent the progression of the disease. For inflammation control, doctors may prescribe a pituitary hormone known as adrenocorticotrophic hormone, or ACTH. This hormone works to stimulate the adrenal glands to produce substances that inhibit inflammation.

Drug Treatment

Steroids
Prednisone (Meticorten). *Function:* decrease inflammation and tissue damage associated with MS. *Side effects:* fat redistribution causing puffiness in the face, acne, thinning of the skin, peptic ulcers, increased susceptibility to infection, metabolism changes.

Immune-System Suppressants
Cyclophosphamide (Cytoxan), azathioprine (Imuran). *Function:* suppress the immune system to slow the course of the disease. *Side effects:* decreases in blood cell counts, increased susceptibility to infection, skin rash, nausea, vomiting.

Beta interferon (Betaseron). *Function:* reduce the progression of MS by minimizing damage in the brain. *Side effects:* fever, chills, fatigue, muscle aches, sweating, depression.

Muscle Relaxants
Dantrolene (Dantrium). *Function:* reduce muscle spasms. *Side effects:* diarrhea, nausea, weakness, liver damage, drowsiness, hallucinations.

Herbal Remedies

Evening Primrose (*Oenethera biennis*), Black Currant (*Ribes nigrum*), Flaxseed (*Linum usitatissimum*) Oils

The omega-3 and omega-6 fatty acids in these oils help maintain the myelin sheath around nerves. Studies show that the oils help control symptoms and prolong remission. *Typical dosage:* 500 to 1,500 milligrams per day of evening primrose or black current seed oils; or 1 tablespoon per day of flaxseed oil. Use pure oils that require refrigeration.

Ginkgo (*Ginkgo biloba*)

This herb, with many time-tested uses in Asian countries, made headlines when studies showed it helped people with Alzheimer's disease. One of the compounds that is likely responsible, ginkgolide, is found in no other plant. Best of all, ginkgolides have been shown to help inhibit flare-ups of MS. Ginkgo is also a strong antioxidant and anti-inflammatory. *Typical dosage:* 3 capsules containing at least 60 milligrams of extract standardized to 24 percent flavone glycosides and 6 percent ginkgolides per day. *Caution:* Rarely, people taking ginkgo may experience gastrointestinal upset, headaches, or skin allergies.

Purslane (*Portulaca oleracea*)

This common, flat, spreading garden "weed" has long been added to salads by those who enjoy slightly bitter wild greens. It turns out that purslane is high in magnesium, one of many minerals that people with MS tend to be deficient in. James A. Duke, Ph.D., author of *The Green Pharmacy,* recommends eating purslane, steamed or raw, along with spinach and other high-magnesium foods. Although purslane is the focus of much new research, it's not yet available in supplement form, so get it fresh from your favorite gardening friend.

Nausea

In any poll of everyone's most hated symptom, nausea would probably rank high. It can dim the joy of early pregnancy. It can make a meal memorable, though undoubtedly for the wrong reason. It can turn an evening of celebration into a morning-after of kneeling before the "porcelain god"—and indeed, you may feel penitent.

But when examined objectively—that is, when you don't have it—nausea, and the vomiting it induces, are simply the body's way of purging itself. If the queasiness comes from microorganisms or toxins, you don't want to completely stop your body from cleansing itself.

Regardless of the cause of nausea, treatment always includes drinking lots of clear liquids (dehydration alone can provoke nausea in some people). Drink small amounts frequently: Sip water, broth, or tea, or suck on chipped ice or frozen herb tea. Drinking sports rehydration fluids helps replace not only water loss but also essential body salts.

If you feel very ill, can't keep down fluids, and haven't urinated within eight hours, or if your nausea and vomiting continue for more than a day, call your doctor. When this happens, you've become dehydrated.

Drug Treatment

Phenothiazines

Prochlorperazine (Compazine), promethazine (Phenergan). *Function:* control nausea and vomiting by acting on the brain. *Side effects:* dry mouth, dry or congested nose, blurred vision, constipation, difficulty urinating, sedation, dizziness, lowered blood pressure, interactions with other drugs.

Other Drugs

Dimenhydrinate (Dramamine). *Function:* decrease nausea, vomiting, and motion sickness. *Side effects:* drowsiness, dizziness, dryness of mouth, nose, and throat.

WHEN NOTHING STAYS DOWN

Sometimes nausea makes it difficult to keep even fluids down. If that's the case, remember to drink liquids in small, frequent sips, not big gulps.

Fortunately, the healing chemicals in many herbs can be absorbed through the skin. This fact comes in handy when nausea makes it hard to drink teas or tinctures. If your stomach turns at the idea of the recommended teas, make one of them but don't drink it. Instead, let it cool, then soak a clean cloth or hand towel with the tea and apply the cloth to your stomach.

Another option: Make a large pot of bath tea by tossing a handful of any of the recommended herbs into a quart of just-boiled water. Allow to steep off heat for 10 to 15 minutes, strain the tea into a warm bath, and soak.

If even tea is too much trouble to make, add 10 to 15 drops of essential oil (not more; essential oils are very concentrated) to a tub of bathwater. Or put the same number of drops into ⅛ cup of vegetable oil and have someone give you a massage.

After one of these topical treatments, you may be able to keep down some much-needed fluids.

Metoclopramide (Reglan, Emex, Clopra, Apo-Metoclop, Maxeran, Octamide, Reclomide). *Function:* relieve nausea and vomiting associated with chemotherapy or surgery. *Side effects:* drowsiness, restlessness, rash.

HERBAL REMEDIES

Ginger (*Zingiber officinale*)

This pungent root has a reputation for controlling nausea of all types. Studies have shown ginger to be especially effective in curbing motion sickness, morning sickness, and postoperative and chemotherapy-induced nausea. You can take ginger in whatever form most appeals—fresh, crystallized, dried, or powdered.

(Do realize, however, that the crystallized form contains sugar.) *Typical dosage:* 2 to 3 cups of tea per day (simmer 1 teaspoon of fresh, grated root or ½ teaspoon of powdered root in 1 cup of water for 10 minutes); or 2 dropperfuls of tincture in water one to three times per day; or four to eight 500-milligram capsules per day. *Caution:* People who have gallbladder disease or a bleeding disorder and those who take blood-thinning medications should consult a physician before taking medicinal doses of ginger. The amounts used to season foods are okay.

Peppermint (*Mentha × piperita*)

Stomach-settling and cramp-easing, peppermint has a well-earned reputation for quelling nausea. It is also a good choice if your nausea comes with a headache or cold, since peppermint is a traditional remedy for both those ailments. Sometimes just sucking on a lozenge that uses peppermint or menthol as a main ingredient can tame nausea. *Typical dosage:* sips of tea as needed (steep 2 to 3 teaspoons of dried leaf in 1 cup of hot water for 10 minutes); or 10 to 20 drops of tincture in water three or four times per day. *Caution:* Avoid peppermint if you have esophageal reflux or heartburn.

Catnip (*Nepeta cataria*)

Another herb that can help unwind intestinal cramping, catnip has a somewhat musky taste. It combines well with peppermint and chamomile and is also a very mild sedative. If your nausea is provoked by nervousness, catnip might be a good choice for settling it. *Typical dosage:* 1 to 3 cups of tea per day (steep up to 1 teaspoon of dried herb in 1 cup of hot water for 10 minutes).

Catnip

Lemon Balm (*Melissa angustifolia*)

This third mint-family member helps expel intestinal gas. It also relieves spasms and works against viruses. Perhaps most important when you're queasy, lemon balm tastes good. *Typical dosage:* one to three cups of tea per day (steep ½ to 4 teaspoons of dried herb or 1 to 3 tablespoons of the fresh herb in 1 cup of hot water). *Caution:* Do not use during pregnancy.

Chamomile (*Matricaria recutita*)

The German Commission E, that country's version of the U.S. Food and Drug Administration, endorses the use of chamomile for relieving intestinal spasms. Chamomile also reduces nausea and helps expel intestinal gas. It's widely used as a sleep aid that's mild enough for children, so if nerves play a role in your bout of nausea, chamomile is an excellent choice. *Typical dosage:* 3 to 4 cups of tea per day (steep 2 to 3 teaspoons of dried flowers in 1 cup of hot water for 5 to 10 minutes); or 10 to 40 drops of tincture in water three times per day.

Lavender (*Lavandula* spp.)

One study has shown that lavender helps decrease motion sickness in animals. Hogs transported in a truck vomited less when they stood on a bed of lavender straw (the people stuck in traffic behind the hog truck probably had less nausea as well). While lavender is safe to take internally, its mere scent helps reduce nausea. You can put a few drops of lavender essential oil in a diffuser, blend 10 drops into an ounce of massage oil, or add 10 drops to a warm bath.

NERVE PAIN

P AIN IS AN ESSENTIAL PART OF LIFE. It provides crucial information about your environment that helps you avoid injury. If you touch something hot or sharp, pain gives you the immediate feedback you need to pull your hand away before damage can occur. Similarly, if you're pulling or twisting a joint or muscle beyond its capacity, pain tells you it's time to stop. And if an artery to your heart becomes clogged, intense chest pain tells you an emergency situation is occurring, one that requires swift action.

Sometimes, however, a nerve or group of nerves that has already been injured continues to send pain signals to the brain. Although removing the cause of the pain might still be important—and you may in fact be in the process of doing so—in this situation the pain itself becomes a problem.

Several medical terms are used to describe this condition, depending on the cause and location of the pain. Neuralgia, neuropathic pain, peripheral neuropathy, and peripheral neuritis all refer to types of nerve pain. In addition, sciatica describes leg pain; lumbago, lower back pain; and trigeminal neuralgia, facial pain.

The cause of the original nerve damage can be any number of events. Nerves can be severed or crushed by blunt trauma, burns, lacerations, or amputations, including surgical ones such as mastectomy. Nerves can be pinched from inside the body by a slipped disc, a vertebra that is out of alignment, a muscle in spasm, or a cancerous growth.

Heavy metals such as mercury or lead can kill nerves. Alcoholism leads to nerve damage, as do persistent elevations in blood sugar from diabetes. Certain medications, such as those used to treat cancer or AIDS, can destroy nerves as well. When no explanation for the pain can be found, doctors refer to it as idiopathic peripheral neuropathy.

Although painkillers (analgesics) may work quite well for short-term aches and pains, they tend to fall short of managing chronic nerve pain. That's because the effects of most painkillers tend to wear off over time. Ongoing use of narcotics can create other problems: drug addiction and dependency.

There's another reason neuropathic pain resists conventional painkillers. Research has shown that an actual "rewiring" of the brain occurs with chronic pain that causes nerve impulses to repeatedly travel back and forth in a loop. It's as if your house were hit by a lightning bolt and the circuit breaker failed to shut off, scrambling all your sensitive electronic devices. When you are "hit" by periods of chronic pain, the brain somehow starts expecting the nerves to send pain messages. You are then dealing with the electrical signals emitted by the damaged nerve plus the brain's heightened awareness of those signals. You become hypersensitive to normal sensations such as light touch, vibration, or slight temperature changes, making it difficult to tell which sensations are reactions to environmental stimuli and which are the result of this rewiring.

With nerve pain, it's important to seek a thorough medical evaluation to rule out any correctable cause of the pain. Fortunately, the development of chronic pain centers around the country has increased the level of expertise in treating these conditions.

DRUG TREATMENT

Nonsteroidal Anti-Inflammatory Drugs (NSAIDs)

Aspirin, ibuprofen, naproxen (Alleve, Naprosyn), ketoprofen (Orudis), indomethacin (Indocin), celecoxib (Celebrex), sulindac (Clinoril). *Function:* decrease production of pain-causing chemicals. *Side effects:* gastrointestinal bleeding, fluid retention, kidney damage, liver damage, allergic reactions.

Other Analgesics

Acetaminophen. *Function:* block production of pain-causing chemicals. *Side effects:* liver damage, allergic reactions.

Narcotics

Codeine (Tylenol #3, Phenaphen with codeine), hydrocodone (Hycodan, Lorcet, Vicoden), oxycodone (Percodan, Percocet, Roxicodone), meperidine (Demerol), morphine, hydromorphone (Dilaudid), pentazocine (Talwin). *Function:* bind to receptors in the brain that control pain, turning them off. *Side effects:* dependency and addiction, impaired breathing (excessive doses can stop breathing), nausea, constipation.

Tricyclic Antidepressants

Amitriptyline (Elavil, Endep), nortriptyline (Pamelor), doxepin (Sinequan). *Function:* modify the processing of pain signals in the brain to decrease hypersensitivity to them. *Side effects:* dry mouth, constipation, lethargy, heart problems.

Anticonvulsants

Phenytoin (Dilantin), carbamazepine (Tegretol), gabapentin (Neurontin), clonazepam (Klonopin). *Function:* stabilize nerve cell membranes to prevent abnormal electrical discharges (seizure-like activity). *Side effects:* lethargy, mental grogginess, reduced white blood cell count, liver damage.

HERBAL REMEDIES

Cayenne (*Capsicum annuum*)

Capsaicin, an extract from cayenne and other peppers, can dramatically reduce chronic nerve pain. Studies have proven its usefulness for arthritis, shingles, trigeminal neuralgia, and diabetic neuropathy. It appears to act by decreasing the concentration of substance P, the primary chemical used by nerve cells to transmit pain signals. This effect can require several weeks of regular use. Unlike regular painkillers, however, capsaicin does not produce a tolerance in the user.

Several commercial capsaicin creams are available, usually in concentrations of 0.025 percent to 0.075 percent. For maximum effectiveness, such creams should be applied four to six times daily. *Caution:* As one might expect from a pepper extract, cayenne creams can cause an intense burning sensation, especially in people with hypersensitive nerves.

Cayenne

Burning does not mean that further injury is occurring, but it can take some getting used to. It is best to start with very small amounts of the lowest concentration cream and gradually build up to the higher strength. Some doctors recommend first applying lidocaine cream (a prescription topical anesthetic) and then applying the capsaicin product once the skin is numb. Continue until you can tolerate the capsaicin by itself.

St.-John's-Wort (*Hypericum perforatum*)

Years before this herb became scientifically accepted as a depression remedy, it was a folk medicine used for many purposes, including wound healing and fighting off infections. Although St.-John's-wort is not an analgesic, it has a calming effect on the nervous system, which helps decrease the sensation of pain. It also helps reduce the muscle tension and spasms that often accompany nerve pain. *Typical dosage:* 900 to 1,200 milligrams of standardized extract per day. *Caution:* May increase skin reactions to sun exposure, especially in high doses. If you decide to try St.-John's-wort, monitor your sun exposure and use sunscreen, especially if you are prone to sunburn.

Corydalis (*Corydalis yanhusuo*)

This tuber is a Chinese herb with potent pain-relieving properties. It is traditionally used for neuralgia, menstrual cramps, and gastrointestinal spasms. Corydalis appears to act like codeine and

OTHER WAYS TO STOP THE PAIN

Here are a few additional healing strategies to try for nerve pain.

◆ **Acupuncture.** This ancient Oriental healing art has now been accepted by the National Institutes of Health as a legitimate therapy for pain. It can sometimes work very well for nerve pain, especially when accompanied by electrical stimulation.

◆ **Physical therapy.** These treatments, including rehabilitative exercise, deep heat, ultrasound, cold packs, and manipulation or massage, can also be very helpful for nerve pain.

◆ **Stress management techniques.** Meditation, yoga, biofeedback, and other stress management techniques can be a central part of your approach to treating chronic pain. Because of the role the brain plays in expecting nerve pain, it may be possible to "rewire" your mental circuits to stop the cycle of pain or at least diminish its effects. Many hospitals and health centers either offer classes in such techniques or can refer you to classes at other locations.

other drugs in the opium family, modifying the perception of pain by specific centers in the brain. It also has antianxiety and sedative effects. Corydalis is usually prescribed by practitioners of Traditional Chinese Medicine as part of a multi-herb formula based on the patient's overall condition. *Typical dosage when taken as a single herb:* ½ teaspoon of powdered herb two or three times daily. *Caution:* May produce fatigue, constipation, and occasional headache.

Jamaican Dogwood (*Piscidia piscipula*)
This tree grows wild in Central America and the northern parts of South America. The bark of its root works similarly to aspirin pain relievers by blocking an enzyme that produces inflammatory and

pain-causing chemicals called prostaglandins. It also has mild sedative and anxiety-relieving properties. *Typical dosage:* one or two 500-milligram capsules of powdered extract every four to six hours as needed.

Obsessive-Compulsive Disorder

Obsessive-compulsive disorder is a fairly common psychiatric disorder—and one that many people harbor misconceptions about. We've all heard the words "obsessive" and "compulsive" used blithely and interchangeably, as in "He's obsessive about keeping his car clean" and "She's a compulsive shopper."

In reality, obsessive-compulsive disorder is a type of anxiety disorder. People who have it experience unwanted, recurrent, insuppressible thoughts that drive them to repeatedly perform ritualized behaviors. The repeated, troubling thoughts are obsessions; the resultant feelings of distress drive the compulsive behaviors. Usually, the behaviors temporarily relieve the thoughts. Then the thoughts recur and demand that the behavior be repeated. It's as though the brain is stuck in a groove, like a phonograph needle caught in a scratch on a record.

In the United States, one in 50 adults has symptoms of obsessive-compulsive disorder. Twice that many have had symptoms at some point in their lives.

No one knows exactly what causes obsessive-compulsive disorder. It can run in families, which indicates a genetic component. In addition, brain scans of obsessive-compulsive patients show actual abnormalities in certain nerve circuits. These circuits use serotonin, a mood-controlling brain chemical, as their messenger, and insufficient serotonin levels seem to play an important role in obsessive-compulsive disorder. In fact, drugs that increase the brain's concentration of serotonin often alleviate symptoms.

If you think you may have this disorder, talk to your health-care provider. Some people with obsessive-compulsive behavior need medication. Others may do well with specific types of psychotherapy. Many people will need to combine drugs or herbal remedies with psychotherapy. Drug treatment usually involves antidepressants, which may take several weeks to reach their full effectiveness.

No herbs have undergone testing in people with obsessive-compulsive disorder. Although anecdotal information and traditional use suggest that some herbs may reduce symptoms, there aren't yet enough statistics for patients to rely on them as a sole treatment.

It is absolutely crucial that people taking prescription antidepressants *do not* add herbs to their regimen or change their medication routine without their doctors' supervision. Some antidepressants, when abruptly discontinued, cause withdrawal symptoms. Others may interact with herbal remedies to produce negative, even dangerous, side effects.

Drug Treatment

Selective Serotonin Reuptake Inhibitors (SSRIs)

Fluoxetine (Prozac), fluvoxamine (Luvox), paroxetine (Paxil), sertraline (Zoloft). *Function:* increase brain levels of serotonin, a mood-controlling brain chemical, to relieve symptoms. *Side effects:* insomnia, anxiety, nervousness, headache, drowsiness, diarrhea, increased sweating.

Tricyclic Antidepressants

Clomipramine (Anafranil), others. *Function:* reduce depression and obsessive-compulsive disorder by influencing brain chemistry. *Side effects:* tremors, headache, dry mouth, unpleasant taste in mouth, excessive sweating, nausea, constipation or diarrhea, fatigue, weakness, drowsiness, nervousness, anxiety, insomnia, cravings for sweets.

Herbal Remedies

St.-John's-Wort (*Hypericum perforatum*)

It's well-known that this herb has been shown in many studies to ease mild to moderate depression. As of this writing, no trials have investigated whether St.-John's-wort can help people with obsessive-compulsive disorder. But some doctors and other health practitioners report that some of their patients have responded positively to the herb. Currently, many products are standardized to contain 0.3 percent hypericin, one of the constituents of St.-John's-wort. *Typical dosage* (based on usual guidelines for depression): 900 milligrams in standardized pills or capsules per day, divided into two or three doses; or 15 to 40 drops of tincture up to three times per day. St.-John's-wort can take as long as six weeks to produce benefits; increasing the dosage doesn't shorten this time. *Caution:* On rare occasions, people who take St.-John's-wort may experience gastrointestinal irritation, allergic reactions, restlessness, dry mouth, fatigue, or increased skin reactions to sun exposure. Do not substitute St.-John's-wort for prescription antidepressants; do not take it with such antidepressants unless under the guidance of a doctor. Consult a doctor before taking this herb if you are pregnant or nursing.

Kava-Kava (*Piper methysticum*)

German doctors commonly prescribe this herb for anxiety and stress. Because obsessive-compulsive disorder is a type of anxiety disorder, kava may help reduce some of the symptoms. *Typical dosage:* up to six 400- to 500-milligram capsules of a nonstandardized product per day, divided into three doses; or 70 milligrams of kavalactones in a standardized extract one to three times per day; or 15 to 30 drops of tincture in water one to three times per day. *Caution:* Large doses of kava can induce a euphoric state, muscle weakness, and dizziness. Do not use if you're pregnant or nursing. Do not combine with alcohol or with drugs that depress the central nervous system, such as sedatives and antidepressants.

Valerian (*Valeriana officinalis*)

Valerian soothes anxiety when given in small doses, while larger doses make most people sleepy. Laboratory tests have shown that components of valerian root bind to the same brain receptors as benzodiazepines, the family of drugs that includes Valium, Xanax, and other tranquilizers. (Remember, however, that you can't substitute valerian for these tranquilizers. Abruptly discontinuing them can produce dangerous withdrawal symptoms.) Some practitioners reserve valerian for evening use and prefer kava for daytime. *Typical dosage:* 300 to 400 milligrams of product standardized to 0.5 to 0.8 percent valeric acid per day; or 20 to 60 drops of tincture per day. *Caution:* May cause stomach upset.

California Poppy (*Eschscholzia californica*)

This herb can decrease anxiety and, in larger doses, insomnia. *Typical dosage:* 2 to 3 cups of tea per day (steep 1 teaspoon of dried herb and/or roots in 1 cup of boiling water for 15 minutes); or 30 to 40 drops of tincture two or three times per day. *Caution:* May interact with monoamine oxidase (MAO) inhibitor antidepressants. Not recommended for use during pregnancy.

Bergamot (*Citrus bergamia*)

The essential oil of this herb, used in aromatherapy, can discourage compulsive behaviors, soothe anxiety, and lift the spirits. So say herbalists

California poppy

Kathi Keville and Mindy Green, authors of *Aromatherapy: A Complete Guide to the Healing Art.* To use bergamot essential oil, put 3 to 5 drops in warm water and inhale; or add about 10 drops to a tub of warm bath water and soak. *Caution:* Can increase skin reactions to sun exposure. Do not take internally.

OSTEOPOROSIS

YOU PROBABLY KNOW SOMEONE WHO led a fairly normal life until an accidental fall caused a hip fracture. Suddenly, this vital person became an invalid. Other people you know may seem to be shrinking as they get older—not from weight loss, but from height loss. And occasionally you'll see an older woman gradually becoming hunched over with a so-called dowager's hump. All of these are hallmarks of the brittle-bone disease known as osteoporosis.

It's estimated that up to 40 percent of Caucasian women over the age of 50 in the United States have osteoporosis. Many experience at least one fracture as a result. But the disease doesn't affect only women—20 percent of osteoporosis cases occur in men.

Osteoporosis is a gradual decrease in bone density that leads to weakness in bone structure. Far from being just the framework for your body, bone is a dynamic living tissue that is constantly changing. Throughout your life, calcium is continually added to and subtracted from your bones. Cells called osteoclasts absorb old bone tissue, while cells known as osteoblasts lay down new bone tissue. Ideally, this process is kept in equilibrium by a number of hormones and other substances that maintain the bones in maximum strength and health.

But with age, bones tend to lose an excessive amount of protein and minerals. Over time, this can lead to osteoporosis, literally "porous bone," a condition of low bone mass and density. People with osteoporosis are susceptible to broken bones and fractures, including severely painful fractures of the vertebrae. Fractures of the spine are most common, but any weak bone can break. Hip fractures are dangerously debilitating, and recovery is often long and uncertain.

A woman is most likely to lose bone, and lose it most rapidly, in the first five to nine years after menopause. But by taking early measures to build bone mass, even people with significant risk factors—male or female—can minimize the effects of aging on their bones.

Drug Treatment

Estrogen Replacement Therapy

Conjugated estrogens (Premarin), dienestrol (Ortho Dienestrol), estradiol (Estrace), others. *Function:* replace dwindling estrogen and thereby maintain bone density. *Side effects:* increased risk of uterine and possibly breast cancer, breast pain, water retention, increased blood pressure and blood clots.

Selective estrogen-receptor modulators (SERMs) such as raloxifene (Evista). *Function:* create estrogen-like effects on bone tissue without stimulating breast or uterine tissue. *Side effects:* hot flashes, sinusitis, weight gain, muscle pain, leg cramps, blood clots.

SHOULD YOU PROTECT YOUR BONES NOW?

Who gets osteoporosis? There are several risk factors that suggest a significantly greater likelihood of developing brittle bones. Women with these risk factors may want to begin watching their bone density while still in their forties.

◆ Smokers are 40 to 50 percent more likely than nonsmokers to experience osteoporosis-related hip fractures. Even if you've smoked for a long time, quitting can improve your health.

◆ Caucasian and Asian women are at greater risk for osteoporosis than Hispanic or African-American women.

◆ Small-statured, thin-boned women, regardless of race, are more likely to develop osteoporosis than other women.

◆ Having a mother or grandmother with osteoporosis increases your risk.

◆ Taking drugs that contribute to loss of bone mass and density raises risk. The most damaging are glucocorticoids or corticosteroids such as cortisone, prescribed for inflammatory diseases such as rheumatoid arthritis, asthma, or certain lung diseases.

◆ Those who have had diseases that interfere with digestion or the absorption of nutrients are more susceptible to osteoporosis. Such disorders include Cushing's disease, diabetes, anorexia nervosa, bulimia, Crohn's disease, irritable bowel syndrome, hyperthyroidism, hyperparathyroidism, liver disease, multiple myeloma, and kidney failure.

Other Drugs
Combination estrogen plus progesterone (Prempro, Premphase). *Function:* decrease rate of bone breakdown and increase bone density. *Side effects:* similar to estrogen replacement therapy with a decreased risk of associated cancers.

Choosing the Right Calcium for You

Many studies prove that taking calcium supplements prevents bone loss. One study from the University of Auckland in New Zealand found that when women who were at least three years past menopause took 1,000 milligrams of calcium per day, they cut their expected bone loss in half.

There are limits, however, to how well calcium supplements can work. And some forms of calcium are more effective than others for some people. Some supplements even have risks or side effects. What form should you take? There are many different forms.

Calcium carbonate, found in many supplements including Tums, requires plenty of stomach acid to break it down. Studies show that about 40 percent of menopausal women have a shortage of stomach acid and can absorb only about 4 percent of this form of calcium. In fact, a study of 241 people found that the use of Tums as a calcium supplement was associated with a higher risk of upper-arm fracture.

Calcium citrate, on the other hand, is very absorbable, even for those with low stomach acid, because it *is* an acid. With sufficient stomach acid, calcium gluconate, lactate, malate, and aspartate are also absorbable forms.

On the other hand, one poorly absorbed form is the in-

Bisphosphonates such as alendronate (Fosamax). *Function:* decrease the amount of bone loss. *Side effects:* stomach pain, diarrhea, constipation, and headache.

Etidronate (Didronel). *Function:* increase bone density. *Side effects:* stomach pain, constipation, diarrhea, muscle aches, headache.

Calcitonin (Calcimar as injection, Miacalcin as a nasal spray). *Function:* reduce the amount of bone reabsorption. *Calcimar side effects:* nausea, flushing, skin rash and redness at site of injection. *Miacalcin side effects:* runny nose, nosebleeds, headache.

creasingly popular calcium hydroxyapatite, derived from bone meal. Moreover, calcium from bone meal, as well as from oyster shell and dolomite, can contain large amounts of lead.

Clearly, charting your path among a wilderness of supplements can be a challenge. Here's what many health care practitioners recommend:

◆ Calcium (as calcium citrate, gluconate, lactate, malate, or aspartate): up to 1,000 milligrams per day for premenopausal women; up to 2,000 milligrams per day for post-menopausal women, taken in two doses per day with meals (and not at the same time as any iron supplements). *Caution:* Consult your doctor before taking such supplements if you have kidney conditions, are prone to kidney stones, or have hyperparathyroidism.

◆ Vitamin D: 400 to 800 IU. *Caution:* Consult your doctor before taking vitamin D if you have heart disease or a circulatory condition.

◆ Magnesium: The appropriate dosage of magnesium is controversial, but what is known is that people who develop osteoporosis are more likely than others to be deficient in this mineral. Some nutritionists recommend that patients take twice as much magnesium as calcium; if you have risk factors for osteoporosis or are entering menopause, check with your doctor or nutritionist to calculate how much magnesium you should take.

HERBAL REMEDIES

Stinging Nettle (*Urtica dioica*)

Herbalists call this plant nature's multivitamin pill because it contains iron, calcium, magnesium, phosphorus, and good-quality protein. But the leaves do sting; drying or cooking removes the stinging compound from their fine hairs. Nettles are often recommended in cases of anemia, which can also be a problem for older women. *Typical dosage:* up to six 500-milligram capsules of dried leaf products per day; up to 3 cups of tea daily

EXERCISE: THE BEST MEDICINE

For women of all ages, the best preventive measure against osteoporosis is exercise. In young adulthood, exercise builds bone density. In later years, exercise not only prevents bone loss but also helps retain the coordination and balance that may help avoid a fall or minimize injury when one occurs.

What's more, exercise enhances agility, strength, and mood. Fear of falling causes many older women to reduce their activity levels, so gaining strength and balance and improving mood can be a real benefit.

For older women, walking is an especially helpful type of exercise. Bones need weight-bearing exercise to build new bone tissue. Studies prove that weight-bearing exercise for 30 minutes daily, or for up to an hour several times a week, slows bone loss.

Strengthening exercises such as weight training are as important as calcium for strong bones, and they can be started at any age. Even someone age 80 or older can be helped by weight training or isometrics—a form of exercise that involves contracting and releasing specific muscles. Your hospital, community recreation center, or senior center is likely to have more information on this exercise technique.

(steep 1 teaspoon of dried herb in 1 cup of hot water for 10 to 15 minutes).

Horsetail (*Equisetum hyemale, E. arvense*)

This traditional diuretic has long been thought to help the body process calcium. It's also nature's source of silica, a compound that helps strengthen bones, nails, and hair. Standardized horsetail products—certified to contain a certain amount of silicic acid, the natural, organic form of silica—are available in capsule form. *Typical dosage:* up to six 400- to 500-milligram capsules per day; or up to 6 cups of tea per day (steep 2 teaspoons of dried herb in 1 cup of hot water for 10 to 15 minutes); or 15 to 30 drops of tincture three times per day.

Red Clover (*Trifolium pratense*)

Commonly grown as cattle fodder, this red-blossomed clover contains compounds called isoflavones that act as a mild form of estrogen. Isoflavones have been getting a lot of notice lately for their ability to help combat symptoms of perimenopause and early menopause; red clover is the richest herbal source of these compounds. *Typical dosage:* up to five 500-milligram capsules per day; or up to 3 cups of tea per day (steep 1 tablespoon of dried herb in 1 cup of hot water for 10 to 15 minutes).

Red clover

Alfalfa (*Medicago sativa*)

Another herb that might seem to offer more benefits to livestock than to people, alfalfa has actually been used for decades as an appetite booster, an aid in the absorption of nutrients, and a general vitality builder. Alfalfa is rich in vitamins and minerals and, like nettle, is considered a "blood builder." *Typical dosage:* up to nine 400- to 500-milligram capsules per day; or 15 to 30 drops of tincture four times per day; or tea as directed by the manufacturer.

A REASON TO SAVOR SOY

Soybeans and many other beans contain natural estrogen-like compounds called phytoestrogens. In one study of soy products, researchers examined 80 post-menopausal women who ate a half-cup of tofu every day. Early results found that the rate of bone loss among the women slowed down.

Phytoestrogens from soy products may be the reason why women living in Asian countries have a much lower rate of hip fractures than women in Western countries. Asian women also eat more seaweed and fish—both rich in minerals.

Siberian Ginseng (*Eleutherococcus senticosus*)

This herb is one of the most commonly used general tonics, or overall health boosters, available. It helps many body systems function and respond to stress. So why use it for osteoporosis? One of the best lifestyle changes a woman at risk for osteoporosis can make is to exercise more; Siberian ginseng helps the body adapt to the increased physical workload. It also helps increase alertness, which may help prevent falls and other mishaps. *Typical dosage:* up to nine 400- to 500-milligram capsules per day; or 20 drops of tincture up to three times per day.

Overweight

You've decided that you want to lose weight. Maybe you're heeding the warnings of health practitioners who tell you that being overweight is bad for your heart, blood pressure, and other body systems. Or maybe you just want to get rid of a few persistent pounds. But when you decide to try products whose names imply that they'll help you slim down and shape up fast, you get frustrated. While such products claim they'll help you burn fat, build muscle, and regain the body of a 20-year-old, they often fail to live up to their promises.

That's because the sleek, muscular bodies of youth are, for the most part, the result of a youthful metabolism. With age, your metabolic rate drops, along with your activity level and your ability to burn fat and build muscle. And there's no product that can completely reverse that process.

So if someone offers to sell you a pill that will reshape your body without exercise—whether it's a drug or an herb—your first instinct should be to walk away. That said, there are some pharmaceuticals that can support a long-term weight-loss program, though many of them have side effects. There also are some herbs that can help.

If you are taking a drug for weight loss and you want to try some natural remedies as well, you *must* consult your doctor. In both the supplement and the pharmaceutical industries, the weight-loss market is an 800-pound gorilla. New products come out rapidly and their interactions with other substances may not be known until someone has a serious reaction.

But what if you have only 5, 10, or 20 pounds to lose? Can herbs alone help you get the trim, toned physique you want? Many health experts believe they can't. Most herbalists and naturopathic doctors approach body composition from a more holistic perspective, examining diet, exercise level, overall build, and other factors before planning a weight-loss program.

So if you want to incorporate herbs into a weight-loss plan, do your research carefully, avoiding products with outlandish claims and sticking with reputable producers. And if you have a lot of weight to lose, don't let anyone tell you it's going to be fast or easy.

THE SECRET OF SPICES

Fat "metabolism" refers to something a little different than how many calories you burn. In this case, metabolism refers to your body's ability to process fats. Lipotropic herbs, such as cinnamon and ginseng, promote the exportation of fat from the liver, which helps the body use fat for energy.

There's good research that these two herbs lower triglycerides and "bad" LDL cholesterol, say some herbalists. When those two measurements go down, it usually means you're metabolizing fats better. It doesn't, however, mean that these herbs will cause your body to release stored fat. Nor will they necessarily increase metabolism. But normalizing the burning and digestion of fat can make a difference in your health.

Some spicy herbs, such as mustard, black pepper, and cayenne, are also marketed as thermogenics. Again, they won't help your body release stored fat. But they do have a real benefit: aiding digestion. They're stimulating, warming, and invigorating. This means you'll get more nutrients from the food you eat. More nutrients means more energy, more metabolic efficiency, and better overall health—which may make it easier to stay on a diet.

Drug Treatment

Nonprescription Sympathomimetics

Phenylpropanolamine (Dexatrim, Acutrim). *Function:* decrease appetite. *Side effects:* irritability, headache, sweating.

Prescription Sympathomimetics

Amphetamine (Biphetamine), phentermine (Fastin, Ionamin), benzphetamine (Didrex), diethylpropion (Tentuate), mazindol (Sanorex). *Function:* stimulate metabolic rate and decrease appetite. *Side effects:* irritability, headache, sweating, dry mouth, increased blood pressure, heart damage.

WHEN IT COMES TO WEIGHT LOSS, IT'S BUYER BEWARE

Stimulants, including some herbs, can help boost a sluggish metabolism by stimulating adrenal hormone production, suppressing appetite, increasing heart rate, improving blood flow to muscles and fat—all activities related to a process called thermogenesis.

Thermogenesis is the process by which the body generates a heat energy that burns fat. The best-known thermogenic herb is ephedra, or ma huang. Studies show that ephedra stimulates thermogenesis. These findings led to the creation of many over-the-counter weight-loss products. They also led many people to abuse and overuse them, resulting in deaths and heart attacks. The U.S. Food and Drug Administration has issued warnings about weight-loss products that contain ephedra, saying that they shouldn't be used by anyone younger than 18 or for more than seven days. And some reputable health food stores refuse to sell such products. In some states, such products cannot be sold.

Other thermogenic herbs include cordyceps, yohimbe, and bitter orange. All should be treated with as much respect—and caution—as ephedra. In fact, the Herb Research Foundation recommends that use of stimulant herbs should be supervised by a health care professional.

Antidepressants

Fluoxetine (Prozac), sertraline (Zoloft). *Function:* increase the amount of serotonin, a mood-controlling chemical, in the brain, decreasing depression and thereby food intake. *Side effects:* anxiety, insomnia, tremor, sweating.

Other Drugs

Sibutramine (Meridia). *Function:* affect brain chemicals to decrease appetite and depression. *Side effects:* increased blood pressure, dry mouth, headache, constipation, insomnia.

Tetrahydrolipstatin (Xenical). *Function:* reduce the amount of fat absorbed in the digestive tract. *Side effects:* abdominal pain, fatty stools, possible decreased absorption of vitamins.

Here are some tips to help you avoid the potential danger zones in the weight-loss product maze:

◆ **Avoid stimulant laxatives and diuretics.** These include senna (*Cassia acutifolia* or *C. senna*), buckthorn (*Rhamnus catharticus*), and aloe (*Aloe vera*). These herbs may help with the occasional bout of constipation, but they won't help reshape your body, and long-term use can cause serious health problems.

◆ **Realize that you're a guinea pig.** Few weight-loss products have undergone rigorous scientific research and most don't have a long tradition of use for body enhancement, so you're experimenting on yourself if you use them. As for specific ingredients, many herbs, especially the culinary kind, are mild. But there are a few to treat with respect, in particular stimulating herbs such as ephedra and caffeine-containing herbs such as guarana (*Paullinia cupana*).

◆ **Buy carefully.** "You do have to be careful with some of these products—they may actually have drugs in them, such as over-the-counter amphetamines," says nutrition consultant and herb expert Leigh Broadhurst, Ph.D. "Go with a brand name. You've got to pay a little more for something from a big company, but if you buy from somebody you've never heard of over the Internet, it's more likely to be doctored up with an amphetamine."

HERBAL REMEDIES

Garcinia (*Garcinia cambogia*)

This is the primary herb sold for enhancing weight loss and boosting your amount of lean muscle. Also known as hila or brindall berry, garcinia is touted as an appetite suppressant that also prevents the body from making fat. Conclusive research is still lacking, however. A single human trial combined garcinia and chromium, resulting in a few more pounds of weight loss in obese volunteers than a low-fat diet alone, but the study's design has led some experts to question whether it's conclusive.

Garcinia is the source of an extract, hydroxycitric acid (HCA), that is marketed as Citrin, CitriMax, and CitriLean. In rats, HCA blocks an enzyme that converts carbohydrates into body fat, but experts point out that this doesn't prove anything about how it works in humans. On the other hand, many herbalists swear by garcinia, and so far, it appears to have no harmful side effects, perhaps because it isn't a stimulant. *Typical dosage:* 1,000 milligrams three times daily, between meals, for the first four weeks of a weight-loss program.

Psyllium (*Plantago spp.*)

If you're looking for appetite suppression, don't forget the less glamorous herbs that provide fiber. Psyllium can help you eat fewer calories and still feel full. Plus it has other health benefits such as lowering cholesterol and fighting constipation. Be sure, though, to drink plenty of water with dietary fibers such as psyllium or glucomannan—without sufficient liquid, these can swell up in your intestine, causing the constipation that they're sometimes taken to cure. *Typical dosage:* up to six 600-milligram capsules per day with a full glass of water; or up to 1 teaspoon of husks or 2 teaspoons of powdered seed in 1 glass of water (drink immediately). For other fiber products, follow package directions for dosage. *Caution:* Take 30 minutes to an hour after meals or taking other drugs.

Siberian Ginseng (*Eleutherococcus senticosus*)

If you're charging into a new exercise program, even if it's only mild walking, a class of herbs called adaptogens may well be helpful. Siberian ginseng is among the foremost of these herbs. It can help your body adapt to the stress of unaccustomed changes. While it won't resculpt your body, you may feel less tired, so you're more likely to stick to your new exercise routine. *Typical dosage:* up to nine 400- to 500-milligram capsules per day; or 20 drops of tincture up to three times per day.

PARKINSON'S DISEASE

WITH 50,000 NEW CASES DIAGNOSED each year, more than a million people in the United States are affected by Parkinson's disease, a progressive disorder of the central nervous system. The incidence of the disease is considerably higher in people over 50, although an unexpected increase has occurred among people between ages 30 and 40.

Parkinson's is caused by unexplained changes in nerve cells in a particular part of the brain, the basal ganglia. These nerve cells degenerate, resulting in reduced production of a crucial chemical that's involved in the transmission of nerve impulses. This chemical is called dopamine.

DON'T SELF-DIAGNOSE OR SELF-TREAT PARKINSON'S

If you think you have symptoms of Parkinson's, your first stop should be your doctor. Parkinson's is a complex and serious disorder. While natural remedies may be very helpful in its early stages, they might also interact with drugs prescribed for Parkinson's. And many of the newer dietary supplements that can be helpful may have side effects yet to be discovered. So seek the care of a qualified professional before venturing to treat this condition with herbs or other natural remedies.

People with Parkinson's disease experience changes in their ability to control their muscles, often—but not always—resulting in a characteristic tremor. The tremor may start in one hand, and progress to the other hand, the arms, and the legs; the jaw, tongue, forehead, or eyelids may also be affected.

Other symptoms include stiffness, a shuffling walk, instability, drooling, and rigidity. Perhaps the most distressing symptom is muscle stiffness in the face and throat, which can make swallowing, talking, and smiling difficult.

FOOD AND SUPPLEMENTS FOR PARKINSON'S DISEASE

It's rare that a simple, humble food turns out to have the same healing compound as a pharmaceutical. But Parkinson's disease is one condition where it happens.

Common in regional Italian cooking, fresh fava beans (or broad beans) are a dietary source of levodopa, which converts to dopamine—exactly what needs to be restored to brain tissue to facilitate normal muscle action. If you've been diagnosed with Parkinson's and want to try fava beans, discuss this choice with your doctor, especially if you're already taking other drugs.

Eating at least one serving per week of cold-water fish such as salmon is also recommended. Fish contains fish oil, which provides essential fatty acids to the body.

Finally, tank up on your antioxidants, which can play a significant role in delaying the progress of Parkinson's. A few to consider:

◆ **Alpha lipoic acid (ALA).** This very powerful antioxidant helps vitamin E and vitamin C do their own antioxidant work. Researchers at the University of Rochester Medical Center found that ALA protected brain cells from certain hazardous chemicals implicated in Parkinson's. *Typical dosage:* 50 to 200 milligrams per day.

◆ **Huperzine A.** This supplement inhibits acetylcholinesterase, a compound that decreases nerve trans-

Usually, the cause of Parkinson's disease is unknown. There is evidence that the disease runs in families. It can be a later complication of viral encephalitis, a rare and dangerous flu-like infection. But there is some speculation that certain medications administered to the elderly, such as stelazine, causes symptoms that may mimic Parkinson's. Exposure to heavy metals and other toxins is also thought to play a role.

Untreated, Parkinson's disease can advance, eventually resulting in severe incapacity. Falls become more frequent late in the disease,

mission. *Typical dosage:* 25 to 50 micrograms two to four times daily. *Caution:* If you are having surgery, be sure to tell your doctor and anesthesiologist that you are taking this compound.

◆ **Velvet bean extract.** Another bean that's high in levadopa, this one has actually been tested on Parkinson's patients and found to be effective. *Typical dosage:* 500 milligrams two or three times per day. Look for products that have a 10 percent L-dopa content.

◆ **Vitamin E and selenium.** Both of these supplements have been shown to slow progression of symptoms in Parkinson's disease. *Typical dosage:* 800 milligrams of vitamin E per day; 200 to 400 milligrams of selenium per day.

◆ **Vitamin C with bioflavonoids.** Tests have shown that vitamin C combined with bioflavonoids, used in the early stages of Parkinson's, may help. It can also help to counteract the side effects of L-dopa therapy. *Typical dosage:* 1,000 to 3,000 milligrams per day.

◆ **Folic acid.** Deficiency of folic acid has been linked to the development of Parkinson's. *Typical dosage:* 400 to 800 micrograms per day.

◆ **SAM-e (S-adenosylmethionine).** Tests conducted on the elderly show that this compound can help alleviate depression and boost mental function. *Typical dosage:* 200 to 1,200 milligrams day.

and intellect may be affected. Understandably, depression is also commonly seen in people with Parkinson's.

Drug Treatment

Dopamine-Affecting Drugs

Levodopa (Dopar, Laradopa, Sinemet). *Function:* supply missing dopamine. *Side effects:* anorexia, nausea, vomiting, irregular heart-beats, tremors, confusion, restlessness.

Bromocriptine (Parlodel), pergolide (Permax). *Function:* mimic the action of dopamine by fitting into the dopamine receptor sites on nerves. *Side effects:* nausea, vomiting, anorexia, decreased blood pressure, irregular heartbeats, tremors, confusion.

Anticholinergic Drugs

Benztropine (Cogentin). *Function:* decrease tremors and rigidity. *Side effects:* dry mouth, nausea, constipation, irregular heartbeats, restlessness, confusion, drowsiness, increased pressure in the eyes.

Antispasmodic Drugs

Trihexyphenidyl (Artane). *Function:* reduce muscle spasms by acting on the parasympathetic nervous system. *Side effects:* dry mouth, blurred vision, dizziness, nausea, nervousness.

Other Drugs

Amantadine (AmanSymmetrel). *Function:* affect the release of dopamine. *Side effects:* headache, restlessness, depression, irritability, insomnia, agitation, confusion.

Herbal Remedies

Ginkgo (*Ginkgo biloba*)

The leaf of this ancient tree boosts microcirculation to the brain, helping deliver more oxygen to all of the brain's cells. This function can inhibit the progress of dementia, a problem in the late stages of Parkinson's disease. *Typical dosage:* 60 milligrams of ginkgo product standardized to 24 percent flavone glycosides, two or three times per day.

Grapeseed (*Vitis vinifera*)

Powerful antioxidant compounds called procyanidins are found in an extract of grapeseeds.
These compounds can help collect harmful
byproducts of the body's chemical processes
that exist in brain tissue. *Typical dosage:*
enough extract to provide 50 to 200 milligrams of procyanidins per day.

Evening Primrose (*Oenothera biennis*)

The brain is composed primarily of unsaturated
fatty acids, giving a clue to potential botanical
medicines for disorders that affect brain chemistry.
The oil from evening primrose seeds is high in an essential fatty acid called gamma-linolenic acid, or GLA.
Canadian researchers have used evening primrose oil as a clinical
treatment for Parkinson's and other tremor-causing disorders. *Typical dosage:* 2 tablespoons of evening primrose oil per day; or 1,500
to 2,400 milligrams in capsules per day.

Grapeseed

PINKEYE AND STIES

PINKEYE, KNOWN AS CONJUNCTIVITIS among medical professionals,
is an inflammation of the conjunctiva—the clear membrane covering the eyelid and much of the eye. When you have the condition,
the white part of your eye appears pink or red; one or both eyes
water and may burn and itch.

Viruses most commonly cause pinkeye; it often comes with
cold symptoms. If pinkeye accompanies a cold sore, however,
check with your physician to make sure that the herpes virus
hasn't infected your eye.

If the organisms causing pinkeye are bacteria instead of viruses,
you'll probably notice a copious yellow-green discharge and the
white part of your eye will turn an angry red. Infectious pinkeye

Eyewash and Compress How-To's

To make an eyewash, first sterilize an eyecup by immersing it in boiling water for 10 minutes (eyecups are usually available in larger drugstores). In another pan, boil 1 cup of water for 10 minutes. Steep 1 teaspoon of the dried herb or herbs of your choice for 5 to 10 minutes. Strain through a coffee filter. Pour this solution—tolerably warm for infections, cool for allergy-reddened eyes—into a sterilized eyecup and lower your eye to the rim. Look left and right and blink in the eyecup for a full minute. Sterilize the eyecup again before treating the other eye. *Caution:* Do not put herbal extracts, no matter whether they contain alcohol or glycerin, directly into your eyes. Doing so causes much burning and stinging.

To make a compress, simply steep 1 teaspoon of the dried herb or herbs as described above. Strain and cool this tea, then use it to moisten a clean, soft cloth. Apply the cloth to closed eyes for 10 minutes at a time as often as needed.

usually starts out affecting one eye but may spread to the other—and to the eyes of family members and close friends. Be sure to wash your hands after touching your eyes and make sure others don't use your towel or washcloth. Better yet, try not to touch your eyes at all.

Mild bacterial and viral eye infections usually go away in several days without treatment.

Drug Treatment

Antibacterial Eyedrops and Ointments
Ofloxacin (Ocuflax), polymyxin B (Neosporin). *Function:* kill bacteria. *Side effects:* temporary blurred vision after using ointments, initial burning or stinging.

Antiviral Eyedrops

Trifluridine (Trifluorothymidine, Viroptic), idoxuridine (Herpex, Stoxil). *Function:* kill the herpes simplex virus when it is a cause of pinkeye. *Side effects:* stinging or burning in the eyes.

Antiallergy Eyedrops

Levocabastine (Livostin), lodoxamide (Alomide), and olopatadine (Patanol). *Function:* interfere with the release of histamine, the

TIPS FOR CHASING AWAY STIES

A stye is basically a pimple at the base of an eyelash. Sties occur when an eyelid oil gland becomes blocked and a bacterial infection (usually staph) develops around the base of the corresponding hair's follicle or root. Sometimes the infection spreads to neighboring follicles. Eventually the lump bursts, relieving the pain. In a day or two, the stye usually heals and disappears.

Sometimes sties result when our eyes simply become irritated by environmental pollen, pollutants, or chemicals. They can also occur in conjunction with allergies such as hay fever.

Sties are not dangerous and almost always go away on their own. You can hasten the process by applying warm compresses—either plain or made with an eyewash tea—for 10 to 15 minutes four times per day. Or you can alternate hot and cold compresses. Apply heat for four minutes, followed by two minutes of cold. Repeat twice, then end with heat.

Don't try to "pop" a stye by squeezing it; this could damage tender eye tissue. Be patient. The stye will burst on its own. Once it does, rinse the eye thoroughly with warm water or with a warm salt-water solution made by dissolving ¼ teaspoon of salt in 1 cup of water that's been boiled for 10 minutes. If your entire eyelid becomes swollen—especially if you also have a fever and generally feel poorly—call your doctor.

body chemical responsible for the itchiness of pinkeye. *Side effects:* brief and mild burning or stinging upon first instilling the drops.

HERBAL REMEDIES

To use any of the following herbs (with the exception of black tea), see "Eyewash and Compress How-To's" on page 454.

Eyebright (*Euphrasia officinalis*)
Eyebright helps any kind of eye irritation, including infectious pinkeye and allergic conjunctivitis. It is astringent, soothing, and antibacterial.

Yarrow (*Achillea millefolium*)
This herb is astringent, antibacterial, and anti-inflammatory, making it a good choice for irritated or infected eyes. *Caution:* If you are allergic to other members of the daisy family, you may also be allergic to yarrow.

Mullein (*Verbascum thapsus*)
The flowers of this common weed are antiviral, healing, and soothing. They make a good addition to an herbal eyewash blend.

Tea (*Camellia sinensis*)
It's easy, it's handy, and it's an almost universally available remedy for pinkeye. Like black tea, green tea contains bioflavonoids that can help reduce inflammation and fight viral and bacterial infection, but it has fewer tannins, the astringent chemicals that help shrink swollen tissue. Whichever kind you use, just moisten a tea bag with warm water and apply to closed eyes for several minutes. You can do the same for a stye. This will improve circulation to the area and can also prevent possible spread of the infection. (If your eye is red or swollen, moisten the tea bag with cool, rather than warm, water.)

Tea

Berberine-Containing Herbs

Berberine fights a broad range of microbes; you can find it in goldenseal (*Hydrastis canadensis*), Oregon graperoot (*Berberis aquifolium*), barberry (*Berberis vulgaris*), and gold thread (*Coptis* species). Berberine can kill staph and strep bacteria, each of which commonly causes bacterial pinkeye. In fact, Murine eyedrops contain berberine as the active ingredient. These are all excellent herbs to look for in commercial formulas or to use in herbal eyewashes.

PNEUMONIA

IT STARTS OUT FEELING LIKE A BAD COLD. But when the symptoms get worse and you wake up with an awful cough that produces ugly, green mucus, you know it's more than a cold. If these symptoms come with exhaustion, fever, shortness of breath, and chest pain, you've probably got pneumonia.

Pneumonia is an infection of the alveoli, the tiny air sacs inside the lungs. Bacteria, viruses, fungi, and other organisms can be at fault; doctors diagnose pneumonia by physical exam, lab tests, and a chest x-ray. The severity of the condition depends on which organisms cause the infection, how much of the lung is infected, and whether there are additional health factors, such as chronic lung disease, immune dysfunction, or age.

Pneumonia is more serious than other lung infections such as bronchitis. Some patients who have it need to be hospitalized.

Fungal infections in the lungs occur primarily in patients with compromised immune systems. Treatment usually involves antifungal drugs such as ketoconazole. For viral pneumonias, specific drug treatments are not available.

DRUG TREATMENT

Antibiotics

Erythromycin, tetracycline, trimethopeim sulfamethoxazole, cephalosporin drugs (Cefalexin). *Function:* rid the lungs of bacte-

MAKING ALLIES OUT OF ANTIBIOTICS

If you have to take antibiotics for your pneumonia, you can prevent the side effects caused by a decrease in normal digestive bacteria. Here are some supplements to try.

◆ **Saccharomyces boulardii.** This beneficial yeast has been used in Europe for decades to prevent side effects of antibiotics. It inhibits yeast overgrowth and also decreases the risk of a certain type of colitis that can be brought on by using antibiotics. This yeast also stimulates production of a part of the immune system that fights infections in mucous membranes, such as in the lungs. *Typical dosage:* one 300-milligram capsule (3 billion viable organisms per capsule) three times per day while on antibiotics and for one week after.

◆ **Acidophilus and bifidus.** These are the two main beneficial bacteria that antibiotics kill. You can begin taking them while on antibiotics, but you need to continue treatment for at least one month after you finish your antibiotic course for complete replacement. Buy the best quality product available (if your health food store has a good sales staff, they can help you select one) and follow directions on the package.

ria. *Side effects:* rash, upset stomach, intestinal upset, yeast infections, severe infection of the colon.

HERBAL REMEDIES

Echinacea (*Echinacea* spp.)

This well-known immune-boosting herb treats infections by bolstering the body's infection-fighting arsenal. It also directly attacks bacteria. *Typical dosage:* 3 to 5 cups of tea per day (simmer 1 to 2 teaspoons of dried root in 1 cup of water for 10 to 15 minutes); or ¼ to 1 teaspoon of tincture three to five times per day; or 500 to

1,000 milligrams in capsules three to five times per day. *Caution*: Some people who are allergic to plants in the aster family, such as ragweed, are also allergic to echinacea.

Goldenseal (*Hydrastis canadensis*) and Oregon Graperoot (*Berberis aquifolium*)

Both of these herbs kill a wide range of bacteria and fungi. They may have mild immune-stimulating effects as well. Wild goldenseal is an endangered plant species due to overharvesting. So look for a product whose source is cultivated goldenseal, or choose Oregon graperoot instead. *Typical dosage:* 3 to 5 cups of tea per day (simmer 1 to 2 teaspoons of dried root in 1 cup of water for 10 minutes); or ¼ to 1 teaspoon of tincture three to five times per day; or 500 to 1,000 milligrams in capsules, divided into three or four doses per day.

TREATING PNEUMONIA AT HOME

During a bout of pneumonia, good nutrition, a healthy diet, and general physical and emotional support are especially important. Get plenty of rest, and if you live alone, try to have a friend or family member stay with you to help you cook, to purchase or prepare your medicines, and to provide all-around TLC.

Stick with a diet of fresh vegetables, fruit, whole grains, legumes, soups, and juices. Stay away from sugar, which suppresses the immune system.

Warm baths or showers may make you feel better. Be sure to drink plenty of fluids; this helps keep respiratory secretions thin and flush toxins out of your body.

If your symptoms are mild, you might be able to treat bacterial pneumonia with herbs. But if you are not feeling better in a few days or if your symptoms worsen, you need to switch to antibiotic drugs. On the other hand, if your doctor believes you have viral pneumonia, the herbs in this chapter are the treatment of choice.

Garlic (*Allium sativum*)

This versatile, highly antimicrobial herb fights bacteria, fungi, viruses, and parasites. To treat infections, eat several raw cloves per day. Can't stomach quite that much fresh garlic? Try thinly slicing or pressing the cloves through a garlic press; then marinate in a combination of equal parts of honey and fresh lemon juice to cover. Store in the refrigerator for up to two days. Eat 1 to 2 teaspoonfuls three or four times per day.

Mullein (*Verbascum thapsus*)

This common wild plant tones the entire respiratory tract. It also fights inflammation, soothes and heals irritated tissues, and helps ease coughs. *Typical dosage:* 2 to 3 cups of tea per day (simmer 1 to 2 teaspoons of dried root in 1 cup of water for 10 minutes); or ⅛ to 1 teaspoon of tincture three times per day.

Elecampane (*Inula helenium*)

In addition to toning the lungs, easing coughs, and having mild antibacterial effects, elecampane offers other advantages. Because it's bitter, it stimulates appetite and supports digestion, meaning you'll get more from the food you are able to eat. *Typical dosage:* 2 to 3 cups of tea per day (steep 1 to 2 teaspoons of dried root in 1 cup of hot water for 10 minutes); or ⅛ to 1 teaspoon of tincture three times per day. *Caution*: Do not use during pregnancy.

Elecampane

Schisandra (*Schisandra chinensis*)

This traditional Chinese lung tonic strengthens the lungs and treats coughs. *Typical dosage:* 2 to 3 cups of tea per day (simmer 1 to 2 teaspoons of dried fruits in 1 cup of water for 10 to 15 minutes); or ⅛ to 1 teaspoon of tincture three times per day. *Caution:* Avoid schisandra if fever is one of your symptoms.

Schisandra

ESSENTIAL OILS FOR LUNG HEALING

Most essential oils have some antibiotic effects. The best way to use them is in a steam inhalation, which takes their healing components deep into the lungs. Eucalyptus oil is especially helpful for pneumonia, because it not only is a decongestant but also helps you cough up mucus. Tea tree oil is another good choice because it's a potent microbe-fighter.

To make a steam with either of these essential oils, carefully pour water (hot enough to steam, but not hot enough to burn your face) in a heat-resistant bowl and place it on a sturdy table. Add a few drops of essential oil, put a towel over your head, and hold your face at least 12 inches away from the steam. Inhale deeply through mouth and nose until you can no longer smell the fragrant oils. Repeat at least three times per day.

You can also apply either of these essential oils directly to the chest after diluting with a vegetable oil (use about 20 drops of tea tree or eucalyptus essential oil per tablespoon of olive, almond, castor, or other neutral oil).

Another option is to make a heat pack. Moisten a thick piece of absorbent cotton or wool flannel with vegetable oil. Warm the cloth in a low-temperature oven. Add 10 to 20 drops of eucalyptus or tea tree essential oil to the cloth and gently rub them in to disperse them. Apply the pack to your chest (the temperature should be comfortable, not hot). Put a piece of plastic over the top of the pack to protect your bedding, and top it with a hot-water bottle if desired. Leave the pack on for 20 to 30 minutes. Repeat one to three times per day.

Castor oil itself, applied topically, increases blood supply and stimulates the immune system. Practitioners of Traditional Chinese Medicine believe that it "moves energy," directing your immune system to the place in your body that needs it. You can simply massage castor oil into the chest area (front and back) once or twice a day. *Caution:* Do not take castor oil or other essential oils internally.

Usnea (*Usnea* spp.)

A medicinal lichen, usnea helps fight the bacteria that are commonly to blame in bacterial pneumonia. But its active ingredients don't dissolve well in water, so tincture is the best way to take it. *Typical dosage:* ¼ to 1 teaspoon of tincture, three to five times per day.

Licorice (*Glycyrrhiza glabra*)

This often-recommended herb has many benefits for the lungs. It is anti-inflammatory and soothing, and it eases coughs. It also nourishes the adrenal glands, which play a role in stress. *Typical dosage:* 2 to 3 cups of tea per day (simmer 1 to 2 teaspoons of dried root in 1 cup of water for 10 minutes); or ⅛ to ½ teaspoon of tincture two or three times per day. *Caution:* Do not take licorice

EXPECTORANT COUGH SYRUP

Any of the herbs described in this chapter can be substituted for the herbs in this recipe, unless you have an allergy or a condition that precludes you from taking them.

- ½   cup water
- ½   cup honey
- 1–2 teaspoons dried mullein leaves
- 1–2 teaspoons dried horehound herb
- 1–2 teaspoons dried rosemary leaves
- 1–2 teaspoons powdered or chopped cinnamon bark
- 1–2 teaspoons dried chopped ginger
- 1   pinch of cayenne

Combine all of the ingredients in a small pot. Bring to a boil, then lower the heat. Simmer, uncovered, until the mixture has reduced by about one-half. Remove from the heat and strain. Cool to room temperature. Take ½ to 1 teaspoonful as often as every two hours. Store in the refrigerator.

if you are pregnant or nursing. Also avoid the herb if you have high blood pressure, are on heart medications, or have liver, kidney, or thyroid disease.

Horehound (*Marrubium vulgare*)

Remember the horehound lozenges carried in old-fashioned pharmacies? The herb that flavors them promotes mucus production and expectoration, but it also relaxes smooth bronchial muscles, helping you breathe more easily. *Typical dosage:* 2 to 4 cups of tea per day (steep 1 to 2 teaspoons of dried herb in 1 cup of hot water for 10 minutes); or ⅛ to ½ teaspoon of tincture three or four times per day.

Coltsfoot (*Tussilago farfara*)

This traditional cough remedy soothes, eases inflammation, and calms lung spasms. *Typical dosage:* 2 to 4 cups of tea per day (steep 1 to 2 teaspoons of dried flowers or leaves in 1 cup of boiling water for 10 minutes); or ⅛ to 1 teaspoon of tincture three or four times per day. *Caution:* Limit use of coltsfoot to no more than four weeks per year.

Hyssop (*Hyssopus officinalis*)

Both a cough suppressant and an antispasmodic, hyssop has been studied for its antiviral properties, mainly in connection with herpes and HIV. It has been used with horehound in folk medicines for lung ailments. *Typical dosage:* 3 to 4 cups of tea per day (steep 1 to 2 teaspoons of dried herb in 1 cup of water for 10 minutes); or ⅛ to ¼ teaspoon of tincture three or four times per day.

Wild Cherry Bark (*Prunus serotina*)

Wild cherry has a powerful suppressant effect on the cough reflex. Because suppressing your cough is actually counter-productive during pneumonia, use this herb only at night when your cough is interfering with much-needed sleep. *Typical dosage:* 1 cup of tea before bedtime (simmer 1 to 2 teaspoons of dried bark in 1 cup of water for 10 minutes); or ⅛ to ½ teaspoon of tincture before bedtime.

Anise (*Pimpenilla anisum*)

This pleasant-tasting seed eases coughs by calming respiratory spasms. *Typical dosage:* 2 to 4 cups of tea per day (steep 1 to 2 tea-

The Good Old-Fashioned Plaster

Herb plasters are a time-honored, highly effective way to treat pneumonia. Herbalists often make plasters with warming herbs such as mustard, ginger, and garlic because they increase blood supply and increase expectoration.

To make a plaster, mix one-half ounce by weight of dried, powdered mustard, ginger, or garlic with one-half ounce of powdered slippery elm or marshmallow root. Add water, a tablespoon at a time, until the mixture forms a thick paste. Spread a thin layer of paste on a piece of thin cloth.

Apply the plaster, cloth side down, on your chest or back and leave it on 15 to 30 minutes. Lift the plaster frequently to make sure your skin is not burning from the heat of the herbs. If you feel pain or if your skin is turning bright red, remove the plaster immediately. It's best to have someone assist you when using a plaster; they're hard to apply on your own. Do not reuse them; make a fresh herbal plaster each time.

spoons of dried seeds in 1 cup of hot water for 10 minutes); or ⅛ to ½ teaspoon of tincture two to four times per day.

Marshmallow Root (*Althaea officinalis*) and Slippery Elm Bark (*Ulmus rubra*)

Both of these herbs are demulcent, which means they contain soothing substances that decrease coughing by coating and protecting irritated tissues. Both work best if taken as a tea. *Typical dosage:* 2 to 4 cups of tea per day (simmer 1 to 2 teaspoons of chopped root or bark in 1 cup of water for 10 minutes).

POISON IVY, OAK, AND SUMAC

IF YOU'RE SENSITIVE TO POISON IVY, oak, or sumac, you probably remember your encounters with these plants in all their morbid details. Maybe as a child you picked a bouquet of shiny reddish leaves for your mom. Maybe your dog ran through poison oak, then trotted back for a big hug. Maybe you slipped while hiking and landed in a patch of the stuff. One to three days later, your skin reddened and itched. Then came the blisters, the oozing, the crusting, the misery of it all.

If you have inhaled smoke from the burning plant, have gotten the oil in your eyes, experience severe itching and discomfort, or find that the rash is becoming infected, call your doctor. Otherwise, you can usually manage this allergic reaction yourself.

Home care begins with removing the powerfully irritating resin of the poison plants as soon as possible after exposure. Flush your skin with lots of water, then wash with soap. Also wash clothes, shoes, gloves, pets, gardening tools, and anything else that might have been in contact with the plant. On your way to washing up, remember that you can spread these resins easily by touch. (That's why pets can spread the itch without getting it themselves—the resin stays on top of their fur.)

The general idea for treating allergic rashes such as those caused by poison ivy, oak, and sumac is to reduce inflammation and dry the skin. That means you want anti-inflammatory and astringent herbs but should avoid ointments and heavy creams that trap moisture. This goes for non-herbal products as well.

DRUG TREATMENT

Antihistamines
Diphenhydramine, taken orally (Benadryl) or as a topical gel (Dermarest). *Function:* reduce itching. *Oral use side effects:* drowsiness, dryness of mouth, nose, and throat.

Calamine products (Caladryl, Ivarest, others). *Function:* dry the rash and relieve itching. *Side effects:* products that combine calamine lotion with a topical anesthetic (benzocaine, lidocaine, pramoxine) may be absorbed in significant amounts through inflamed skin and cause an allergic reaction.

Corticosteroids

Hydrocortisone, topically (Cortaid, Lanacort, and others) or orally, dexomethasone (Decadron), prednisone (Orosone). *Function:* reduce itching and cool inflammation. *Short-term topical use side effects:* none. *Oral use side effects:* acne, indigestion, nausea, vomiting, gas, headache, dizziness, insomnia, increased appetite.

Herbal Remedies

Grindelia (*Grindelia squarrosa, G. robusta*)

Also known as gumweed, this plant exudes a gummy resin. To use it on a rash from a poisonous plant, mix a tincture of grindelia with an equal quantity of cool water. Moisten a cloth with this solution and apply as a compress. You can repeat the application as often as needed.

Jewelweed (*Impatiens capensis*)

This plant has a strong reputation for quelling poison ivy, oak, and sumac rashes. Apply either the crushed fresh leaves or a compress made from tea or a fluid extract. To make a tea, steep 1 heaping teaspoon of dried leaves or 2 teaspoons of fresh leaves in 1 cup of hot water for 10 minutes; strain and cool. To use a fluid extract, add 1 teaspoon to 1 cup of cool water. Wet a clean cloth with either liquid and apply to the rash. Repeat as needed.

Plantain (*Plantago* spp.)

A common lawn weed, plantain contains a soothing substance called allantoin. It's anti-inflammatory, antimicrobial, and as a bonus, it speeds wound healing. So if you get poison ivy or other such rashes often, let plantain keep its spots in your lawn. When you get a rash—or a mosquito bite—pick a few leaves, wash them, mash them, and apply as a poultice to your rash. Repeat as necessary.

Aloe (*Aloe vera*)

This well-known sunburn remedy is soothing, anti-inflammatory, and antibacterial, and it hastens healing, so it's great for the poison itchies. Slice a leaf, scoop out the gel, and apply as needed. You can also look for commercial aloe vera gel product, but check the label to make sure that it contains mostly pure aloe vera.

Witch Hazel (*Hamamelis virginiana*)

This herb is soothing, cooling, and drying—perfect for weepy rashes. The easiest way to use it for poison rashes is to buy the fluid extract carried in most drugstores. Simply apply it as needed to the rash—splash it on or saturate a clean washcloth and drape it over the rash.

Cucumber (*Cucumis sativus*)

This cool customer is just what you want on inflamed skin. You can apply slices of cucumber directly to your rash; or puree cucumber in the blender, apply this mash to your skin, cover with a loosely woven cloth, and lie down for a bit. Repeat as often as you like.

Oats (*Avena sativa*)

This time-honored anti-itch remedy is easy to use. Add oats to a cool bath. Put ½ to 1 cup of cut oats in cheese-cloth or a clean athletic sock, tie, and use the cloth- or sock-bound oats as a washcloth. You can also add 3 to 5 drops of essential oil of peppermint to your oatmeal bath for an extra cooling touch. *Caution:* Don't be tempted to go overboard and add more than a few drops; essential oils are very concentrated and can irritate skin if used in more than minute quantities.

Tea (*Camellia sinensis*)

If you break out with poison ivy unexpectedly on a camping trip, it's good to be a tea drinker. Tea is antioxidant-rich, and its tannic acids contract inflamed tissue and relieve itching. Just grab a tea bag (black or green tea will work), moisten it, and apply to the skin. Repeat as necessary.

Oats

Time-Tested Itch Relievers

Getting your first bad case of poison ivy as an adult can be distressing if you're not familiar with the flaming itch. Luckily, the commonsense cures you've heard about for years really do work. Try these:

◆ **Take a bicarb bath.** Put ½ cup of baking soda in a tepid bath. (Avoid hot water, which generally increases itching and hives.)

◆ **Play games with paste.** Not the kind of paste you used to eat in kindergarten, but a paste of baking soda and water. Finger-paint the paste on affected areas.

◆ **Create a cure with clay.** Simply mix water and green clay powder to make a remedy that's a favorite of Sunny Mavor, coauthor of *Kids, Herbs, and Health.* Clay draws oils, including the resin that's causing your itch, away from the skin and feels pleasantly cooling. Many health food stores stock this powder.

◆ **Put the itch on ice.** Relief will be quick, though temporary. Use a commercial cold pack or simple cubes in a resealable bag.

◆ **Plan for prevention.** Before you accidentally tangle with these plants again, learn to identify them. Know how and where they usually grow and what they look like in different seasons. If they're on your property, your county extension office can give you advice on safely removing them.

PROSTATE ENLARGEMENT

FOR A GLAND THE SIZE OF A WALNUT, the prostate manages to cause men a lot of trouble. Basic anatomy explains the problem: The prostate wraps around the base of the urethra, the tube that transports urine from the bladder to the penis. Consequently, when the gland enlarges, it obstructs the flow of urine.

Early symptoms of prostate enlargement commonly affect men in their mid to late forties, though symptoms can occur earlier. A little urinary hesitation is often the first sign that something is amiss, and what once happened effortlessly seems to require a few minutes of straining to get started. A chronic sensation of pressure or urgency may develop, and over time, it becomes increasingly difficult to fully empty the bladder. This means an increased risk of bladder infection as well as restless nights from frequent trips to the bathroom. In severe cases, urine can back up into the kidneys and damage them.

When the prostate gland enlarges for reasons other than cancer or infection, doctors call the condition benign prostatic hypertrophy (BPH). BPH is one of the most common of all health problems experienced by men. In fact, it has been estimated that 50 to 60 percent of men between the ages of 40 and 60, and up to 90 percent of men over 80, have some degree of BPH. The cost of treatment is staggering: In the United States alone, more than $1 billion a year is spent on surgery and hospital care for BPH.

Why is BPH so common? Experts believe that two things are to blame: normal hormonal changes that occur as men age and environmental factors.

Hormone levels shift for men in mid-life just as they do for women. Research shows that testosterone—the predominant male hormone—begins to decline while estrogen and prolactin—the "female" hormones—show a relative increase. As blood levels of testosterone drop, however, the rate of this hormone's conversion into a compound called dihydrotestosterone (DHT) actually increases, es-

EATING FOR A HEALTHY PROSTATE

Herbs are only one alternative to drug treatment for prostate enlargement. Here are a few others.

◆ **Zap problems with zinc.** This mineral has been shown to inhibit an enzyme that fosters prostate enlargement. Rich dietary sources of zinc include oysters and other shellfish, red meat, ginger, eggs, nuts, seeds, and grains. Experts usually recommend that men with benign prostatic hypertrophy (BPH) take 25 to 60 milligrams of zinc per day.

◆ **Push the protein.** High protein diets (in which 45 percent of daily calories come from protein) have been shown to block the same enzyme that zinc affects, while diets containing less than 10 percent protein can increase DHT (dihydrotestosterone), the "bad" testosterone. Soy protein is especially helpful. It's high in hormone-like substances called isoflavones that block the effects of excessive estrogen as well as inhibit compounds that build DHT. It also contains compounds called phytosterols that have been shown to increase urinary flow. For optimal results,

pecially in the prostate gland. Enlarged prostates can have four to six times the normal amount of DHT. And there lies the problem: DHT makes prostate cells grow.

Certain toxic organic chemicals appear to make DHT build up in the prostate. Many of these toxins are residues of industrial solvents and pesticides. Cadmium, a toxic heavy metal, has been shown to increase prostatic DHT. So has elevated cholesterol. Fortunately, this increased production of DHT can be blocked by dietary changes, some drugs, and herbs.

DRUG TREATMENT

Alpha Adrenergic Receptor Antagonists

Terazosin (Hytrin), doxazosin (Cardura), prazosin (Minipress). *Function:* relax the smooth muscles of the prostate and bladder eat 3 to 4 ounces of soybeans, tofu, tempeh, or powdered soy protein every day.

◆ **Go fish or go flax.** Essential fatty acids derived from salmon, mackerel, haddock, cod, or flaxseed can alleviate the symptoms of BPH. These oils appear to work by decreasing inflammation, which may be a contributing cause of prostate enlargement. Flaxseed is best consumed as a meal made from the fresh ground seeds. *Typical dosage:* mix 2 to 4 tablespoons into a shake or smoothie or sprinkle it on food daily. If you just want to eat fish instead, 3 to 4 servings per week is recommended.

◆ **Turn on to tomatoes.** These red wonders may turn out to be the miracle food for keeping your prostate healthy. Tomatoes are very high in lycopene, an antioxidant pigment similar to beta-carotene, but much more potent, at least where the prostate is concerned. The lycopene in fresh tomatoes does not appear to be absorbed very well, but cooking increases its absorbability, especially when it is combined with oil. Particularly good dietary sources of lycopene include organic catsup and organic tomato paste. Lycopene is also available in tablet form. *Typical dosage:* 10 to 30 milligrams per day.

neck to allow easier urination. *Side effects:* fatigue, dry mouth, headaches, dizziness, low blood pressure.

Other Drugs

Finasteride (Proscar). *Function:* decrease blood levels of dihydrotestosterone and the size of the prostate gland; effective in only about 30 percent of men. *Side effects:* loss of libido, impotence.

HERBAL REMEDIES

Saw Palmetto (*Serenoa repens*)

Although this plant grows wild in the coastal regions of Florida, South Carolina, and Georgia, most of the research on its clinical effects has occurred in Germany, France, and Italy. Urologists in these countries have been successfully treating BPH with an ex-

Don't Self-Diagnose This Condition

The symptoms of an enlarged prostate can strike fear into the hearts of grown men. Yet many cases of benign prostatic hypertrophy (BPH) are mild and respond well to simple preventive treatments early on. Nevertheless, an enlarged prostate gland, because of its location, can hide prostate cancer by making it more difficult to diagnose. That's why, if you have BPH symptoms, it's crucial not to suffer in silence—no matter how much you hate going to the doctor. Don't put off that visit: Chances are the news will be good.

Saw palmetto

tract of saw palmetto berries for many years, but only recently has the herb achieved acceptance in the United States. More than 17 studies confirm its effectiveness and safety; one compared it to Proscar and found that the herb worked just as well as the drug but with fewer side effects. *Typical dosage:* 160 milligrams of a fat-soluble extract standardized to contain 85 to 95 percent fatty acids and sterols, two times per day, for several months. (It may take that long before the saw palmetto's full effect is achieved, but it can safely be taken indefinitely.)

Pygeum (*Prunus africanum*)

This evergreen prune tree grows in the mountains of Africa. Extracts made from its bark have been used in Europe for more than 30 years to treat BPH. The bark appears to contain compounds that work together to decrease swelling and inflammation in the prostate and to block the detrimental effects of testosterone. At least nine published studies involving hundreds of men have demonstrated that pygeum improves urinary flow, decreases nighttime urination, and enhances quality of life for those with BPH. While the herb appears to work well, especially in combination with saw palmetto, one concern is that pygeum has been overharvested and is on the verge of becoming an endangered species. So some herbalists recommend saving pygeum for when other herbs haven't worked. *Typical dosage:* 50 to 100 milligrams of a product standardized to contain 14 percent triterpenes and 0.5 percent n-docosanol two times per day. *Caution:* Some men may experience mild stomach upset when taking pygeum.

Stinging Nettle (*Urtica dioica*)
Herbalists have long used this common weed as a diuretic. While it has not been studied as thoroughly as saw palmetto or pygeum, research in Europe has shown that extracts of the root do have anti-inflammatory properties and can relieve symptoms of an enlarged prostate. Since stinging nettle root does not appear to shrink an enlarged gland, it is best used in combination with saw palmetto. *Typical dosage:* 300 to 600 milligrams of nettle root extract per day; or ½ to 1 teaspoon of tincture per day. *Caution:* May cause mild upset stomach or occasional diarrhea.

Pumpkin Seed (*Curcubita pepo*)
Ever roast these seeds after carving your pumpkin? The raw seeds have long been a popular folk remedy for expelling intestinal worms and parasites. In the Ukraine, they are also used to treat prostate inflammation. In Europe, pumpkin seed oil is often combined with saw palmetto in formulas for BPH. Researchers have found that pumpkin seed oil increases urine flow; it also contains other ingredients that might help BPH. *Typical dosage:* about 3 tablespoons of ground seeds per day; or 500 to 600 milligrams of pumpkin seed oil in capsules per day.

RAYNAUD'S PHENOMENON

W E ALL EXPERIENCE COLD HANDS AT TIMES. What makes people with Raynaud's phenomenon different? Cold and sometimes emotional stress cause the small blood vessels of their fingers and toes to constrict, drastically reducing blood circulation. These extremities first turn white or blue, then sometimes red. Pain, numbness, and tingling often accompany episodes. Sometimes the skin at the fingertips ulcerates. Sometimes the same thing happens to the tongue and tip of the nose.

In cold, damp climates, Raynaud's affects 20 to 30 percent of women but only 4 to 13 percent of men. In what's called primary Raynaud's phenomenon, the cause isn't known. Symptoms usually develop during a person's late teens or early twenties. Both hands are affected and often both feet.

In secondary Raynaud's phenomenon, an underlying problem such as rheumatoid arthritis, scleroderma, or mechanical trauma (such as repeated use of a vibrating tool) causes the circulatory problem. The disorder begins later in life, and often only one extremity is affected.

For severe cases of Raynaud's that don't respond to drugs, a surgery called sympathectomy, in which the nerves that cause constriction of the blood vessels in the hands are cut, may provide some relief. Newer methods involve cutting these nerves in the hands, not near the spinal cord. If your symptoms are mild, you can probably avoid both drugs and surgery.

DRUG TREATMENT

Calcium Channel Blockers
Nifedipine (Procardia, Adalat), amlodipine (Lotrel, Norvasc), diltiazem (Cardizem, Dilacor-XR), felodipine (Lexxel, Plendil, Renedil), isradipine (Dyna Circ). *Function:* inhibit small blood vessels from constricting; reduce the accumulation of platelets to min-

SIMPLE STRATEGIES FOR RAYNAUD'S

The primary management of Raynaud's is simple and cheap: Avoid getting cold, and if emotional upsets trigger symptom flare-ups, learn to manage stress. The former entails doing whatever it takes to keep your hands and feet warm. Gloves and warm socks are particularly important, and a hat helps conserve body heat. On chilly days, bundle up before you go out the door, not halfway down your front walk. Put on your gloves even if you're going straight from your home to your car. Some people with Raynaud's have to wear gloves to remove things from the refrigerator. If you enjoy winter sports, you might want to invest in battery-warmed gloves and boots or chemically activated hand- and foot-warming packets. If you experience symptoms anyway, immerse your hands in warm (not hot) water or put them in your armpits or between your thighs.

   If stress seems to make your fingers and toes go cold and white, consider getting relaxation training or learning yoga and meditation. And stay away from tobacco products, as nicotine causes constriction of peripheral blood vessels.

imize the clogging of small vessels. *Side effects:* tiredness, dizziness, headache, numbness or tingling in hands and feet, swelling of ankles and feet, nausea, constipation, shortness of breath.

HERBAL REMEDIES

Ginkgo (*Ginkgo biloba*)
An extract of the leaves of the ginkgo tree improves circulation to the brain and extremities by dilating small blood vessels. It also protects cells from low-oxygen situations (which is what occurs during a Raynaud's attack), and inhibits platelets from sticking together and clogging small vessels. Ginkgo is also an antioxidant.

Several studies have shown that ginkgo can help with circulation. Studies focusing on ginkgo's possible benefits for people with Raynaud's have yet to be done, but practitioners are suggesting this herb to their patients. *Typical dosage:* 120 to 160 milligrams of extract standardized to contain 6 percent terpene lactones and 24 percent ginkgo flavone glycosides, divided into two or three doses per day. *Caution:* Do not take ginkgo if you routinely take aspirin or blood thinners such as warfarin.

Bilberry (*Vaccinium myrtillus*)

This herb contains flavonoids called anthocyanosides that function as potent antioxidants, inhibit the release of inflammatory compounds, help maintain the health of capillaries, and relax small blood vessels—all good things for people with Raynaud's. It also

SUPPLEMENTS TO KILL THE CHILL

Though there's not a lot of research on the use of vitamins and minerals in treating Raynaud's, many of them influence blood flow. Also, some people with the disorder have been found to be deficient in these nutrients.

◆ **Inositol hexanicotinate.** This form of niacin won't cause skin flushing, as other forms can. Two studies involving people with Raynaud's have shown a positive effect. One study found that a dose of 4,000 milligrams per day during cold weather reduced Raynaud's attacks. *Typical dosage:* 500 milligrams three times daily for the first two weeks, then 1,000 milligrams three times per day.

◆ **Magnesium.** Deficiency in this mineral appears to play a significant role in Raynaud's phenomenon. Even in people without Raynaud's, decreased magnesium levels can induce small arteries to constrict. Though research is continuing on whether supplements can help, you'd be wise to make sure you're getting the daily value of magnesium: 350 milligrams for men and 280 helps preserve the small vessels after circulation has been temporarily and drastically curtailed, which happens upon exposure to cold. Although yet to be studied in people with Raynaud's, this herb has been shown to be effective in the treatment of capillary fragility, varicose veins, and other vascular disorders. *Typical dosage:* 240 to 480 milligrams of capsules or tablets standardized to 25 percent anthocyanosides, divided into two or three doses per day.

Garlic (*Allium sativum*)

Like ginkgo, garlic has been shown to improve intermittent claudication, another circulation disorder. Garlic inhibits platelets from clumping, breaks up clots, lowers blood pressure and cholesterol, and acts as an antioxidant. Any of these properties can help pa-

milligrams for women (320 if you're pregnant). Good food sources include kelp, wheat bran, wheat germ, molasses, brewer's yeast, nuts, peanuts, tofu, buckwheat, and other whole grains.

◆ **Essential fatty acids.** By increasing your intake of the right essential fatty acids, you can combat processes of inflammation that sometimes play a role in disorders such as Raynaud's. So far, essential fatty acid treatment has shown a mild positive effect in relieving Raynaud's. Flaxseed oil, though not yet studied, may be a good choice as it's rich in two main types of essential fatty acids and is also inexpensive. *Typical dosage:* 1 to 2 tablespoons of flaxseed oil per day. Animal studies have shown that evening primrose oil can reduce blood-vessel constriction, so it may also be worth a try; follow manufacturer's suggestions for dosage.

◆ **Antioxidants.** Theoretically, this group of nutrients should help people with Raynaud's. When circulation slows significantly, tissue-damaging substances called free radicals are generated. Antioxidants can mop up these free radicals to prevent injury. Dietary supplements that might help include vitamin C (500 milligrams once or twice per day) and vitamin E (400 IU per day).

tients with Raynaud's by maintaining healthy blood vessels. *Typical dosage:* up to three 500- to 600-milligram capsules per day; or two raw cloves per day minced and blended into foods. *Caution:* If you already take a blood-thinning medication, consult your doctor before taking garlic.

Cayenne Pepper (*Capsicum annuum*)

This powerful antioxidant reduces blood cholesterol and platelet stickiness. It also warms you up! Add as much of this spice to foods as you can stand. You can also apply an ointment containing cayenne or its active ingredient, capsaicin, to hands and feet; such creams are now available in most pharmacies. *Typical dosage:* up to three 400- to 500-milligram capsules per day; or 5 to 10 drops of tincture in water one to three times per day. *Caution:* Be sure to wash your hands after applying cayenne to avoid getting it in your eyes or on other sensitive areas. Excessive internal doses can cause gastrointestinal irritation in some people.

Ginger (*Zingiber officinale*)

Another warming spice, ginger is antioxidant and reduces platelet stickiness and cholesterol. It also reduces inflammation and relieves pain. *Typical dosage:* up to eight 500- to 600-milligram capsules per day; or ½ to 1 teaspoon per day of the ground powder mixed into foods; or 1 to 2 teaspoons of grated fresh root per day; or 10 to 20 drops of tincture in water three times per day. *Caution:* If you take a blood thinner, consult your doctor before taking therapeutic doses of ginger.

Hawthorn (*Crataegus* spp.)

This herb acts as a tonic for the heart and blood vessels. It increases the strength of both the vessels and the heart's contractions, thereby increasing circulation to the extremities. Although this herb is usually used in congestive heart failure, many practitioners feel it has value for people with Raynaud's as well. Most research has focused on hawthorn's leaves and flowers, and most capsules, tablets, and tinctures are made from them. But a tea made from the berries is a traditional remedy for improving circulation. *Typical dosage:* up to nine 500- to 600-milligram capsules per day of nonstandardized herb; or 160 milligrams three times per day of a product standardized for oligomeric procyanidins; or 10 to 30 drops of tincture three times per day; or 3 to 4 cups of tea per day (simmer 1 teaspoon of dried berries in 1 cup of water for 10 to 15 minutes).

Gotu Kola (*Centella asiatica*)

Best known as a wound-healer, this herb acts to maintain the health of the skin and underlying connective tissue. In one study, people with scleroderma who took 20 milligrams of gotu kola extract three times per day decreased their symptoms, including joint pain, skin hardening, and immobility of the fingers. People with scleroderma often develop Raynaud's. If you have one or both conditions, this may be an herb to try. *Typical dosage:* up to eight 400- to 500-milligram nonstandardized capsules per day, divided into three doses; or 20 to 40 drops of tincture two times per day; or 20 milligrams of standardized product three times per day.

Gotu kola

SCABIES

IF YOUR MOTHER USED TO TUCK YOU IN with the rhyme, "Sleep tight, don't let the bed bugs bite," you may not have known what she meant. She was referring to scabies, a microscopic mite that burrows into the surface of the skin to lay its eggs. Infected bedding or clothing transmits the mite; the resulting constant itch can rival chiggers and poison ivy in intensity.

Scabies mites cause lesions that occur in lines most likely to turn up on the hands, wrists, armpits, genitalia, inner thighs, and elbows. The mites and their eggs can be seen with a microscope or magnifying glass. Scabies outbreaks are common where people are in close proximity, such as in schools, summer camps, and nursing homes. Those with compromised immune systems, such as AIDS patients, tend to get scabies more often. Crusted or Norwegian scabies is a special type that's more difficult to treat.

If you or a family member has scabies, make sure to thoroughly clean all bedding before, during, and after treatment to prevent reinfestation. Keep an eye on your pets, as they could be the source of the scabies.

Treatment of scabies is designed to kill the mites and to control the itching that can last after all mites have died. You'll also want to prevent bacterial infection of the lesions.

Researchers have not yet tested herbal remedies for scabies, although people have been using herbs for this purpose for years. The best way to use most of the following herbs is to make a strong tea and use it as a skin wash, then apply an essential oil preparation.

Drug Treatment

Insecticides
Gamma benzene hexachloride (Lindane). *Function:* kill the mites with an insecticide applied to the skin. *Side effects:* nerve damage, skin irritation.

Permethrin 5 percent cream (Nix, Elimite), crotamiton cream or lotion (Eurax), benzyl benzoate 20 to 30 percent lotion (generic), and sulfur preparations (generic). *Function:* kill the mites. *Side effects:* skin irritation.

Corticosteroids
Triamcinolone (Aristocort, Kenacort, Atolont). *Function:* heal the skin after scabies mites are eliminated and quell itching. *Side effects:* acne, redness, thinning of the skin.

Other Drugs
Oral ivermectin (Mectizan). *Function:* kill scabies mites. *Side effects:* anorexia, lethargy.

Herbal Remedies

Neem (*Azadiracta indica*)
This tree's essential oil has pesticide properties and may be useful against scabies when applied to the skin. The oil also has antibac-

terial and antifungal activity. But little research has tested dosages for neem products. So follow the manufacturer's recommendations on how to use a product containing neem for scabies. *Caution:* Use externally only.

Clove (*Syzygium aromaticum*)

This spice has traditionally been used on the skin to treat scabies. Clove essential oil has analgesic and anti-inflammatory properties, plus antimicrobial activity, which is important to prevent a bacterial infection from occurring in any broken skin that the rash's itching may have produced. But clove oil can also irritate skin, so try a test patch first. If irritation results, use a lower concentration. You can apply a mixture of 10 drops of clove oil and 1 cup of vegetable oil such as olive or almond oil to the rash before bedtime. You can also try adding the clove oil to a mixture of half honey and half water; apply in the same way. *Caution:* Do not use clove oil during pregnancy.

USING OILS TO FOIL SCABIES

After washing the infested area with an herbal skin wash, apply a generous amount of essential oil prepared from your herbs of choice. In addition to any mite-killing power that the preparation may have, the oil helps to smother the pests.

It's important to dilute essential oils before applying them to the skin. For most oils, mix no more than 1 teaspoon of essential oil with 1 cup of what's called a carrier oil—you can use any neutral vegetable oil such as almond, olive, sesame, or even corn oil.

Another herbal oil technique is the infused oil. Herbal expert James A. Duke, Ph.D., author of *The Green Pharmacy,* recommends applying oil of St.-John's-wort extracted in evening primrose oil. To make it, combine a cup or so of fresh St.-John's-wort flowering tops in enough evening primrose oil to cover them. Steep for two weeks. Strain out the herbs and apply the oil to scabies lesions up to three times per day.

Tea Tree (*Melaleuca alternifolia*)

The essential oil from this plant fights a number of parasites, including the mite that causes scabies. To use, combine 1 teaspoon of tea tree oil with 5 teaspoons of vegetable oil. Apply liberally to the skin, especially before bedtime. *Caution:* If skin irritation results, further dilute the oil more or discontinue use.

Rosemary (*Rosmarinus officinalis*)

This herb fights many parasites and may help stop an infestation of scabies. *Typical dosage:* 1 cup of boiling water poured over 1 to 2 teaspoons of dried herb. Allow to cool; use it to wash infested skin as often as three times per day.

Tea tree

Tansy (*Tanacetum vulgare*)

A strong tea made of tansy has been traditionally used for scabies. The dried herb itself has a long history of use for shooing away insects, so it may work on mites. To make the tea, simmer 2 teaspoons of dried herb in 1 cup of water for 10 minutes. Strain, cool, and use to wash the infected skin one or more times per day. If you apply it only once, do so before bedtime. *Caution:* Do not take internally.

SHINGLES

BLAME CHICKEN POX. That mostly harmless illness we get as children can come back to haunt us decades later. Herpes zoster, the other name for shingles, is the illness that occurs when the chicken pox virus, which goes dormant in the nerves along the spine, becomes active again.

The reason the virus reactivates isn't clear, but it may have to do with a weakening of the immune system, which can occur with age. Stress can also impair immunity temporarily. Chronic illnesses, especially those that attack the immune system, such as AIDS or certain cancers, can lower resistance. So can medications that suppress the immune system, such as cortisone taken long-term or drugs used after a transplant or during chemotherapy.

When the chicken pox virus multiplies within the nerves, it produces a burning, tingling, or intensely painful sensation in the area serviced by those nerves. Pain may follow a line that wraps from the back around one side of the ribs. Or it may travel down an arm or a leg or spread across one side of the face. The affected skin may be extremely sensitive to touch. The person may also feel lousy in general, with slight fever and headache.

When the virus migrates along the nerves to the skin, it produces a rash of many clustered blisters. The rash, like the pain, involves only one side of the body. The blisters are often painful and sometimes itchy and take about ten days to crust, scab, and heal. About 10 percent of people have pain that lingers several months after the rash clears. The rash can become infected; if this happens, if the discomfort is severe, or if your immune system is suppressed and you get shingles, see your doctor.

In general, patients with compromised immune systems, whether due to chronic illness or immune-suppressing medications, receive more aggressive treatment for shingles because the outbreak can cause such people to develop more severe illness.

DRUG TREATMENT

Analgesics

Acetaminophen, aspirin, ibuprofen, naproxen (Aleve). *Function:* reduce pain, fever, and (except acetaminophen) inflammation. *Acetaminophen side effects:* not common with short-term use and regular doses. *Aspirin side effects:* heartburn, indigestion, stomach irritation, mild nausea or vomiting. *Ibuprofen and naproxen side effects:* dizziness, nausea, stomachache, headache.

Antiviral Drugs

Acyclovir (Avirax, Zovirax), famciclovir (Famvir), valacyclovir (Valtrex). *Function:* kill viruses. *Side effects: rare.*

Vidarabine (Vira-A). *Function:* kill viruses. *Side effects:* decreased appetite, nausea, vomiting, diarrhea, tremor, dizziness, confusion, hallucinations, headache.

Tricyclic Antidepressants

Amitriptyline (Elavil, Emitrip, Endep, Enovil, Limbitrol), desipramine (Norpramin). *Function:* help reduce pain. *Side effects:* tremor, headache, dry mouth, unpleasant taste in mouth, constipation, diarrhea, nausea, fatigue, weakness, drowsiness, nervousness, excessive sweating, insomnia.

Corticosteroids

Prednisone (Deltasone, Meticorten, Orasone, others). *Function:* reduce pain. *Side effects:* increased appetite, weight gain, fluid retention, indigestion, nausea, vomiting, dizziness, insomnia, acne, poor wound-healing, decreased immune function.

Herbal Remedies

Cayenne or Chili Pepper (*Capsicum* spp.)

Why not fight fire with fire? Hot peppers contain capsaicin, which depletes substance P, a chemical involved in the nerve transmission of pain. Several studies have shown capsaicin-containing creams effective in easing the pain of shingles. You can buy a commercial cream or you can make your own by blending a small amount of cayenne powder into body lotion or aloe vera gel. Aloe has its own benefits and may soothe the burning of cayenne, which might be too irritating during the blister phase of shingles. Try combining 1 tablespoon of aloe gel with up to ⅛ teaspoon of cayenne pepper. Apply to a test patch of normal skin; if it burns, add more aloe gel. Use as often as necessary. *Caution:* When you use cayenne products, wash your hands afterward to avoid spreading the oil to your eyes or other sensitive areas.

Lemon Balm (*Melissa officinalis*)

Who would think that this leafy, lemon-scented herb would be an ally against viruses? One study has proven lemon balm's effectiveness against the herpes simplex virus, a relative of the one that causes shingles. So it's worth a try, especially since it's very safe. Commercial creams containing it are widely available. If you have access to fresh lemon balm leaves, moisten them, wrap them in a loosely woven damp cloth such as cheesecloth or thin T-shirt cotton, and apply to the blisters. To make a compress, make tea (steep 1 to 2 teaspoons of dried leaves in 1 cup of hot

SHINGLES ◆ 485

GO TO THE PANTRY, GET THE BOX

The basic home remedies for shingles are the same ones you or your mother may have used for chicken pox, poison ivy, and other itchy rashes: cool compresses, calamine lotion, and simple pastes made of cornstarch or baking soda and water.

Resist those commercial appeals to buy goopy ointments and corticosteroid creams. Ointments can impede the drying and crusting of the shingles lesions that healing requires and may increase the risk of a crust falling off prematurely and producing a scar. Once the scabs loosen on their own, ointments and salves are fine. Creams containing corticosteroids (such as hydrocortisone) may decrease the inflammation of shingles, but they also interfere with your skin's local immune response.

Keep in mind that the virus responsible for shingles is contagious. Wash your hands after touching the rash, and take other precautions to avoid spreading it. Be especially cautious around those who are pregnant; the virus can be dangerous to pregnant women who have never had chicken pox.

water for 10 minutes), then strain and allow to cool. Dampen a clean cloth with the tea and apply to the rash three to five times per day. You can also take lemon balm internally. *Typical dosage:* 3 or more cups of tea per day (use the same recipe as above).

Licorice (*Glycyrrhiza glabra*)

One of this root's virus-fighting, active ingredients inhibits the herpes simplex virus. Licorice also coaxes the body to produce more interferon, a natural antiviral substance. Plus it fights inflammation without the side effects of cortisone drugs. Because licorice tea is intensely sweet, you may want to blend it with some of the other herbs listed in this section. Good choices would be lemon balm, ginger, St.-John's-wort, and mullein. *Typical dosage:* 2 to 3 cups of tea per day (simmer 1 teaspoon of dried chopped root in 2 cups of water for 15 minutes); the tea can also be cooled to use in a compress. *Caution:* Limit use to not more than six weeks. Do not use if you have high blood pressure, diabetes, or a disease of the thyroid, kidney, liver, or heart. Do not use licorice if you're pregnant or nursing.

Baikal Skullcap (*Scutellaria baicalensis*)
This Chinese herb works against both viruses and bacteria, so it's a good one to apply topically to shingles. Grind the dried root to a powder in a coffee mill or food grinder; then mix a tablespoon of powder with enough water to form a paste and apply just as you would a paste of baking soda, up to six times per day as needed.

Mullein (*Verbascum thapsus*)
This flower can inhibit the herpes simplex virus; it can also gently reduce pain. Used in a compress, a tea made from mullein leaves calms inflammation and soothes irritated skin. *Typical dosage:* 4 to 6 cups of tea per day (steep 1 heaping teaspoon of dried flowers and leaves in 1 cup of water for 10 minutes); the tea can also be cooled and applied to the rash as a compress as needed.

St.-John's-Wort (*Hypericum perforatum*)
Used externally, St.-John's-wort has a long history of healing wounds. It can also help reduce pain and itching, which makes it a good choice for shingles. Most commercial products that you'll see for external use are infused oils, meaning an oil in which the flowers have been steeped for a few weeks. But during the blister and crust stages of shingles, you don't want to apply an oil. Avoid these products until the scabs have dropped off, and use a compress made with tea instead. *Typical dosage:* 15 to 40 drops of tincture three times per day; or 300 milligrams of standardized capsules or tablets three times per day. Or you can apply a compress made with a tea of St.-John's-wort (steep 2 teaspoons of flowering tops in 1 cup of hot water for 10 minutes; then strain and cool). Dampen a clean cloth with the tea and apply for 15 minutes, up to three times per day. *Caution:* May increase skin reactions to sun exposure.

Turmeric (*Curcuma longa*)
This spice contains curcumin, which has potent anti-inflammatory properties. Topical curcumin, like capsaicin from cayenne, is

ALOE-AND-HERBS SHINGLES GEL

If you have access to fresh leaves of lemon balm or flowering tops of St.-John's-wort, double the quantities of them in this recipe. (Flowering tops are the flowers in bloom, plus about 3 to 5 inches of the stem.)

- 2 cups aloe vera gel
- ¼ cup lemon balm leaves
- ¼ cup St.-John's-wort flowering tops
- ⅛ cup cut dried licorice root
- 2 tablespoons cayenne or turmeric
- 8 drops of bergamot, lemon, tea tree, or lavender essential oil

Blend the first five ingredients in a quart-sized jar. Let sit for 24 hours at room temperature. Strain through a tightly woven cloth into a clean jar. Add the essential oil and cap tightly. Store in the refrigerator.

Apply to a test patch of normal skin. If it burns on contact, add more aloe vera gel. If it doesn't, you can try blending in a bit more cayenne. Apply to the rash three to five times per day as needed.

After applying the gel, be sure to wash your hands with soap to avoid spreading the compounds that burn.

For most people with shingles, cayenne may be too irritating to apply during the blister phase. In addition, some people with pain that lingers after the shingles rash has healed find that cayenne burns too much. If this is true for you, you can still use this gel; just omit the cayenne.

thought to ease pain by depleting substance P, the nerve transmitter of pain. See "Aloe-and-Herbs Shingles Gel" above to use turmeric topically. *Typical dosage:* one 250- to 500-milligram standardized capsule, up to three times per day; or 10 to 30 drops of tincture up to three times per day. *Caution:* Do not take turmeric internally if you have gastritis, stomach ulcers, gallstones, or bile duct obstruction.

Aloe (*Aloe vera*)

Antibacterial and anti-inflammatory, aloe vera gel soothes irritated skin and makes a great vehicle for other herbs. If you grow this plant, slice the leaf lengthwise, scoop out the gel, and slather on the rash. Or you can use a commercial preparation of pure aloe vera gel, ideally one without artificial colorings and preservatives. Apply as often as needed to the rash during any of its stages.

Sinus Infections

You've had a bad cold, and after 10 days or so you're ready to get back to your normal life. Unfortunately, your cold isn't finished with you. The congestion, sinus pain, headache, fever, and fatigue won't go away.

That's when you begin to suspect you may be dealing with a sinus infection. You have all the telltale symptoms: Your headache is worse when you lean over or lie down, your nasal discharge has changed from clear to yellow-green, your breath is bad, and a decreased sense of smell has sandbagged your appetite.

Like many other maladies, sinus infections come in two main varieties: acute and chronic. An acute sinus infection often follows on the heels of a cold or a bout of hay fever. In fact, one study found that nearly 40 percent of people whose common colds lasted seven days or longer developed signs of sinus infection that showed up on x-rays. Viruses are the most common cause of acute sinus infections.

Chronic sinus infection is a low-grade inflammation that persists for three months or longer. The same viruses cause it, but other factors—stress, air pollution, allergies, or an overtaxed immune system—make chronic sinus infection tough to get rid of. Compared with an acute infection, symptoms of a chronic infection are less dramatic, but they include the usual annoyances: headache, congestion, varying degrees of nasal discharge, postnasal drip (with or without a cough), fatigue, bad breath, impaired ability to concentrate, and a diminished sense of smell. Fever is uncommon.

Chronic sinus infection has become one of the most prevalent chronic illnesses in the United States. According to the National Center for Health Statistics, more than 37 million Americans have the condition.

Since medical science offers no foolproof cure, many people with chronic sinus infection get the message that they have to learn to live with their misery. Fortunately, an array of simple home remedies and alternative treatments can keep the infection at bay.

Drug Treatment

Oral Decongestants

Pseudoephedrine (Sudafed, many combination products), phenyl-propanolamine (Contac, Dimetapp, Sinarest), phenylephrine combination (Nasahist, Nalgest, many others). *Function:* decrease mucous membrane swelling, which can help improve sinus drainage. *Side effects:* insomnia, jitters, increases in heart rate and blood pressure.

TAKING THE WATERS

If you have a sinus infection, one of your primary goals is to thin nasal secretions, which makes them easier to expel. One way to do this is by drinking lots of fluids, especially warm liquids such as herb teas and brothy soups.

Another way is to inhale steam. Breathing warm steam—from a hot shower, steam shower, commercial inhaler, or a simple pot of hot water—helps loosen mucus, soothe dry membranes, and decongest. It may even relieve sinus headache. Adding antiseptic, decongesting herbs such as eucalyptus and thyme gives steam treatments an extra punch.

Two other water tips: A damp, hot-to-tolerance towel placed over the face can increase blood flow to the sinuses and decrease discomfort. Warm baths can help banish that all-over sick feeling. For an herbal bath, you can simply strain the herbal infusion from your steam inhalation pot into the tub.

Decongestant Nasal Sprays

Phenylephrine (Dristan, Neo-Synephrine), oxymetazoline (Afrin, Sinex), xylometazoline (Neo-Synephrine II). *Function:* decrease mucous membrane swelling, which can help improve sinus drainage. *Side effects:* rebound congestion, risk of dependency and abuse.

Intranasal Corticosteroids

Beclomethasone (Vancenase, Beconase), budesonide (Rhinocort), fluticasone (Flonase), triamcinolone (Nasacort), mometasone (Nasonex). *Function:* shrink swollen mucous membranes to allow drainage ducts from the sinuses to open; used when allergies such as hay fever underlie the infection. *Side effects:* burning or drying of the nose, sneezing.

Antibiotics

Trimethoprim-sulfamethoxazole, ampicillin-clavulanate, cefaclor, clarithromycin, amoxicillin, erythromycin-sulfisoxazole (many brand names). *Function:* kill bacteria that cause the sinus infection. *Side effects:* diarrhea, nausea, vomiting, headache, vaginal yeast infection, allergic reactions; other side effects depend upon the specific antibiotic used.

HERBAL REMEDIES

Echinacea (*Echinacea angustifolia, E. purpurea, E. pallida*)

This herb is well-known for its ability to rev up the immune system, which may help fight off a bout of sinus infection. Most herbalists recommend taking echinacea every one to two hours at the beginning of an infection, then stopping once symptoms resolve. With sinus infections, your immune system has already been challenged by the cold or allergy that caused it, so frequent dosing is especially important. *Typical dosage:* up to nine 300- to 400-milligram capsules per day; up to 60 drops of tincture three times per day until symptoms cease. *Caution:* People allergic to

Echinacea

other members of the aster family, such as ragweed, may be allergic to echinacea. Not for use by those with autoimmune diseases such as lupus.

Astragalus (*Astragalus membranaceus*)

This Chinese herb may soon be known as "the other immune herb." Whereas echinacea stimulates the immune system when taken in frequent, large doses for a short period of time, astragalus gradually rebuilds the immune system's strength. It may be of particular help to people who get sinus infections often and tend to hold on to them for a long time. *Typical dosage:* eight or nine 400- to 500-milligram capsules per day; or 15 to 30 drops of tincture twice per day.

Shiitake (*Lentinus edodes*)

You might call this mushroom the cook's immune-boosting herb. It's delicious in soup, stock, or stir-fry, but to fight an illness, take it in capsule form. *Typical dosage:* 500 milligrams of standardized extract capsules or tablets two times per day.

Oregon Graperoot (*Mahonia aquifolium*)

You'll probably be hearing a lot about Oregon graperoot in the years to come. Its broad-spectrum antimicrobial, astringent, and anti-inflammatory properties are useful for a number of conditions, including sinus infections. *Typical dosage:* 15 to 30 drops of tincture, three times per day.

Garlic (*Allium sativum*)

The same compounds that make garlic pungent also fight bacteria. Cooking deactivates the critical ingredients, though, so you'll need to take garlic in capsules, eat it raw, or add it during the last minutes of cooking. *Typical dosage:* up to three 500- to 600-milligram capsules per day (look for products that deliver up to 5,000 milligrams of allicin daily). *Caution:* Some people experience digestive problems.

Usnea (*Usnea barbata*)

This lichen fights streptococcus bacteria, a frequent cause of bacterial sinus infection. Because usnea extracts poorly into water, you need to take it as a tincture. *Typical dosage:* 15 to 30 drops of tincture, three times per day.

Peppermint (*Mentha × piperita*)

This popular garden herb contains the decongestant menthol. In one study people who inhaled menthol said they felt as if they had less nasal congestion, although their measurable air flow didn't increase. You can use peppermint in teas or add the leaves or essential oil to steam inhalation treatments. Blend a few drops of peppermint essential oil in a tablespoon of vegetable or nut oil and rub this blend into your temples (don't get it in your eyes). *Typical dosage:* tea throughout the day as needed (steep 1½ teaspoons of dried leaf in 1 cup of hot water for 15 minutes); or a few drops of essential oil in hot water for steam inhalation.

Horseradish (*Armoracia rusticana*)

This condiment gives you that welcome sensation of instant sinus relief. Both regular ground horseradish and a dab of Japanese wasabi work well, but start with small amounts and work up. *Caution:* Use these condiments carefully if you have ulcers or other digestive problems.

Feverfew (*Tanacetum parthenium*)

Best known for its ability to prevent migraines, this herb is also recommended by herbalists to ease headaches—including those that may accompany a sinus infection. *Typical dosage:* up to three 300- to 400-milligram capsules per day; or 2 average-sized fresh leaves per day.

ANTIHISTAMINES: NO ANTIDOTE FOR SINUS TROUBLE

Beware over-the-counter sinus remedies because many contain antihistamines. Antihistamines thicken mucus, making it harder to expel, and can cause drowsiness. Commonly used antihistamines are diphenhydramine, brompheniramine, chlorpheniramine, and phenyltoloxamine. Studies have failed to find that combination antihistamine-decongestant drugs do any good for sinus infections.

Meadowsweet (*Filipendula ulmaria*) and Willow Bark (*Salix* spp.)

Both of these herbs contain salicin, the pain-relieving precursor to aspirin, and both have traditionally been used for headache and other types of pain. Both taste bitter, which by itself resolves some types of headache pain. *Typical dosage:* up to six 400-milligram capsules per day; or up to 3 cups of tea per day (steep ½ teaspoon of powdered bark or dried herb in 1 cup of hot water for 10 minutes).

Ginger (*Zingiber officinale*)

This root's anti-inflammatory and pain-relieving powers make it a natural for relieving headaches. Because ginger tends to make those who eat it feel warm, it's great for infections that make you feel chilled. But you'll want to avoid it if fever comes with your sinus infection. *Typical dosage:* up to eight 500- to 600-milligram capsules per day; or ½ to 1 teaspoon of chopped fresh root per day; or 10 to 20 drops of tincture in water three times per day. *Caution:* Do not use if you have gallbladder disease.

SMOKING ADDICTION

Admit it: You really do want to quit because you know smoking is bad for your health. Just in case you need a little extra encouragement, here are the facts: Smoking is the major preventable cause of death in the United States. It causes cancer and heart disease. It gives smokers raspy voices and nagging coughs. And it makes smokers' mouths smell and taste like ashtrays. So why are you still smoking?

It's because nicotine is highly addictive—as addictive as heroin, according to some researchers. Nicotine binds to specific receptor sites in the brain, causing changes in mood. That's why heavy smokers who attempt to quit experience withdrawal symptoms such as nervousness, irritability, insomnia, and even mild depression. No wonder it can be hard! But it *can* be done.

Several drugs are available for smokers trying to quit. Most are aimed at helping smokers gradually wean themselves from nicotine instead of going "cold turkey."

Those who are quitting smoking with the help of a doctor may be prescribed other medicines, among them antianxiety drugs, adrenergic-blockers, and antidepressants. See the chapters on anxiety and depression for details on these medications.

Cigarette smoke irritates cells in the airways, paralyzing the tiny hairs, or cilia, which move impurities out of the lungs. When you quit smoking, you may notice increased coughing and mucus production. This phase may last a few weeks to a few months, depending on how long and how much you have smoked. While it may be irritating, this reaction is a good sign— it means your lungs are beginning to recover. Lung tonics and expectorants can help you expel the yucky junk and heal the lung tissues.

In addition, calming herbs and herbs that provide support in times of stress can reduce anxiety and insomnia. Herbs that alleviate depression can be especially helpful for people who smoke as a way of coping with this mood disorder. And several types of herbal medicine can help alleviate the symptoms of nicotine withdrawal.

Drug Treatment

Nicotine Supplements
Transdermal nicotine (skin patches) and nicotine chewing gum (Habitrol, Nicotrol, Prostep). *Function:* alleviate symptoms of nicotine withdrawal. *Patch side effects:* insomnia, headache, nausea, vertigo, muscle aches, stomach upset, skin irritation. *Gum side effects:* mouth irritation, hiccups, excess salivation.

Herbal Remedies

Mullein (*Verbascum thapsus*)
This herb tones the mucous membranes of the respiratory tract, soothes irritated lungs, and speeds healing of damaged tissues. It also helps thin mucus secretions so they can be coughed up more easily. *Typical dosage:* 2 to 3 cups of tea per day (steep 1 to 2 teaspoons of dried leaves in 1 cup of hot water for 10 minutes); or ½ to 1 teaspoon of tincture three times per day.

A Chinese Herbal Inhaler

You've likely seen commercials for a nicotine inhaler. An herbal version of this product has been used in China for decades. Smoker's Aroma is a commercial product that uses a combination of aromatic herbs; those wishing to quit smoking sniff the product for two minutes three times per day, plus whenever the craving for a cigarette hits them. The herbs contain molecules that attach to nicotine receptors in the brain. After users have successfully quit, they keep the bottle of herbs with them for occasional cravings that occur when their resolve is low. To find Smoker's Aroma, see "Herbs and Herbal Products for Buying" at the end of this book.

Coltsfoot (*Tussilago farfara*)

Here's another herb that helps soothe inflamed lung tissue, loosen secretions, and tone the lungs. *Typical dosage:* 2 to 3 cups of tea per day (steep 1 to 2 teaspoons of dried leaves in 1 cup of hot water for 10 minutes); or ¼ to 1 teaspoon of tincture three times per day. *Caution:* Limit use of coltsfoot to no more than four weeks per year.

Coltsfoot

Lobelia (*Lobelia inflata*)

This cough-easer gently relaxes bronchial muscles and the entire nervous system. Lobelia may have some binding action on nicotine receptor sites, which could decrease cravings. *Typical dosage:* 2 to 3 cups of tea per day (steep ¼ to ½ teaspoon of dried leaves in 1 cup of hot water for 10 minutes); or 6 to 10 drops of tincture three times per day. *Caution:* Lobelia can cause nausea and vomiting. If this occurs, discontinue use.

Skullcap (*Scutellaria lateriflora*)

This sedative herb can help alleviate the anxiety that sometimes accompanies giving up cigarettes. *Typical dosage:* 2 to 6 cups of tea per day (steep 1 to 2 teaspoons of dried leaves in 1 cup of hot water for 10 minutes); or ¼ to 2 teaspoons of tincture two to six times per day.

Valerian (*Valeriana officinalis*)

Can't sleep without a last puff? Valerian relaxes tense muscles; it can be used as a sleep aid if insomnia is one of your quitter's symptoms. *Typical dosage:* 2 to 6 cups of tea per day (steep 1 to 2 teaspoons of dried root in 1 cup of hot water for 10 minutes); or ⅛ to 2 teaspoons of tincture up to six times per day. *Caution:* Avoid during pregnancy.

Kava-Kava (*Piper methysticum*)

This South Pacific ceremonial herb relieves anxiety without causing drowsiness or decreasing mental function. *Typical dosage:* up to 6

MAKING YOUR QUIT DAY STICK

Kicking the cigarette habit starts with small steps. Although there is no perfect time to quit, it is probably best not to try during especially stressful times—when you're moving into a new home, for example, or starting a new job. When the time is right for you, here are some tips that can help you snuff the cigarette habit.

◆ **Make the commitment.** Before having that last drag, set a quit date and make it public, possibly even signing a contract with family and friends. Mark your quit date on your calendar.

◆ **Reduce your intake.** Once you've determined your quit date, gradually reduce the number of cigarettes you smoke each day. On the day you set as your quit date, you must stop smoking completely.

◆ **Avoid smoking cues.** Get rid of all your cigarettes, lighters, and ashtrays, and avoid situations where you would normally smoke. Spend time in places that do not allow smoking.

cups of tea per day (simmer 1 to 2 teaspoons of dried root in 1 cup of hot water for 10 minutes); or ¼ to 2 teaspoons of tincture up to six times per day; or 3 or 4 capsules of extract standardized to 30 percent kavalactones per day (a daily total of 250 to 300 milligrams). *Caution:* Do not use kava if you're pregnant. Do not combine with alcohol; do not operate heavy machinery or drive when taking kava. If you suffer from depression, check with your doctor before taking kava.

Passionflower (*Passiflora incarnata*)

This gently sedating herb can be used as a sleep aid. If your daytime anxiety is severe, it can also be taken during the day. *Typical dosage:* ¼ to 1 teaspoon of tincture or glycerin extract three or four times per day; or up to 2 teaspoonfuls at bedtime to relieve insomnia.

◆ **Occupy your mouth and hands.** Chew on straws or carrot sticks, eat sugarless candy, or chew gum. Fiddle with rubber bands or paper clips; carry around a small rubber ball and squeeze it vigorously whenever a craving occurs. When a craving is strong, do something incompatible with smoking, such as taking a shower or going for a brisk walk around the block.

◆ **Reward yourself.** Make a list of all the benefits you enjoy when you don't smoke and review it frequently. On your quit day, give yourself a special treat—a new pair of shoes, a dinner at your favorite restaurant, a bouquet of roses. Save the money you would have spent on cigarettes and at the end of the first month, buy something frivolous.

◆ **Exercise.** Taking a brisk walk or working out at a health club channels some of the nervous energy many ex-smokers feel when they quit. Exercise also helps prevent weight gain, which is common while quitting.

◆ **Seek out help.** Hypnotherapy, acupuncture, and support groups seem to help some people quit successfully, although no controlled clinical studies have evaluated the effectiveness of such interventions.

St.-John's-Wort (*Hypericum perforatum*)

One of the most popular herbal remedies, St.-John's-wort has proven to help in cases of mild to moderate depression. If a blue mood plays a role in your smoking habit, you should begin taking St.-John's-wort two to four weeks before your quit date. *Typical dosage:* 900 milligrams of standardized extract capsules per day; or ½ to 1 teaspoon of tincture per day. *Caution:* May cause increased skin reactions to sun exposure.

Licorice (*Glycyrrhiza glabra*)

Stress is one reason that many people smoke. The act of quitting is itself stressful for both the emotions and the body. Licorice nourishes the adrenal glands, the ones most worn out by stressful conditions. It also eases lung symptoms by fighting inflammation, soothing irritated tissues, and helping expel mucus. *Typical dosage:* 1 to 3 cups of tea per day (simmer 1 to 2 teaspoons of dried, chopped root in 1 cup of water for 10 minutes); or ⅛ to ½ teaspoon of tincture two or three times per day. You can also buy long pieces of whole licorice root and chew on them throughout the day—this gives you something to do with your hands and mouth. If you notice darkening of the teeth, discontinue using the herb in this way. *Caution:* Do not use licorice for more than six weeks. Avoid the herb if you have high blood pressure, if you're on heart medications, if you're pregnant or nursing, or if you have heart, liver, or kidney disease.

Schisandra (*Schisandra chinensis*)

This herb supports the whole body in times of stress and has the added advantage of toning the lungs and easing coughs. *Typical dosage:* 1 to 3 cups of tea per day (simmer 1 to 2 teaspoons of dried fruit in 1 cup of water for 10 minutes); or ⅛ to ½ teaspoon of tincture three times per day.

Turmeric

Turmeric (*Curcuma longa*)

This bright yellow spice has been shown to help remove the carcinogens that smoking puts in your body. If you're overwhelmed by the number of herbs recommended here, just put turmeric on your spice shelf where it's handy and add it to food several times a week. *Typical dosage:* 250 to 500 milligrams in capsules two or three times per day, with meals; or ⅛ to ½ teaspoon of tincture two or three times per day.

SORE THROAT

A H, THAT RAW, SCRATCHY FEELING. Where did it come from this time? Many things can make your throat sore: hay fever, postnasal drip from a sinus infection, smoky air, a too-hot beverage, mouth-breathing while sleeping, shouting, and infections by viruses and bacteria. The most common type of sore throat comes with viral illnesses such as colds and flu. Viral sore throats typically last three to four days. They go away without any medical treatment, but antibiotics don't make them go away faster. Herbs, however, can soothe the symptoms of sore throats, boost immune function, and fend off viruses.

DRUG TREATMENT

Analgesics
Acetaminophen, aspirin, ibuprofen, naproxen. *Function:* relieve pain and (except acetaminophen) inflammation. *Acetaminophen side effects:* chronic use or dosages higher than recommended commonly cause liver damage, with symptoms of jaundice, nausea, vomiting, and an all-over ill feeling; long-term use can also damage kidneys. *Aspirin side effects:* heartburn, indigestion, stomach irritation, mild nausea or vomiting. *Ibuprofen and naproxen side effects:* dizziness, nausea, stomachache, headache; with continuous use, stomach lining irritation.

Narcotic Analgesics
Codeine combinations (Aceta with Codeine, APA with Codeine, Tylenol with Codeine), acetaminophen with hydrocodone (Allay, Co-Gesic, Duocet). *Function:* relieve severe sore throat pain. *Side effects:* dizziness, drowsiness, headache, nausea, vomiting, stomachache, constipation.

Antibiotics
Penicillin (Pen Vee, Ledercillin-VK, many others), erythromycin (E-Mycin, Erybid, Ery-Tab, Erythrocin, others), clarithromycin (Blaxin), azithromycin (Zithromax). *Function:* kill bacteria in cases of strep throat. *Side effects:* mild nausea, vomiting, diarrhea, vaginal yeast infection.

HERBAL REMEDIES

Echinacea (*Echinacea purpurea, E. angustifolia, E. pallida*)

Anti-inflammatory echinacea helps thrust your immune system into all-systems-alert mode. It also can numb inflamed throat tissues. In studies, echinacea kills some of the viruses that commonly infect the upper respiratory tract. It's also weakly bacterial, but it shouldn't be

COULD IT BE STREP?

Although it's children who often come down with strep throat, adults do, too. Strep accounts for about 15 percent of sore throats for all ages. It most commonly strikes during the late winter and early spring.

Signs that you may have strep include fever greater than 101.3°F, white coating on the tonsils, and tender lymph nodes in the neck. Some people, particularly children, also have headache, stomachache, and vomiting. The usual symptoms that accompany a cold—cough and runny nose—are commonly absent in strep.

If you think you have strep, go to your doctor to be tested. While it isn't life-threatening, strep is contagious. Left untreated, it can progress to complications including abscess formation in the throat and spread of infection to the blood, middle ear, sinuses, or mastoid bone (the bony bump just behind the ear). Even more rarely, untreated strep can lead to rheumatic fever and a kidney disease called acute glomerulonephritis.

Your doctor will likely prescribe antibiotics for strep. If you have allergies, work with your doctor to find an antibiotic that has the fewest side effects for you. Take *all* of the medication.

There are things you can do to help antibiotics do their work (see "Can You Use Herbs with Antibiotics?" on page 502). You can also minimize the antibiotic's effect on the "good" bacteria in your digestive tract by eating plenty of active-culture yogurt and kefir or taking a supplement of *Lactobacillus acidophilus* bacteria.

relied upon to knock off strep bacteria. Liquid echinacea products produce a somewhat numbing tingle when swallowed. Depending on your symptoms, this property may be soothing or irritating.

You can take echinacea along with antibiotics for strep. A German study found that this combo led to faster healing time and fewer recurrent infections. *Typical dosage:* up to nine 300- to 400-milligram capsules per day; or 60 drops of tincture every two to three hours while you're awake the first two days of illness. Then decrease to 60 drops of tincture three times per day. Discontinue when symptoms are gone. *Caution:* If you're allergic to ragweed, you may be allergic to echinacea.

Shiitake (*Lentinus edodes*)

These culinary treasures have antiviral and immune-stimulating effects. You can cook with them or take encapsulated products. *Typical dosage:* up to five 400-milligram capsules a day.

Licorice (*Glycyrrhiza glabra*)

Whole-root licorice reduces inflammation, soothes the throat, stimulates the immune system, and increases the body's production of the antiviral substance interferon. But the deglycyrrhizinated, or DGL, licorice that's used to treat ulcers doesn't contain the components you want for cold- and flu-fighting. *Typical dosage:* up to 3 cups of tea per day (simmer ½ teaspoon of dried chopped root in 1 cup of water for 10 to 15 minutes); or up to six 400- to 500-milligram capsules per day; or 20 to 30 drops of tincture three times per day. *Caution:* Do not take for longer than six weeks. Do not use if you're pregnant or nursing. People with high blood pressure, diabetes, or diseases of the thyroid, kidney, liver, or heart should not take licorice unless advised to do so by their physician.

Marshmallow (*Althaea officinalis*)

This root soothes inflamed mucous membranes. It also has a mild stimulating effect on the immune system. *Typical dosage:* up to six 400- to 500-milligram capsules a day; or 20 to 40 drops tincture up to five times per day; or 3 cups of tea per day (simmer 1 teaspoon of dried root in 1 cup of water for 10 minutes).

Mullein (*Verbascum thapsus*)

Soothing mullein fights flu viruses. *Typical dosage:* up to 6 cups of tea per day (steep 2 teaspoons of dried leaves and flowers in 1 cup of hot water for 10 to 15 minutes); or 25 to 40 drops of tincture every three hours.

Plantain (*Plantago lanceolata, P. major*)

Another tissue-soother, plantain is demulcent, anti-inflammatory, and antibacterial. The German Commission E, that country's equivalent of the U. S. Food and Drug Administration, endorses it as safe and effective for throat inflammation. *Typical dosage:* up to 4 cups of tea per day (steep 2 teaspoons of dried leaves in 1 cup of hot water for 10 to 15 minutes); or 3 to 6 grams in capsules per day.

CAN YOU USE HERBS WITH ANTIBIOTICS?

With all of the bad publicity antibiotics have gotten recently, some people wonder if they should use them at all. But antibiotics have their place: fighting bacterial infections that herbs can't vanquish.

So are herbs worthless in fighting bacteria? Probably not. With respect to strep, however, most of the research on the antimicrobial abilities of herbs involves studies done on cultures in test tubes. None have compared herbs to either placebos (fake pills) or conventional antibiotics in humans.

Such research *does* suggest that applying these herbs directly to the infection site might do some good. For strep throat, this means you can gargle with a tincture dissolved in water or squirt a liquid extract onto the back of the throat.

Herbs can also help boost your immune system while the antibiotic kills the bacterial infection. One German study found that adding echinacea to the antibiotic treatment of strep throat helped patients get well faster and reduced the chance of relapse.

Until studies confirm that herbs are effective in fighting strep infections, don't substitute them for antibiotics. Instead, use them *with* whatever antibiotics your doctor prescribes.

Slippery Elm (*Ulmus rubra*)

The inner bark of this tree has a long tradition of soothing all manner of sore throats. *Typical dosage:* 2 to 3 cups of tea per day (steep ½ teaspoon of powdered bark in 1 cup of hot water for 10 minutes). You might also find lozenges made with slippery elm. Take them according to the manufacturer's directions.

Eucalyptus (*Eucalyptus globulus*)

This fragrant herb has the Commission E's blessing as a remedy for easing sore throat. Its aromatic oils are antiseptic and cooling, and its tannins have an astringent action that shrinks in-flamed, swollen tissues. *Typical dosage:* up to 3

Eucalyptus

cups of tea per day (steep 1 teaspoon of crushed leaves in 1 cup of hot water for 10 minutes). You can also suck on one of the many commercially available types of eucalyptus lozenges. *Caution:* Do not take eucalyptus internally if you have a serious liver disease or inflammatory condition of the gastrointestinal tract or bile ducts.

Garlic (*Allium sativum*) and Onion (*A. cepa*)

These two pungent herbs possess antiviral and antibacterial activity. Garlic fights streptococcus. *Typical dosage:* up to three 500- to 600-milligram capsules per day; or 1 or 2 raw cloves per day minced into food. As for onions, try including them in food daily.

Oregon Graperoot (*Mahonia aquifolium*)

This herb and its berberine-containing cousins, goldenseal (*Hydrastis canadensis*), gold thread (*Coptis chinensis*), and barberry (*Berberis vulgaris*), all fight bacteria. Berberine even has some activity against streptococcus. These plants are also mucous membrane tonics, meaning they help to ease the irritation of sore throat. *Typical dosage:* 60 drops (about two dropperfuls) of tincture three times per day; or up to six 500- to 600-milligram capsules per day. *Caution:* Do not take if pregnant or nursing.

Lemon Balm (*Melissa officinalis*)

This mint-family member works against a variety of viruses and bacteria including streptococcus. It works well as a tea or as a gargle. *Typical dosage:* 3 to 4 cups of tea per day (steep 1 teaspoon of dried leaves in 1 cup of hot water for 10 minutes); or gargle with this tea as needed.

Usnea (*Usnea barbata*)

Also known as old man's beard, this lichen fights streptococcus and has anti-inflammatory and immune-stimulating actions. *Typical dosage:* 60 drops of tincture three times per day.

SPORTS INJURIES

IF, LIKE MOST WORKING PEOPLE, you spend the majority of your time chained to a desk, occasional athletics likely provide your primary avenue of exercise. The information age may have saved you from being injured falling under the tractor. But instead, you twist your back trying to knock a few points off your golf handicap or you sprain an ankle trying to keep up with teenage swing dancers at a nephew's wedding.

Here are some common injuries you might experience, nearly all of which come from overdoing it.

◆ Muscle cramps occurring during or after exertion. These cramps are often triggered by dehydration. The best prevention is to drink ample fluids before, during, and after exercise. Don't wait to become thirsty; it's too difficult to catch up on your fluid losses. If you plan to exercise for more than an hour, switch from plain water to a sports drink such as Gatorade. These products help replace carbohydrates and salts. If you develop a cramp, stop and gently stretch the affected muscle. Sometimes gentle massage helps. So does heat. Once you're home, you can soak in a hot bath or apply a hot, damp towel or hot water bottle.

◆ Sore muscles while exercising. Dehydration may be the culprit here, too, along with depletion of muscle fuels and accumulation of the waste product lactic acid. Part of the solution lies in consuming sufficient amounts of the many nutrients exercising muscles require. Try eating a banana or other fruit a half-hour before exercising.

◆ Stiff and sore muscles after exercising. This type of pain signals that you've overdone it. Edmund R. Burke, Ph.D., director of

EASING THE PAIN OF A STRAIN

If you experience significant pain or limited range of motion because of a sports injury, see a doctor. You can treat mild sprains and strains at home, starting with RICE — an acronym for rest, ice, compression, and elevation.

◆ **Rest** means just that. Sounds easy, but if you must keep active, gently exercise the parts of your body that don't hurt. Swimming and yoga can often be tolerated.

◆ **Ice** is also simple—apply a plastic bag of cubed or crushed ice, a bag of frozen peas or corn, or a commercial cold pack. Protect your skin by covering it with a damp cloth. The day of the injury, ice the area for 20 to 30 minutes, three or four times per day. Continue ice compresses until a couple of days after the injury begins to feel better. Because heat increases swelling, some experts don't recommend using it within the first two weeks—unless the primary problem is tight muscles, in which case heat helps muscles relax. Others say you can alternate hot and cold applications as long as you end with cold.

◆ **Compression** entails wrapping the injured limb with an elastic bandage, but only as snugly as, say, a trouser sock. You don't want to cut off the circulation and increase swelling below the injury. Remove and rewrap the bandage at least twice a day.

◆ **Elevation** means raising the injured area above the heart—not just propping your ankle, if that's what you've hurt, on a footstool. Instead, lie flat and prop your leg or other injured area on pillows. This improves the return of blood and other fluids to the heart to reduce swelling.

the Exercise Science Program at the University of Colorado at Colorado Springs, calls it an athletic hangover.

Such muscle strains arise from tiny tears in the muscle. Intense exercise can generate unstable molecules called free radicals, which contribute to this muscle damage. Increased blood flow makes the muscle actually swell. For these aches, try a hot tub soak, a sauna session, gentle stretching, or massage. As long as the muscles are only stiff, not injured, heat acts to loosen and relax them. It also promotes better circulation to carry away the muscles' waste products. Dr. Burke says the most important remedy is rest. If you use prevention and increase your training level gradually, you may not need a remedy! Forget the "no pain, no gain" adage. Getting right back on the exercise bike after muscle tears, Dr. Burke cautions, can do more harm than good.

Drug Treatment

Analgesics
Acetaminophen, aspirin, ibuprofen, ketoprofen (Orudis). *Function:* reduce pain and (except acetaminophen) inflammation. *Acetaminophen side effects:* with high dosage, liver damage, as evidenced by jaundice, nausea, vomiting, and an all-over ill feeling. *Aspirin side effects:* heartburn, indigestion, stomach irritation, mild nausea or vomiting. *Ibuprofen and ketoprofen side effects:* dizziness, nausea, stomachache, headache; with continuous use, stomach lining irritation.

Herbal Remedies

Turmeric (*Curcuma longa*)
Long prized as an anti-inflammatory and antioxidant agent, turmeric is now turning up in research studies that examine the effect of its active ingredient curcumin. Experiments confirm that curcumin is a potent anti-inflammatory agent. In Ayurvedic medicine, turmeric is used both topically and internally for sprains and other musculoskeletal inflammations. *Typical dosage:* 400 to 600 milligrams three times per day. You'll see some products that in-

VITAMINS FOR WEEKEND WARRIORS

Vitamins C and E are both antioxidants, a class of chemicals that help mop up the free radicals that contribute to tissue damage after an athletic injury. Vitamin C is also critical for production of collagen, a major component of the musculoskeletal system. For sports injuries, try a daily dose of 800 to 3,000 milligrams of vitamin C and 200 to 1,000 IU of vitamin E. Because vitamin C is rapidly excreted, it's best to divide the total into 500-milligram doses and take it frequently.

clude bromelain with turmeric for better absorption. You can boost absorption yourself by taking curcumin with a little fat, such as flaxseed oil, another good anti-inflammatory. *Caution:* High doses of curcumin may irritate the lining of the stomach and intestines. Do not take if you are pregnant or have ulcers, gastritis, gallstones, or bile duct obstruction.

Ginger (*Zingiber officinale*)

This spice has a wealth of beneficial effects, including anti-inflammatory, antioxidant, and analgesic properties. Ginger inhibits the production of inflammatory chemicals called prostaglandins and leukotrienes. Meanwhile, the component 6-shogaol mildly reduces pain, probably by blocking the nerves' transmission of pain signals. *Typical dosage:* up to eight 500-milligram capsules per day; or 10 to 20 drops of tincture three times per day; or ½ to 1 teaspoon of dried ground root per day; or ⅓ ounce fresh root (about a quarter-inch slice) per day.

Kava-Kava (*Piper methysticum*)

This herb from the South Pacific has a long tradition of use in relieving pain and relaxing tight muscles. *Typical dosage:* up to six 500-milligram capsules per day; or 15 to 30 drops of tincture three times per day. *Caution:* Not for use during pregnancy or nursing.

Do not combine with alcohol or sedatives. Do not exceed the recommended dose.

Cayenne (*Capsicum annuum*)

Topical use of capsaicin, the active compound in cayenne, has been the focus of much pain research. When first applied to the skin, capsaicin activates pain nerves. It then renders them unresponsive. Although this can relieve pain on the skin, it may not do much for deeper musculoskeletal pain. It does, however, increase local blood flow and produces a sensation of warmth. Taken internally, cayenne acts as an antioxidant and anti-inflammatory agent. *Typical dosage:* three 500-milligram capsules a day; or 5 to 10 drops of tincture in water three times per day. *Caution:* Excessive doses may irritate a sensitive gastrointestinal tract.

Peppermint (*Mentha × piperita*)

The aromatic oil menthol in peppermint is a "counterirritant," a substance that causes an irritation that blocks another irritation. Simply put, the cooling sensation of mint oil interferes with the sensation of pain. Many commercial and herbal liniments contain menthol. Look for them at your health food store or pharmacy, and apply them topically as the manufacturer directs. *Caution:* Some people develop an allergic skin rash when they contact peppermint oil or pure menthol. Heat seems to aggravate possible skin reactions. Try a test patch before you slather on a menthol-containing ointment. If you use peppermint essential oil for massage or in a warm bath, dilute it first—about 10 to 15 drops in 1 ounce of vegetable oil.

Boswellia (*Boswellia serrata*)

The gum resin extract of this tree has anti-inflammatory and analgesic properties. Commercial products are used in India for the treatment of arthritis and have become available in Europe and the United States. Because they are so new, little research has explored dosage. Follow the manufacturer's instructions.

Arnica (*Arnica montana*)

This lovely wildflower helps heal bruises and the swelling associated with sprains. To use it externally as a compress, add 1 tablespoon of tincture of arnica to 2 cups of water; soak a clean cloth and apply it to the strain or bruise. Several commercial creams, gels, and ointments contain arnica either alone or in combination with other remedies. Apply these topically as the manufacturer recommends. *Caution:* Arnica is also used internally in homeopathic preparations for trauma, but the doses used are minuscule. Don't confuse homeopathic use with taking the whole herb internally; the latter is not recommended. Also, do not apply arnica products to open wounds.

Comfrey (*Symphytum officinale*)

Applied externally, comfrey can relieve pain, swelling, and inflammation. You can buy commercially made comfrey salve and ointments and apply them as needed. To make a poultice of the dried leaves, coarsely chop them, then dampen them with a little hot water. Allow to cool before applying to the painful area. Cover with gauze or clean cloth. Leave on for at least 15 minutes. Reapply four times per day or as needed.

Horse Chestnut (*Aesculus hippocastanum*)

The bark, seeds, and leaves of this tree have a long history of use as a remedy against bruises, sprains, and swelling. Horse chestnut contains astringent tannins and the anti-inflammatory compound aescin, which has been shown to slow the leakage of fluid from stressed or irritated blood vessels. (It's this "leakage" that causes tissue swelling after an injury.) You can apply a gel containing horse chestnut extract; just follow the manufacturer's instructions.

STRESS

STRESS IS AN UNAVOIDABLE FACT OF LIFE. We should be glad for its presence, because without it we would surely die of boredom. When doctors speak of stress, however, they're referring to the body's nonspecific response to any demand—emotional, psychological, mental, or physical. Extreme grief and extreme joy both bring stress, and both trigger the same physical responses to it.

On the other hand, people in general often complain about being stressed. Usually they're talking about the fact that their lives are over-scheduled and they have little time to relax. Oddly, many people say "I'm so stressed out" with a paradoxical mix of exasperation and pride—as if stress were a modern-day badge of courage, and people who are *not* stressed don't lead important enough lives.

But living in a constant harried state saps energy. You may feel exhausted and nervous, your immune system may sputter and falter, your sleep may become disrupted, and your moods may deteriorate into fits of irritability and depression.

DRUG TREATMENT

No single drug cures stress. Many drugs are designed to ease its symptoms: pain drugs for headaches, a variety of drugs for stomach ulcers, vasodilators for high blood pressure, antidepressants for depression, sedatives for anxiety. To read more about these medicines, refer to the chapters on each specific condition. But to really *cure* stress, you need to take an honest look at your overall lifestyle and health habits.

HERBAL REMEDIES

Siberian Ginseng (*Eleutherococcus senticosus*)
Also known as eleuthero, this herb supports the health of the adrenal glands and bolsters the body's resistance to stress-related illnesses. Studies confirm that Siberian ginseng stimulates the immune system, improves athletic performance, and sharpens mental alertness. In one large study, people exposed to increased workload, exercise, heat, and noise improved their mental alertness and physical performance by taking Siberian ginseng. *Typical dosage:* 20 drops of tincture up to three times per day; or up to nine 400- or 500-milligram capsules per day.

Panax Ginseng (*Panax ginseng, P. quinquefolius*)
This "true" ginseng enhances immune function, increases mental alertness and concentration, facilitates motor coordination, and improves the ability to cope with both mental and physical stress. Germany's Commission E, that country's equivalent of the U. S.

ABOUT HERBS FOR STRESS

The herbs that can help you cope with stress and its effects are a diverse group. You'll see stress supplements and other stress products on the market, but if you read their labels carefully, you'll see that they contain completely different ingredients. That's why it's important to have a basic understanding of the different types of herbs that can help with stress symptoms.

◆ **Adaptogens.** These are substances that, over time, help the body cope with stress. They cause minimal side effects, generally improve immune function, and help balance various organ systems. Most of them also support the adrenal glands, the organs that pump the "fight or flight" hormones into a stressed system. Some increase mental alertness, physical stamina, and athletic performance.

◆ **Adrenal gland tonics.** Stressful situations stimulate the release of hormones such as adrenaline and cortisol from the adrenal glands. When you're under duress most of the time, the adrenal glands can become exhausted, and you start to feel fatigued, nervous, and irritable. Adrenal gland tonics gradually restore the health of these glands.

◆ **Liver herbs.** When you're under stress, you're more likely to smoke, drink, and otherwise not watch your safety. Exposure to pharmaceutical drugs, alcohol, herbicides, pesticides, and other toxins stresses the liver; so do excess hormones. With any kind of chronic stress, it's a good idea to include liver herbs in your routine.

◆ **Sedatives and calmatives.** This group of herbs calms frayed nerves, settles anxiety, and induces sleep. A calmative is a milder version of a sedative; for most people it isn't strong enough to induce sleep, but it can help dispel that frantic feeling. Some herbs are calmatives when taken in smaller doses and sedatives when taken in larger doses.

Food and Drug Administration, endorses Panax ginseng as a "tonic for invigoration and fortification in times of fatigue and debility." In a study of nurses who switched from day to night shifts (a stressful and exhausting feat for most people), those taking Panax ginseng adapted better in terms of mood and mental and physical performance. *Typical dosage:* up to four 500- to 600-milligram capsules per day; or 100 milligrams of product standardized to between 5 and 7 percent ginsenosides, one or two times per day. Many practitioners recommend taking ginseng for two or three weeks, followed by a one- to two-week break. *Caution:* Do not combine with caffeine, do not exceed recommended dosage, do not take during pregnancy, and do not take if you have high blood pressure or diabetes, or if you are taking blood thinners unless under a doctor's supervision.

Schisandra (*Schisandra chinensis*)
These berries are valued by practitioners of Traditional Chinese Medicine for their properties as a general tonic and for their ability to counter stress and fatigue. Although weaker than Siberian and Panax ginsengs, schisandra is both safer and tastier. Studies show that it helps improve work capacity and mental efficiency, tones the nervous system, and increases endurance. It's also a strong antioxidant and protects the liver from toxic exposure. *Typical dosage:* up to six 580-milligram capsules per day; or 15 to 25 drops of tincture in water two times per day; or 2 cups of tea per day (simmer 2 heaping teaspoons of dried fruit in 2 cups of water for 10 to 15 minutes).

Reishi (*Ganoderma lucidum*)
This medicinal mushroom can help calm anxiety, ease insomnia, and tone the immune system. *Typical dosage:* up to five 420-milligram capsules per day; or up to three 1,000-milligram tablets up to three times per day; or up to 2 teaspoons of tincture 2 or 3 times per day; or 1 teaspoon of syrup per day.

Gotu Kola (*Centella asiatica*)
Another traditional remedy, this one from the Ayurvedic medicine of India, gotu kola is considered to be rejuvenating to the nervous system. Preliminary studies suggest that this herb improves mental functions such as memory, improves the ability to cope with stress and fatigue, gently relieves anxiety, and might even increase longevity. *Typical dosage:* 2 to 3 cups of tea per

ANTI-STRESS INHALER

To make this inhaler, you'll need a small, clean glass vial with a tight-fitting lid.

1 teaspoon salt

5 drops of essential oil (blend any two of the following: lavender, Roman or German chamomile, bergamot, rose, geranium, lemon balm, clary sage)

Pour the salt and essential oil into the vial and cover. Open and sniff as needed. *Caution:* Not for internal use.

day (steep 1 teaspoon of dried herb in 1 cup of hot water for 10 minutes); or 20 to 40 drops of tincture two times per day; or up to eight 400- to 500-milligram capsules per day.

Ashwaganda (*Withania somnifera*)

Also called Indian ginseng, this herb has been used in Ayurvedic medicine for more than 2,500 years. Studies show that it reduces anxiety, bolsters the immune system, and relieves the pain and swelling associated with inflammation. Like the ginsengs, it seems to enhance the body's ability to cope with stress and to generally enhance mental acuity, reaction time, and physical performance. *Typical dosage:* there's no consensus on a therapeutic dose. Follow manufacturer's or practitioner's recommendations.

Milk Thistle (*Silybum marianum*)

It may not win herbal beauty contests, but milk thistle is one of the best-researched herbs for protecting the liver and stimulating regeneration of liver cells after injury. This herb makes a good choice for people who frequently indulge in alcohol or who are exposed to other toxins. *Typical dosage:* 1 to 3 cups of tea per day (steep 2 teaspoons of dried, powdered seed in 1 cup of hot water for 10 to 15 minutes); or 10 to 25 drops of tincture in water up to three times per day; or standardized products equal to 140 milligrams of silymarin, three times per day for 6 weeks, then reducing to 90 milligrams three times per day for as long as stress symptoms persist. You can also use the seeds as a condiment; just roast them for 2 minutes in a dry pan, cool, grind, and add to meals as needed.

Kava-Kava (*Piper methysticum*)

This South Pacific root calms and takes the edge off nerves, but it does so without the loss of alertness that accompanies sedative medications and without the side effects associated with common antianxiety drugs. In the South Seas, people consume kava as a beverage, much as Europeans drink (and revere) wine. At low doses, kava creates a sense of tranquility. Herbal practitioners also find it useful for relaxing tight muscles and relieving pain. *Typical dosage:* up to six 400- to 500-milligram capsules of non-standardized product per day, divided into 3 doses; or 1 to 3 doses of product standardized to 45 to 70 milligrams of kavalactones per day; or 15 to 30 drops of tincture in water one to three times per day. *Caution:* Do not exceed recommended dosages; do not operate a car or heavy machinery while taking kava until you learn how it affects you. Do not take kava if you're pregnant or nursing. Also, do not take the herb with alcohol or drugs that depress the central nervous system, such as sedatives and antidepressants, or with dopamine prescribed for Parkinson's disease.

STRESS-BUSTER TEA

This tea combines an adaptogen with several calming herbs. It's sweetened with orange peel and stevia, so you won't even need to add sugar.

- **1 tablespoon Siberian ginseng root**
- **2 teaspoons linden flowers**
- **2 teaspoons oatstraw**
- **1 teaspoon kava-kava root**
- **1 teaspoon orange peel**
- **¼ teaspoon stevia herb or to taste**
- **3 cups water**

Simmer all ingredients in a covered pot 10 minutes. Remove from heat and steep an additional 15 minutes. Strain and drink as needed, up to 5 cups per day.

Valerian (*Valeriana officinalis*)

One of the stronger herbal sedatives, valerian soothes anxiety, relaxes tight muscles, and relieves pain when given in low doses. Because valerian has sedative properties, some practitioners reserve it for evening use and prefer kava for daytime. *Typical dosage:* 300 to 400 milligrams per day of product standardized to contain 0.5 to 0.8 percent valeric acid; or 20 to 60 drops of tincture one to three times per day. For insomnia, take valerian one hour before bedtime. *Caution:* May cause stomach upset.

California Poppy (*Eschscholzia californica*)

In low doses this herb decreases anxiety, and in larger doses it promotes sleep. German physicians prescribe it for anxiety. A commercial product that combines California poppy and corydalis (*Corydalis yanhusuo*) is used in Europe to treat insomnia, agitation, and anxiety. California poppy also mildly relieves pain and calms cramps. *Typical dosage:* 2 to 3 cups of tea per day (steep 1 teaspoon of dried herb or roots in 1 cup of boiling water for 15 minutes); or 30 to 40 drops of tincture two or three times per day. *Caution:* May interact with monoamine oxidase (MAO) inhibitor antidepressants. Do not take it if you're pregnant.

St.-John's-Wort (*Hypericum perforatum*)

Shown in many studies to ease mild and moderate depression, this herb also eases premenstrual tension and anxiety and helps relieve nerve or muscle pain. Although the exact way this herb affects brain chemistry isn't completely understood, studies show that it can act in the same way as Prozac and other antidepressants. If you feel overwhelmed and hopeless, St.-John's-wort may help. *Typical dosage:* 3 cups of tea per day (steep 1 teaspoon of flowering tops in 1 cup of hot water for 10 minutes); or 60 drops of tincture in water two or three times per day; or one 300-milligram capsule standardized to 0.3 percent hypericin, one to three times per day. *Caution:* Do not take with antidepressant drugs unless under the guidance of a doctor. The herb may increase skin reactions to sun exposure.

Passionflower (*Passiflora incarnata*)

Extracts of this flower have been shown in a study to decrease anxiety and induce sleep. Germany's Commission E, approves passionflower's use for "nervous restlessness." Herbalists consider it

WHEN TO CONSULT A PROFESSIONAL ABOUT STRESS

Stress isn't all in your head, and it's not something you can continually ignore. If you feel chronically tense, anxious, and nervous and have persistent versions of any of the symptoms below, you should seek professional help, whether from an internist, family doctor, naturopathic doctor, practitioner of Traditional Chinese Medicine, psychiatrist, psychologist, another mental health worker, or someone trained in relaxation therapy. If you don't know whom to consult, start with your family doctor.

Physical Symptoms

◆ Nail biting

◆ Hair twirling, tugging, or pulling

◆ High blood pressure

◆ Upset stomach, ulcer pain, diarrhea, or constipation

◆ Insomnia or restless sleep

◆ Teeth clenching or grinding or waking in the morning with a sore jaw

◆ Fatigue

Psychological Symptoms

◆ Irritability

◆ Depression with feelings of hopelessness

◆ An urge to withdraw

◆ Feeling that no one appreciates or understands you

◆ Emotional outbursts of anger or frustration

◆ Inappropriate or uncontrolled fits of laughter or crying

a toning, strengthening herb for the nervous system and a helpful remedy against worrying, particularly when an overactive mind interferes with sleep. *Typical dosage:* 2 to 3 cups of tea per day (steep ½ to 1 teaspoon of dried herb in 1 cup of hot water for 10 minutes); or 30 to 40 drops of tincture three or four times per day. *Caution:* Passionflower may contain minute amounts of chemicals that can reduce the effects of monoamine oxidase inhibitor (MAO) antidepressants. Some experts advise against using the herb during pregnancy.

Hops (*Humulus lupulus*)

This herb, which is used in making beer, helps you sleep. It has a somewhat bitter taste, so you might want to blend it with peppermint, spearmint, or lemon balm. Germany's Commission E approves it for restlessness, anxiety, and sleep disturbances. *Typical dosage:* 2 to 3 cups of tea per day (steep 1 heaping teaspoon of the strobiles, or fruiting bodies, in 1 cup of hot water for 10 minutes); or 30 to 40 drops of tincture in water two or three times per day. *Caution:* Some experts recommend that people with depression should not take hops regularly.

Hops

Chamomile (*Matricaria recutita*)

This herb has an age-old reputation for calming nerves and gently aiding sleep. It's also anti-inflammatory and antispasmodic. *Typical dosage:* 2 to 3 cups of tea per day (steep 1 teaspoon of dried flowers in 1 cup of hot water for 10 minutes); or 30 drops of tincture in water three times per day. *Caution:* If you're allergic to other members of the daisy family, such as ragweed, you might also be allergic to chamomile.

Lavender (*Lavandula angustifolia*)

Just the smell of it can calm and relax. Lavender also eases headaches and relaxes tight muscles. *Typical dosage:* 10 to 15 drops of essential oil in a tub of warm bathwater; or make a massage oil by adding 10 to 15 drops of lavender essential oil to 1 ounce of almond, sesame, or avocado oil.

Lemon Balm (*Melissa officinalis*)

This sweet-smelling member of the mint family has mild sedative properties. *Typical dosage:* 2 to 3 cups of tea per day (steep 1 teaspoon of dried leaf in 1 cup of hot water for 10 minutes); or 60 drops of tincture in water three or four times per day.

Linden (*Tilia europea*)

The flowers of this tree have historically been used for their mild sedative, antispasmodic, and pain-relieving properties. Modern herbalists use infusions internally or in warm baths to reduce nervousness. *Typical dosage:* 2 to 3 cups of tea per day (steep 1 teaspoon of dried flowers in 1 cup of hot water for 10 to 15 minutes); or 1 teaspoon of tincture in water three or four times per day. Or add 4 cups of tea to a warm bath (use the same recipe as above).

STROKE

NOTHING IS MORE FRIGHTENING THAN A STROKE. You are visiting with friends in your living room and suddenly you are unable to feel the right side of your body. You can't move, and one side of your face droops. You can't speak or the words come out garbled. If help is handy, you are rushed immediately to the emergency room.

Strokes are caused by a sudden decrease in blood supply and oxygen to part of the brain. The exact symptoms depend on which part and the degree of damage. Damage to the brain, with the loss in feeling or function that results, could be permanent. Severe strokes can even cause death.

How does a stroke happen? Several different components of blood can play a role, including blood clots, cholesterol plaques, and a type of blood cell called platelets, among other substances. Fragments of these break off from an artery. These fragments, or emboli, then travel into arteries in the brain. Because the arteries in the brain are smaller, these fragments can become stuck and block circulation.

Who is at risk for stroke? You're automatically a candidate if you have high blood pressure, diabetes, heart disease, narrowing of the carotid arteries due to cholesterol-based plaques, or a specific type of arrhythmia called atrial fibrillation—or if you smoke. Doctors can predict an impending stroke when they detect abnormal sounds over the carotid artery, known as carotid bruits, or if you've had what doctors call a transient ischemic attack (TIA). These attacks are brief episodes of temporary, limited brain dysfunction, lasting less than 24 hours and usually less than 10 minutes. Between 50 and 75 percent of those who experience full-blown strokes have already had a TIA at some time.

Once you have a stroke, little can be done to reverse the resulting

ADOPTING HEART-HEALTHY HABITS

Your risk of stroke is closely related to the health of the coronary and other arteries, so lifestyle changes that benefit these body systems automatically reduce your chances of experiencing a stroke. Among the changes you have the power to make:

◆ Stop smoking.

◆ Exercise regularly.

◆ Eat a high-fiber, low-cholesterol, low-animal-fat diet. Include soy products and a rich variety of fruits, vegetables, whole grains, and legumes, and look for food with a high bioflavonoid content. Whole books are written about foods that promote a healthy heart and circulatory system; for a start, check out the recommendations in the chapters on heart disease and high cholesterol.

◆ Consider supplementation. If you're otherwise healthy, you are probably leading a busy life that makes it hard to get enough essential fatty acids and other essential nutrients in your diet, no matter how many vegetables you eat. Check supplement recommendations in the chapter on heart disease.

SUPPLEMENTS FOR AVOIDING STROKE

Bromelain, made from proteolytic enzymes found in pineapple, fights inflammation, inhibits platelet clumping, and has been shown to break down atherosclerotic plaques. *Typical dosage:* 250 to 500 milligrams three times per day on an empty stomach. *Caution:* Occasionally causes upset stomach.

brain damage. So if you have risk factors or a family history of stroke, you should focus on doing what you can to lower your risk and improve the health of your circulatory system. If you have these conditions, review the chapters on cholesterol, heart disease, high blood pressure, and diabetes.

Most people who have strokes are hospitalized. If they are admitted soon enough, they can be given intravenous drugs that dissolve emboli or clots to limit brain damage. Once a stroke happens, doctors may prescribe anticoagulants, but treatment focuses mainly on supporting the patient's return to health.

If you're at risk for stroke based on your medical history, a previous TIA, or the presence of bruits, doctors may prescribe the drugs listed below or cholesterol-lowering drugs.

If you are taking medications of any kind for heart disease or atherosclerosis, anticoagulants or drugs that affect platelet function, do not use herbs without consulting your doctor and/or an experienced herbalist. Some heart medications interact with herbs. Never stop any medication without supervision, and always keep your doctor informed of all other substances you take.

DRUG TREATMENT

Clot Reducers

Dipyradamole (Persantine). *Function:* prevent clumping of platelets. *Side effects:* dizziness, abdominal pain, headache, rash.

Toclopidine (Ticlid). *Function:* prevent clumping of platelets. *Side effects:* decrease in white blood cells or platelets, elevated cholesterol.

Other Drugs

Aspirin. *Function:* reduce clots or emboli. *Side effects:* heartburn, indigestion, stomach irritation, mild nausea or vomiting.

Warfarin (Coumadin). *Function:* prevent blood clots by inhibiting vitamin K-dependent coagulation. *Side effects:* bleeding, allergic reactions, interactions with other drugs and foods.

HERBAL REMEDIES

Ginkgo (*Ginkgo biloba*)

An extract of the leaves of this tree benefits the nervous system, the brain, the heart, and the arteries. It may even prevent stroke. In people who have experienced a stroke, ginkgo improves the functioning of nondamaged areas of the brain and helps ease depression, a common result of stroke. *Typical dosage:* 40 to 80 milligrams of capsules standardized to 24 percent heterosides three times per day. *Caution:* Rarely, individuals may experience gastrointestinal discomfort, headache, and dizziness.

Garlic (*Allium sativum*) and Onion (*A. cepa*)

Each of these delicious, aromatic herbs contains substances that decrease clumping of platelets, lower blood cholesterol, and increase HDL, the "good" cholesterol. Garlic promotes the breakdown of fibrin-based clots, which can form stroke-causing emboli.

FRESH GINGER-HONEY CHUTNEY

Here's one tasty way to take your daily ginger, which lowers blood cholesterol and prevents platelet clumping.

2 tablespoons grated or finely chopped ginger
2 tablespoons honey
1 teaspoon fresh lemon juice or to taste

Combine ingredients and stir. Store in an airtight container in the refrigerator. Take up to 2 teaspoonfuls per day, before meals or with food.

Typical dosage: at least 1 clove of garlic or ½ of a small onion per day; or enough garlic capsules to provide 10 milligrams of allicin per day.

Hawthorn (*Crataegus* spp.)

This traditional European herb helps prevent stroke by treating heart disease and atherosclerosis. It is antioxidant and anti-inflammatory. It lowers serum cholesterol and blood pressure and stabilizes collagen, thus strengthening the wall of arteries. *Typical dosage:* 2 to 3 cups of tea per day (simmer 1 to 2 teaspoons of dried berries in 1 cup of water for 10 minutes); or ½ to 1 teaspoon of tincture three times per day; or 100 to 250 milligrams of capsules standardized to 20 percent procyanidins three times per day.

Ginger (*Zingiber officinale*)

Another delicious, aromatic herb, ginger is a good stroke preventive because of its benefits to the arteries. It lowers blood cholesterol, prevents platelet clumping, and produces anti-inflammatory effects. It works best when eaten fresh and taken on an empty stomach. *Typical dosage:* ⅓ ounce by weight (a slice about ¼ inch thick) of fresh ginger root per day; or 150 to 300 milligrams of freeze-dried ginger in capsules three times per day. *Caution:* May cause stomach upset in susceptible people, especially at higher doses.

Alfalfa (*Medicago sativa*)

The leaf from this grain may help decrease blood cholesterol and shrink plaques already present. *Typical dosage:* eight or nine 400- to 500-milligram capsules per day; or 15 to 30 drops of tincture four times per day; or follow manufacturer's directions.

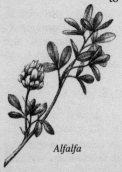

Alfalfa

SUNBURN

B Y NOW, MOST PEOPLE ARE AWARE of the long-term effects of excessive sun exposure: wrinkles, loss of skin elasticity, and skin cancer. But it's still not uncommon to be surprised by an accidental sunburn. Hazy skies don't filter the rays that burn. Water and snow reflect the sun, increasing your chances of turning uncomfortably pink. High altitudes and southern locations increase risk of sunburn. And sometimes, because the warm rays of spring just feel so good after a long winter, it's easy to forget about SPFs and bask a half-hour too long, resulting in a good bit more healthy glow than you had planned on.

DRUG TREATMENT

Analgesics
Aspirin, acetaminophen, ibuprofen, naproxen. *Function:* relieve pain and (except acetaminophen) inflammation. *Aspirin side effects:* heartburn, indigestion, stomach irritation, mild nausea or vomiting. *Acetaminophen side effects:* chronic use or higher dosages may damage the kidneys or liver. *Ibuprofen and naproxen side effects:* continuous use may irritate stomach lining; long-term use at high doses may damage the kidneys or liver.

Topical Anesthetics
Lidocaine plus antiseptic (Bactine), benzocaine (Solarcaine, Americaine, Unguentine), benzocaine and menthol (Dermoplast), benzocaine and chloroxylenol (Foille), benzocaine and aloe (Lanacane). *Function:* soothe local sunburn pain. *Side effects:* increased skin reactions to sun exposure.

HERBAL REMEDIES

Aloe (*Aloe vera*)
This plant's ability to soothe burn pain is so well-known that drug and discount stores stock it right next to the sunscreen. You may

not have known that aloe is also anti-inflammatory, antibacterial, and antifungal, and it speeds healing. If you have an aloe plant, simply slice the leaf lengthwise, scoop out the inner gel, and apply to burned skin. If you buy your aloe vera gel, try to pick one without artificial colorings or preservatives.

Aloe

Tea (*Camellia sinensis*)

Both green and black teas are cooling to sunburns. And the antioxidants in tea can mop up the harmful unstable molecules called free radicals that result from any injury, including sunburn. Just wet a tea bag with cool water and apply to a small sunburned area. For larger areas, toss the tea bag in a cup of hot water, steep for 5 minutes, and remove the bag. Put the tea in the fridge for a half hour or so, and apply it with a clean cloth as you would any other herbal compress.

Witch Hazel (*Hamamelis virginiana*)

This astringent tightens swollen tissues, decreases inflammation, and soothes sunburns. You can find a liquid form of witch hazel in almost any drugstore. Simply apply to sunburned skin with a washcloth as often as needed.

Calendula (*Calendula officinalis*)

Anti-inflammatory, astringent, antiseptic, and cooling, calendula promotes healing of mild burns. You can make a tea by steeping 1 to 2 teaspoons of dried calendula flowers in 1 cup of hot water for

HELP FROM THE PANTRY

Vinegar is a time-tested remedy for sunburn. You can dilute it with an equal part of water and splash over mild burns. You can also put a cup of vinegar in a tub of tepid water and have a soak. Any kind of vinegar works, but apple cider vinegar is more strongly scented and wine vinegars can stain clothes, so either distilled or white vinegar is usually the best choice.

10 minutes. Strain and chill; use as with any other compress. You can also find calendula in many forms in health food stores.

Echinacea (*Echinacea purpurea, E. angustifolia, E. pallida*)

When applied to the skin, tea made with this herb improves the healing of wounds and burns. To make a tea, simmer 2 teaspoons of minced root in 2 cups of water for 10 minutes, or steep 1 teaspoon of dried leaf in 1 cup of hot water for 5 to 10 minutes. Strain, cool, and apply to the skin with a clean cloth.

Plantain (*Plantago* spp.)

Antimicrobial and anti-inflammatory, plaintain contains the tissue-knitting substance allantoin. Best of all, it grows nearly everywhere as a common garden weed. To use it, simply crush a fresh leaf and apply directly to a burn. If you're traveling where you can't get to a drugstore, this is a good emergency remedy for minor burns and bug bites.

St.-John's-Wort (*Hypericum perforatum*)

You may have heard of this herb in connection with depression, but it is also anti-inflammatory, reduces pain, and speeds healing of wounds and minor burns. Make a tea by steeping 1 to 2 teaspoons of dried flowering tops in 1 cup of hot water for 10 minutes. The water will turn red. Strain, cool, and apply to your skin.

TOOTHACHE

A TOOTHACHE CAN BE ONE OF THE worst pains you ever experience. It's your tooth's way of telling you that something is very wrong and needs attention. It is no exaggeration to say that toothache usually occurs when the nerve of the tooth is either damaged or dying.

Since the bacteria that attack teeth can get into the bloodstream and infect other parts of the body, it's important to get professional

If You Can't Get to the Dentist Right Away

Most dentists don't make house calls, and yours may or may not be able to see you just when a toothache strikes. Or you may be traveling when a tooth decides to act up. In these cases, here's what to do until you can get to see a dentist.

◆ Stay away from the extremes. Do not eat very hot or very cold foods. You can try a warm or cold pack applied to the outside of the mouth, but if the pain begins to increase, remove it immediately.

◆ Do not eat hard foods. Sometimes a toothache results from a hairline fracture in the tooth. Biting on something hard can increase the fracture and bring the pain to a new level.

help for a toothache. Even if your pain subsides—which may mean that the tooth's nerve is dead—the bacterial infection might remain.

Drug Treatment

Analgesics
Aspirin, acetaminophen, ibuprofen, naproxen (Aleve). *Function:* relieve toothache pain and (except acetaminophen) inflammation. *Aspirin side effects:* heartburn, indigestion, stomach irritation, mild nausea or vomiting. *Acetaminophen side effects:* chronic use or high doses may damage the liver or kidneys. *Ibuprofen and naproxen side effects:* continuous use may irritate the stomach lining; long-term high-dose use may damage the liver and kidneys.

Herbal Remedies

Clove (*Syzygium aromaticum*)
The essential oil of these fragrant buds is one of the best natural pain relievers. It's also antibacterial. Simply place some oil on a cotton swab and gently apply it to the affected area. You should

feel numbness fairly quickly, and it should last for at least an hour. In a pinch, when no other relief can be had, you can chew or crush whole cloves and apply them directly to the site of the pain.

Garlic (*Allium sativum*)
Like clove, this common kitchen remedy is a powerful bacteria-fighter. Simply bruise a clove of garlic and hold it next to the infected tooth. It may sting a little; remove it if it hurts too much.

Turmeric (*Curcuma longa*)
Used in many natural tooth products, this bright yellow spice is a healing powerhouse; it's antibacterial and anti-inflammatory, for starters. It also stimulates circulation, which helps bring more immune cells to the site of an infection. And in the middle of the night, with a tooth throbbing so badly that you can't bear to drive to the drugstore, you can mix a teaspoon of turmeric with enough water to make a paste and just dab it on the sore tooth.

Chamomile (*Matricaria recutita*)
If you have an aching tooth, chances are your nerves are frayed as well. Chamomile can help with both problems; it's used in Europe to treat mouth and gum irritations and is known worldwide as a gentle sedative. It also fights infection, promotes healing, and is one of the safest herbs known. *Typical dosage:* up to 3 cups of cooled tea per day (steep ½ to 1 teaspoon of dried flowers in 1 cup of hot water for 10 minutes).

TOOTH PAIN PACK

This recipe combines the pain-fighting components in clove bud oil with the infection-fighting ingredients in both chamomile and goldenseal.

- 1 drop of clove bud essential oil
- 2 drops of German chamomile essential oil
- ½ teaspoon goldenseal powder

Mix the goldenseal and essential oils with a few drops of water until a thick paste forms. Dab onto the affected area with a cotton-tipped swab. Apply not more than four times per day until you can see your dentist.

Ulcers

Iᴛ's ᴀ ᴅᴇᴇᴘ, ᴀᴄʜɪɴɢ, ɢɴᴀᴡɪɴɢ ᴘᴀɪɴ over your stomach that may ease a little bit right after you eat. Taking a few of the antacids you keep in your medicine chest helps a little, too. But the pain keeps coming back. And it gets worse every time you become upset, drink a cup of coffee, or have a cocktail. Could you have an ulcer?

Peptic or gastric ulcers are raw sores in the upper gastrointestinal tract—either in the stomach or in the duodenum, where the stomach connects with the small intestine. A certain amount of hydrochloric acid and the digestive enzyme pepsin are necessary for the stomach to do its work of digesting food and absorbing some nutrients. But when the balance of these substances goes awry, you can get an ulcer.

A variety of factors can tip this balance the wrong way. Your body may produce excess stomach acids; smoking, alcohol, coffee, and stress can aggravate such overproduction. Drugs such as aspirin, ibuprofen, and other anti-inflammatories can cause ulcers. The bacterium *Helicobacter pylori* is found in up to 95 percent of patients with recurrent ulcers, which is why doctors sometimes

USING TINCTURES FOR ULCERS

People with ulcers are often advised to avoid alcohol. But alcohol-based tinctures are one of the easiest ways to take many of the herbs that help ulcers. If you're using tinctures rather than teas, put the recommended dose in a cup, add boiling water, and allow the mixture to sit for 10 minutes. This helps evaporate some of the alcohol, which can worsen ulcers. You can also substitute glycerin extracts, known as glycerites; use the same dosages. (The best way to take ulcer herbs, however, is in a tea.)

ANTIBIOTIC ALTERNATIVES

If your ulcer is caused by the *Helicobacter pylori* bacterium and you prefer to not take antibiotics, preliminary scientific studies show good results using a combination treatment of licorice, vitamin C, and manuka honey. (This honey is made by a specific type of bee. You can find it in some health food stores.) Take licorice in the following dosage: 3 cups of tea per day (simmer 1 teaspoon of dried root in 1 cup of hot water for 10 minutes); or ⅛ to ½ teaspoon of tincture three times per day; or chew 1 or 2 tablets of deglycyrrhizinated (DGL) licorice three times per day before meals. Add 3,000 to 10,000 milligrams of vitamin C plus 1 tablespoon of manuka honey three or four times per day. If you experience diarrhea or burning in the stomach, reduce the dose.

Continue the treatment for two months. After that, you should be retested for the bacteria. If it is still present, go for the antibiotics.

prescribe antibiotics for them. Heredity, food allergies, lack of fiber in the diet, and deficiencies of vitamins A and E may also contribute to the formation of an ulcer.

If you have blood in your stool or any chronic or recurrent upper abdominal pain, you may have an ulcer. Get a medical exam to rule out other causes.

Although drug treatment of ulcers is very effective, drugs that block the production of acid in the stomach can cause digestive problems, nutritional deficiencies, and increased risk of gastrointestinal infections, including *candida,* when used long-term.

Fortunately for people with ulcers, many safe, effective herbs exist that can help these wounds heal. First among them is licorice, with a number of clinical studies confirming its usefulness in treating ulcers. In addition to licorice, there are several anti-inflammatory, ulcer-healing, stomach-soothing herbs. All are pleasant-tasting and safe for long-term use. Using them in combination can be especially helpful.

DRUG TREATMENT

Antacids

Maalox, Mylanta, Tums, and others. *Function*: temporarily ease ulcer pain by neutralizing stomach acid. *Side effects*: may eventually cause production of more acid; may cause kidney stones, calcium and phosphorus depletion, headache, and coordination and concentration problems with excessive use.

Hydrochloric Acid Blockers

Cimetidine (Tagamet), ranitidine (Zantac), famotidine (Pepcid), nizatidine (Axid). *Function:* block production of hydrochloric acid. *Side effects:* nausea, vomiting, headache, confusion, breast swelling, sexual dysfunction; when used long-term, may cause di-

STOMACH-SOOTHING TEA

This tea combines four stomach-soothing, ulcer-healing herbs. You can carry it with you and sip it frequently throughout the day—the more the better. It can be drunk hot or cold.

To blend:

½ cup dried chamomile flowers

½ cup dried calendula flowers

½ cup dried meadowsweet herb

½ cup dried, chopped, or powdered slippery elm bark

Combine the herbs and store the mixture in a glass jar away from heat and light.

To brew:

3–6 tablespoons tea blend

3–6 cups boiling water

Add the herbs to a teapot, pour boiling water (as many cups as tablespoons of tea) over the herbs, and let steep for 10 minutes. Strain into a jar or vacuum bottle. The unused tea can be refrigerated and kept for up to three days.

OTHER ULCER TREATMENTS

Cabbage juice is one food treatment that studies have shown may be helpful for ulcers. Cabbage juice is high in a chemical called glutamine, which may stimulate the stomach to produce more of a protective compound called mucin. To achieve this protective effect, you need to drink about four cups of juice a day in divided doses.

Other ulcer strategies:

◆ Avoid foods that worsen symptoms.

◆ Take supplements of vitamins A and E if you think you may not be getting enough of these vitamins. You need 10,000 IU of vitamin A (or 15,000 to 25,000 IU of beta-carotene) per day and 400 to 800 IU of vitamin E per day.

◆ Boost your fiber intake.

◆ Avoid smoking and coffee (including decaf).

◆ Avoid aspirin, ibuprofen, and other anti-inflammatory drugs.

gestive problems, nutritional problems, skin conditions, and gastrointestinal symptoms.

Other Drugs

Omeprazole (Prilosec). *Function:* inhibit stomach acids. *Side effects:* interactions with other drugs; increased production of gastrin, a stomach hormone.

Misoprostol (Cytotec). *Function:* inhibit ulcer-causing compounds called prostaglandins. *Side effects:* gastrointestinal upset; may cause miscarriages in pregnant women.

Sucralfate (Carafate). *Function:* form a barrier at the base of the ulcer, inhibit pepsin, and bind bile salts. *Side effects:* constipation, interference with absorption of other drugs, low phosphate, excess aluminum levels in the blood.

Antibiotics, often in combination with bismuth subsalicylate (Pepto-Bismol). *Side effects:* vary with antibiotic type and combination used, but all diminish healthy intestinal bacteria.

Herbal Remedies

Licorice (*Glycyrrhiza glabra*)

The premier ulcer-healing herb, licorice seems to work as well as ulcer-treating drugs, but with fewer side effects. Instead of inhibiting acid production, it strengthens the stomach's normal protective mechanisms and induces healing. It may even help eliminate *H. pylori*, the bacteria at fault in many ulcers. Licorice has also been shown to decrease ulcer formation caused by drugs such as aspirin. Unlike whole licorice, a form of the herb called DGL, or deglycyrrhizinated licorice, can be taken by people with high blood pressure and those who take heart or blood pressure drugs. *Typical dosage:* 3 cups of tea per day (simmer 1 teaspoon of dried root in 1 cup of hot water for 10 minutes); or ⅛ to ½ teaspoon of tincture three times per day; or 1 or 2 tablets of DGL licorice chewed three times per day before meals. (Because DGL licorice is activated by saliva, it does not work as well if you simply swallow it; chew it instead.) *Caution:* DGL licorice may cause diarrhea in some people. Whole licorice should not be used if you're pregnant or nursing, if you have heart disease, liver disease, or diabetes, or if you are taking heart or blood pressure drugs. Limit use of whole licorice to six weeks unless under the supervision of a qualified health practitioner.

Chamomile (*Matricaria recutita*)

This lovely, old-fashioned herb promotes healing, decreases inflammation in the stomach, and can ease the anxiety that may be perpetuating the ulcer. *Typical dosage:* 3 to 6 cups of tea per day (steep 1 to 2 teaspoons of dried herb in 1 cup of hot water for 10 minutes); or ¼ to 1 teaspoon of tincture or glycerite three or four times per day.

Calendula (*Calendula officinalis*)

These beautiful orange or yellow flowers are anti-inflammatory and wound-healing. They are also mildly astringent, which helps reduce bleeding. So if bleeding is one of your ulcer symptoms, calendula is a good choice. *Typical dosage:* 3 to 6 cups of tea per day (steep 1 to 2 teaspoons of dried flowers in 1 cup of hot water for 10 minutes); or ¼ to 1 teaspoon of tincture or glycerite three or four times per day.

Meadowsweet (*Filipendula ulmaria*)

This remedy for the gastrointestinal tract contributes to ulcer healing by decreasing inflammation, protecting and soothing the stomach lining, and reducing excess acidity. It is also mildly astringent. *Typical dosage:* 3 to 6 cups of tea per day (steep 1 to 2 teaspoons of dried herb in one cup of hot water for 10 minutes). *Caution:* Avoid meadowsweet if you are allergic to aspirin; it contains a chemical relative of aspirin.

Marshmallow Root (*Althaea officinalis*)
When water is added to this soothing root, a rich mucilage, or slippery substance, forms that helps it coat and soothe an irritated ulcer. *Typical dosage:* 3 to 6 cups of tea per day, sipped frequently throughout the day (steep 1 to 2 teaspoons of dried root in 1 cup of hot water for 10 minutes or steep the same amount in cold water overnight); or ¼ to 1 teaspoon of tincture or glycerite 3 or 4 times per day. *Caution:* The mucilage in marshmallow may absorb other drugs taken at the same time, so if you are using other drugs, ask your practitioner's advice about a dosage routine.

Slippery Elm (*Ulmus rubra*)
The bark of this tree is another herb that forms mucilage to protect, soothe, and heal the stomach lining. *Typical dosage:* 3 to 6 cups of tea per day (steep 1 to 2 teaspoons of dried bark in 1 cup of hot water for 10 minutes or steep in cold water overnight); or ¼ to 1 teaspoon of tincture or glycerite three or four times per day.

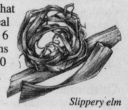

Slippery elm

Mallow (*Malva sylvestris*)
Another mucilage-former, this herb can be prepared the same way as marshmallow or slippery elm. *Typical dosage:* 3 to 6 cups of tea per day (steep 1 to 2 teaspoons of dried bark in 1 cup of hot water for 10 minutes or steep the same amount in cold water overnight); or ¼ to 1 teaspoon of tincture or glycerite three or four times per day.

Plantain (*Plantago major*)
A common garden weed that grows almost everywhere in the world, plantain has soothing, astringent, and wound-healing properties. *Typical dosage:* 3 to 4 cups of tea per day (steep 1 to 2 teaspoons of dried leaves or 1 tablespoon of fresh herb in 1 cup of hot water for 10 minutes); or ¼ to 1 teaspoon of tincture or glycerite three or four times per day.

Vaginal Infections

M OST WOMEN GET A VAGINAL INFECTION at least once—but how many of them talk about it? Ten years ago you couldn't bring up such a topic on television. But now, commercials for vaginal creams seem to be everywhere.

What causes vaginal infections and the burning and itching that accompany them? It can be anything that disrupts the normal pH of the vagina: tampons, spermicidal creams and gels, IUDs, douches, stray feces, or even sex. Antibiotics are common culprits, because while they're combating bacterial infection elsewhere in the body, they tend to kill off the beneficial microbes that keep the vaginal environment healthy. Other factors that can predispose a woman to vaginal infections include heavy sugar intake, postmenopausal hormonal changes, hormone replacement therapy, diabetes, pregnancy, and oral contraceptives.

Drug Treatment

Antifungal Creams
Nystatin (Micostatin, Nilstat), miconazole (Monistat), clotrimazole (Gyne-Lotrimin), butoconazole (Femstat3). *Function*: soothe irritated tissues and kill offending microorganisms. *Side effects*: itching, burning, and skin rash.

Antibacterial Creams
Clindamycin (Cleocin Vaginal Cream), metronidazole (Metro-Gel). *Function*: kill organisms that cause bacterial vaginosis. *Side effects*: itching and burning on the skin, rash, ringing in the ears, diarrhea.

Oral Antibiotics
Clindamycin (Cleocin), metronidazole (Flagyl, Femazole). *Function:* eliminate protozoa or bacteria that can cause vaginitis. *Clindamycin side effects:* ringing in the ears. *Metronidazole side effects:* nausea, diarrhea, headache, increased sensitivity to alcohol.

IF INFECTIONS KEEP COMING BACK

For recurring vaginal infections, your immune system needs a different type of help than echinacea. Think of echinacea as high-octane gasoline for your body's disease-fighting engine. It helps the machine rev fast and hard, but it doesn't fix accumulated wear and tear—in fact, it can worsen it.

If yeast or other vaginal infections keep coming back, your best bet is to see a natural health practitioner who'll recommend an herbal tonic program that you'll use for a series of months. It will likely include herbs such as astragalus, reishi, shiitake, nettles, or burdock—botanicals that gently and gradually rebuild the immune system and the many organs it involves. Such a program will likely include some diet changes as well, such as cutting down on caffeine and sugar.

It's a lot of work, but following an herbal tonic program faithfully is likely to do more for your health than just curing infections. You may find yourself losing weight, gaining energy, and responding to stress better than before your recurring infections began.

HERBAL REMEDIES

Garlic (*Allium sativum*)

Garlic is the premier antibacterial and antifungal herb. When taken internally, it helps fight vaginal infections no matter what their cause may be. Many naturopathic doctors also suggest using a whole, peeled garlic clove as a suppository. *Typical dosage:* one or more fresh cloves added to food per day; or up to three 500- to 600-milligram capsules daily. Look for products that deliver at least 5,000 micrograms of allicin daily.

Echinacea (*Echinacea angustifolia, E. purpurea, E. pallida*)

This herb is an immune supercharger that enhances the action of white blood cells and other specialized infection-fighters throughout your body. If your infection is a sudden one, not one that keeps recurring, echinacea can help your body mobilize its defenses to fight it. *Typical dosage:* up to nine 300- to 400-milligram capsules per day; or up to 60 drops of tincture three times per day.

Oregon Graperoot (*Berberis aquifolium*)

This herb contains berberine, one of the best botanical infection-fighters. Suppositories and creams containing Oregon graperoot are available over the counter at natural food stores. The herb can also be taken internally as part of your immune-system regimen. *Typical dosage:* 15 to 30 drops of tincture once per day. *Caution:* Not for use during pregnancy.

Pau d'Arco (*Tabebuia impetiginosa*)

Pau d'arco

This is a South American tree with a reputation for combating yeast infections. Its bark has long been widely available in prepackaged teas and combination products. *Typical dosage:* up to four 500- to 600-milligram capsules, or nine 300-milligram capsules, per day; or 20 to 50 drops of tincture up to four times per day; or two to three cups of tea per day (simmer 2 to 3 teaspoons of inner bark in 2 to 3 cups of water for 15 minutes, then divide into two or three doses).

Goldenseal (*Hydrastis canadensis*)

Goldenseal is another of the berberine-containing bacteria- and yeast-fighting herbs. It also stimulates digestion and the liver's secretion of bile. If you've taken antibiotics to fight an infection, your liver is responsible for clearing residues of these drugs from your body. *Typical dosage:* up to six 500- or 600-milligram capsules per day; or 20 to 50 drops of tincture once daily. *Caution:* Not for use during pregnancy or while nursing.

Milk Thistle (*Silybum marianum*)

As long as you're taking care of your liver, add some of these liver-repairing seeds to your regimen. They've been shown to protect it and stimulate its own capacity to generate new cells, especially important after a round of antibiotics. *Typical dosage:* 140 milligrams of standardized silymarin extract three times per day; or 10 to 25 drops of tincture up to three times per day.

Tea Tree (*Melaleuca alternifolia*)

Essential oil made from the leaves of this tree contains a potent antifungal agent. But it is also so strong that for vaginal infections and itching, it's best to seek it as an ingredient in manufactured products. Use according to manufacturer's instructions.

COMMON AND HARMLESS, OR CAUSE FOR CONCERN?

Although drugstores now boast several competing brands of over-the-counter yeast infection cures, it's important to be sure what kind of vaginal infection you have. Why? Some infections can be transmitted sexually, so your partner could inadvertently reinfect you. And some microorganisms can travel up the fallopian tubes, causing painful pelvic inflammatory disease or PID, which can have an impact on fertility and future health.

The most common vaginal infections are:

◆ **Yeast infections**—caused by the yeast organism *Candida albicans*. Once you've had one of these, you seldom forget the symptoms—white curdish discharge and a miserable itch. If you are experiencing your first yeast infection, however, it's a good idea to consult a doctor for a diagnosis so you'll know your own symptoms in case of a recurrence.

◆ **Trichomoniasis**—caused by a protozoan. This infection produces yellowish discharge and a burning itch, occasionally accompanied by frequent, burning urination.

◆ **Bacterial vaginosis**—another common vaginal infection often caused by the bacterium *Gardnerella vaginalis*. This infection can spread to the uterus and fallopian tubes. It's usually accompanied by a thin, gray or greenish discharge.

Varicose Veins

With each beat, your heart sends oxygen-rich blood coursing through your arteries to all parts of your body. Once the oxygen is used up, the blood must return to your lungs for replenishing. It makes the return trip via flexible yet delicate veins, whose muscular walls contract to move the blood along.

The veins in your legs must work against gravity to push great volumes of blood back to your heart. A series of valves stops the blood from flowing backward. But the weight of the blood, along with other factors, can cause the valves to malfunction. When the blood flows backward, it stretches the veins, especially if they are already weakened by poor circulatory health.

This process is what produces those bulging, blue varicose veins, which appear most often on the legs. You are more likely to develop varicose veins if you sit or stand for long periods. Changing position frequently and exercising helps prevent them.

Varicose veins are very common. They tend to run in families, and they affect women more than men. Hemorrhoids are a specific type of varicose vein; if you have them, you may have the conditions that cause varicose veins to develop in your legs.

The symptoms of varicose veins vary. They can make your legs feel tired, achy, and hot; yet some women don't feel them at all. Small, superficial varicose veins, called spider veins, rarely produce symptoms. The larger veins that lie near the surface of the leg are unattractive but pose little risk.

Varicose veins deep in the leg can cause serious trouble. When the veins are weak, fluids can leak through the porous vein walls. Eventually, the vein can burst and create slow-healing ulcers just under the skin. Or blood clots may form; if a clot breaks loose, it can travel to the brain, heart, or lungs and cause serious, potentially life-threatening problems.

Drug Treatment

Doctors most often perform surgery to remove the weakest veins. Another treatment, sclerotherapy, involves injecting a salt solution into the vein. It makes a clot that pinches off the vein, damaging and destroying it. Compression bandages are then wrapped around the leg from the toes up to the injection site and left in place for at least three weeks. There is no known drug therapy that cures varicose veins.

HERBAL REMEDIES

Horse Chestnut (*Aesculus hippocastanum*)

Several studies have demonstrated the effectiveness of horse chestnut extract in reducing varicose veins and relieving the itching and pain such veins can produce. In one three-month study, horse chestnut extract improved the condition as effectively as the combination of a diuretic medication and compression stockings. How does the herb work? A compound in horse chestnut effectively seals off tiny openings in blood-vessel walls. *Typical dosage:* 30 to 150 milligrams per day of commercial extract; you can also find topical horse chestnut creams in many health food stores. *Caution:* Don't try to make your own products; the crude herb can be toxic. Use only manufactured extracts.

Butcher's Broom (*Ruscus aculeatus*)

Compounds in this well-known European medicinal herb inhibit inflammation and constrict the blood vessels. The herb is also high in vitamin C and other compounds that tone vein walls. *Typical dosage:* 20 to 40 drops of tincture two or three times per day; or 2 to 3 cups of tea per day (steep 1 teaspoon of dried herb in 1 cup of water for 10 to 15 minutes); or two to three 500-milligram capsules with a little water two or three times per day. You can also purchase butcher's broom in a formula that combines it with other herbs. Take these formulas according to the manufacturer's directions.

Butcher's broom

Hawthorn (*Crataegus* spp.)

The leaves, flowers, and fruits of this plant are wonderful for strengthening and protecting the whole cardiovascular system. Studies show that its combination of antioxidant compounds helps lower blood pressure and prevent clotting. Hawthorn can be taken as a tea, tincture, or standardized extract; the berries, or the leaves and flowers, or all three parts are used. *Typical dosage:* up to nine 500- to 600-milligram capsules per day; or up to 3 cups of tea per day (steep 1 teaspoon of dried berries in 1 cup of hot water for 10

Two Vein Foods: Bromelain and Buckwheat

Bromelain, an enzyme derived from pineapple, is recommended for many heart and circulatory conditions. You can simply treat yourself to fresh pineapple several times a week, or take bromelain as a supplement. *Typical dosage:* 500 milligrams twice per day between meals.

If you're focusing on the health of your circulatory system, you'll certainly want to eat a balanced diet with lots of fiber-rich beans, vegetables, fruits, and whole grains. But be sure to give buckwheat a try; it not only has plenty of fiber but also is loaded with the healthy flavonoid rutin, which can strengthen blood-vessel walls. You can find rutin in supplement form, sometimes combined with other bioflavonoids. Aim for a daily dosage of 500 milligrams of total bioflavonoids. If you like green tea, it's another good source of bioflavonoids. Try to drink two to three cups per day.

Another set of nutrients to emphasize is the anthocyanidins. These colorants give bilberries, blueberries, purple grapes, and many other fruits and vegetables their deep coloring. Anthocyanidins protect blood-vessel walls and prevent leakage. They strengthen the connective tissue that supports blood vessels. Anthocyanidins are available in pill form. Proanthocyanidins, derived from either grapeseed or pine bark, have similar properties and are available in supplement form. *Typical dosage:* 150 milligrams of proanthocyanidins per day.

to 15 minutes); or 10 to 30 drops of tincture up to three times per day. *Caution:* If you are taking any digitalis- or digoxin-based drugs, consult your doctor before using hawthorn or products that contain it.

Gotu Kola (*Centella asiatica*)

Traditionally used for memory improvement and stress reduction, gotu kola strengthens connective tissue and the integrity of the protective sheath around the veins. Studies show that the herb effectively relieves weak veins and foot and ankle swelling. *Typical dosage:* up to eight 400- to 500-milligram capsules per day; or up to 3 cups of tea per day (steep 1 teaspoon of dried herb in 1 cup of hot water for 10 to 15 minutes); or 20 to 40 drops of tincture up to two times per day.

Ginkgo (*Ginkgo biloba*)

Compounds in ginkgo help increase blood flow to the brain, peripheral arteries, and heart. Ginkgo's antioxidant properties make it a fine heart tonic as well. Numerous clinical trials have been performed with standardized ginkgo extract in the last 15 years; they show that ginkgo not only improves circulation but also protects blood vessels, preventing abnormal leaking from tiny veins. Some research suggests that ginkgo may reduce the risk of abnormal clotting—a major factor in heart attacks and stroke. *Typical dosage:* 3 capsules, each containing at least 40 milligrams of standardized extract, per day. *Caution:* Rarely, people who take ginkgo may experience gastrointestinal upset, headaches, or skin allergies as a result.

WARTS

FORGET THAT OLD YARN ABOUT TOADS giving you warts. It just doesn't happen. Rather, these unsightly, embarrassing growths are caused by the human papillomavirus. Some 75 strains of this virus exist. Various strains can cause common warts, plantar warts, and plane warts.

Common warts usually grow on the hands, but they can also turn up on the feet, face, and neck. Plantar warts, on the other hand, occur on the soles of the feet and can cause pain. Plane or flat warts grow in clumps and usually occur on the face. They're flesh-colored, and as their name implies, flat.

Doctors sometimes deal with warts by destroying them or removing them surgically. Methods include freezing them with liquid nitrogen, vaporizing them with a laser beam, or manually cutting them away (though surgery is usually reserved for deep, persistent plantar warts).

Of the herbs discussed in this chapter, only piñon blanco has been tested on humans for its ability to expel warts. On the other hand, the remaining herbs are backed by years of traditional use and anecdotal evidence of successful cures. Whether you choose drugs or herbs, know that it can take weeks of persistent, daily application of the substance to get rid of the wart. Small warts, not surprisingly, are easier to treat than large ones.

DRUG TREATMENTS

Salicylic Acid Preparations
Liquids, gels, or plaster pads (Compound W, Mediplast, Wart-Off, others). *Function:* dissolve the wart. *Side effects:* localized warmth, peeling, stinging.

Cantharidin (Cantharone, Verr-Canth) alone or in combination with podophyllin and salicylic acid (Cantharone-Plus). *Function:* causes the area to blister so that the wart sloughs off. Treatments are applied by a doctor and repeated weekly, after removing dead tissue. *Side effects:* local stinging, redness, tenderness, and blistering.

THE TRIED-AND-TRUE WART REMOVER

Plain old salicylic acid, available over the counter, is an inexpensive home treatment for warts. To use it, first soak the area in water to soften the wart. Then apply the salicylic acid—but because it is an acid, apply it to only the wart, not to any irritated or infected skin, mucous membranes, moles, or birthmarks. (Also don't use it on warts with hair, genital warts, or facial warts.) The next morning, you can use a nail file to remove dead skin from the wart. Then repeat the process as often as directed on the label. *Caution:* If you have diabetes or a circulatory disorder, consult your doctor before using salicylic acid on your own.

Soaking the area in water between treatments can further soften a wart. Each morning, you can file away the dead skin with a nail file. Afterward, wash the file with soap and plenty of hot water.

HERBAL REMEDIES

Celandine (*Chelidonium majus*)

This herb is a member of the poppy family that grows in moist soil along the edges of roads and forests. The orange-yellow sap contained in both the roots and above-ground parts provides a remedy for warts and other skin problems. Scientific research has focused on the ability of some of its chemical constituents to fight viruses, bacteria, fungi, tumors, and inflammation. *Typical dosage:* squeeze the sap onto the wart once or twice a day until the wart disappears. If you don't have access to the fresh plant, make a strong tea by simmering 2 teaspoons of minced, dried root in 2 cups of water for 10 to 15 minutes. Strain and dab on with a cotton ball.

Black Birch Bark (*Betula lenta*)

This bark contains antiviral compounds and salicylic acid. In other words, it contains the same active ingredient used in many over-the-counter wart-removal remedies, only in lower concentrations. If these birch trees grow in your neighborhood, remove a one-inch square of the moist, inner bark and tape it to the wart, inner side down. (Be sure to take your square from a different tree each time; don't remove a patch that goes all the way around the tree's circumference or you may kill the tree.) You can also buy powdered birch bark from your health food store, add enough water to make a paste, apply to the wart, and cover with gauze. Keep the bark or powder in place for 10 minutes; if no irritation develops, leave it on for an hour the first day. Gradually increase the time each day for a week; then switch to an overnight treatment. You can also make a tea by simmering 2 teaspoons of chopped birch bark in 2 cups of water for 15 minutes. Strain and let cool. Dab this liquid on with a cotton ball once a day.

Bloodroot (*Sanguinaria canadensis*)

This herb yields a rust-colored sap that European settlers used for removing warts. It contains chemicals that both irritate skin and dissolve tough, warty tissue. Andrew Weil, M.D., author of *Spontaneous Healing,* says that he's seen a bloodroot paste help get rid of warts. *Typical dosage:* apply the sap from the fresh plant or a paste made from mixing the dried, powdered root with water once or twice a day. Cover with a gauze bandage.

Piñon Blanco (*Jatropha curcas*)

This Peruvian shrub has antiviral properties. In one study, sap from this plant worked better in removing warts on humans than a placebo (a fake pill). It worked more slowly, however, than treatment with liquid nitrogen; remember that both pharmaceutical and herbal wart treatments can take weeks to produce results. Apply the sap to your wart once or twice a day until it goes away. If skin irritation occurs, stop using the herb.

Bloodroot

Dandelion (*Taraxacum officinale*)

The stems and leaves of this common weed produce a milky latex that has worked to rid some people of their warts. Just pick a dandelion and squeeze the white stuff from the stem onto your wart two or three times per day until it disappears.

White Cedar (*Thuja occidentalis*)

This tree has antiviral compounds and a reputation for removing warts. You can buy a tincture and paint it on the wart two or three times per day. *Caution:* Don't use this herb internally if you're pregnant.

Pineapple (*Ananas comosus*)

In theory, the protein-dissolving enzyme bromelain, which is derived from pineapples, may help soften and remove tough, warty tissue. You can try cutting a piece of pineapple husk large enough to cover your wart and taping it over the wart overnight. Remove in the morning and reapply each night as needed.

Banana (*Musa paradisiaca*)

According to Montana herbalist Sunny Mavor, coauthor of *Kids, Herbs, and Health,* banana peel has helped a number of people make their warts go away—and it's a bit less sticky than pineapple. Cut a small circle from the peel, lay the inner surface against the wart, and tape in place. Apply fresh peel every 24 hours until the wart disappears.

PART IV

HERB PROFILES

A Close-up Look at the Most Common Herbs

IN THIS SECTION, YOU'LL READ MORE about the herbs most frequently used for a variety of conditions. You'll find basic information on each herb: its other common names; where it is harvested; the plant parts used; available forms of the herb; the conditions it is used for; any cautions or reasons that you shouldn't take it; and, when applicable, "conscious consumer information" to guide your buying decisions. Some herbs are now endangered in their wild form, and should be purchased from reputable sources that specify that the herb was harvested from cultivated plants.

Much of this information is also available in the condition chapters. However, the herb descriptions there are specifically tailored to the herb's use for that specific condition and its recommended dosages. How much you'll need to take of an herb depends on what you want it to do. There are no dosages in this section, which is mainly for readers who want to compare information on one herb with information on another herb. You may want to see how many disorders that you're prone to can be helped by a particular herb, or to compare which herbs for a single condition come from which countries. The list of other common names for herbs may remind you of a remedy that your grandparents swore by.

If, in this section, you see that an herb is used for a particular condition, you should read the chapter on that condition before purchasing or taking the herb. Sometimes condition chapters offer additional cautions for specific conditions—for example, possible bad interactions of herbs and drugs. It's also important not to self-treat some disorders, while others are best treated by a professional who creates a program of herbal remedies especially for you.

ALOE (*ALOE VERA*)

Also called: Cape aloe.

Source: Native to Africa; grown commercially in southern Texas and Mexico.

Parts used: Leaf gel, juice.

Forms available: Various concentrations of the gel, powdered dry juice. The gel is incorporated into ointments, creams, lotions, and the like. Some of aloe's active compounds deteriorate in storage, so use the fresh gel for maximum potency.

Uses: Externally, aloe gel has long been valued for healing minor burns, wounds, and abrasions, and relieving associated pain and inflammation. Aloe juice may hold promise for treating diabetes and reducing levels of triglycerides and blood sugar.

Caution: Don't use this herb if you have intestinal obstruction, abdominal pain of unknown origin, diarrhea, inflamed intestines (colitis, Crohn's disease, irritable bowel syndrome). Aloe juice may produce a laxative effect if taken in a higher dose than recommended. Don't use for more than 10 days.

ARNICA (*ARNICA MONTANA, ARNICA* SPP.)

Also called: Leopard's bane, mountain tobacco.

Source: Native to Europe; most species occur in the mountains of western North America.

Parts used: Whole plant, flower.

Forms available: Creams, ointments, gels, tinctures, homeopathic preparations.

Uses: Externally as an anti-inflammatory, pain reliever, and antiseptic for sprains, bruises, acne, injuries, and swelling caused by bone fractures, insect bites, rheumatic pains, and chilblains. Seldom used internally because its primary active constituents are considered toxic.

Caution: Avoid during pregnancy. Use only on short-term basis for acute conditions. May cause allergic dermatitis in sensitive persons or with prolonged use. Do not apply to open wounds or broken skin, except under the advice of a health care practitioner. Taken internally, low doses can cause gastroenteritis; high doses may damage the heart and in rare cases can induce cardiac arrest.

Conscientious consumer information: May be at risk in the wild; needs further study.

ASTRAGALUS (*ASTRAGALUS MEMBRANACEUS*)
Also called: Huang qi.
Source: Native to northeast China, where it is also grown commercially.
Part used: Root.
Forms available: Capsules, tablets, extracts, tinctures, and in many traditional Chinese formulas.
Uses: Colds, flu, minor infections. Many studies confirm immune-boosting, antiviral, antibacterial, and tonic properties. Shows promise in restoring T-cell function in cancer patients and preventing growth of cancerous cells.
Caution: None known.

BEARBERRY (*ARCTOSTAPHYLOS UVA-URSI*)

Also called: Uva-ursi, kinnikinnik, mountain box.
Source: Cool temperate regions from northern Europe to northern Asia, Japan, and North America.
Part used: Leaf.
Forms available: Teas, capsules, tinctures. Some products are standardized to 2 percent arbutin.
Uses: Mild urinary tract infections.
Caution: Do not use while you're pregnant or if you have a kidney disorder or irritated digestive condition. Bearberry may interact with herbs or drugs that acidify the urine. Discontinue its use after one week, except under the supervision of a health care practitioner. Overuse may promote liver damage. Not recommended for children.

Bearberry

BILBERRY (*VACCINIUM MYRTILLIS*)
Also called: Whortleberry, huckleberry.
Source: Woods and forest meadows of Europe; commonly wild-harvested.

Part used: Fruit (berries).

Forms available: Capsules, tablets. Some products are standardized to 25 percent anthocyanosides.

Uses: Narrowing of the arteries, diarrhea, bruises, varicose veins, hemorrhoids, mouth and throat inflammations, eye conditions such as night blindness, cataracts, macular degeneration, and diabetic retinopathy.

Caution: May interact with anticoagulant drugs.

Black Cohosh (*Cimicifuga racemosa*)

Also called: Black snakeroot, sheng ma, bugbane, rattleweed.

Source: Open woodlands from southern Ontario south to Georgia, west to Arkansas, and north to Wisconsin. Most of the root is wild-harvested; some is grown commercially in Europe.

Part used: Root.

Forms available: Capsules, tablets, tinctures.

Uses: Premenstrual syndrome, menopausal symptoms such as hot flashes, and menstrual cramps.

Caution: Avoid during pregnancy or when nursing. May cause stomach upset.

Conscientious consumer information: Threatened in the wild; purchase from reputable sources.

Burdock (*Arctium lappa, A. minus*)

Also called: Lappa, beggar's buttons.

Source: Throughout Europe, western Asia, and the United States.

Parts used: Root, leaf.

Forms available: Capsules, tablets, liquid extracts, tinctures.

Uses: Water retention, detoxification.

Caution: No hazards are known. It's thought that one case of human poisoning attributed to burdock was caused by contamination with or mistaken use of belladonna root.

Calendula (*Calendula officinalis*)

Also called: Pot marigold.

Source: Native to south-central Europe and northern Africa.

Part used: Flower.

Forms available: Tea (for gargle, mouthwash, or internal use), ointments, creams, spray, tinctures, extracts.

Uses: Mild burns, sunburn, mouth infections, sore throat, wounds. Extracts may be beneficial in treating duodenal ulcers.

Caution: Persons allergic to the pollen of other members of the aster family, such as ragweed, may be allergic to calendula.

CASCARA SAGRADA (*RHAMNUS PURSHIANA*)

Source: From a small tree native to the Pacific Northwest.

Part used: Bark.

Forms available: Tea, capsules, liquid extracts. Some products are standardized to 20 to 30 percent anthraquinones.

Uses: Constipation.

Caution: May interact with heart drugs, corticosteroids, and licorice root; consult your doctor. Don't use cascara sagrada if you have intestinal obstruction, abdominal pain of unknown origin, diarrhea, inflamed intestines (colitis, Crohn's disease, irritable bowel syndrome). Limit use to 10 days or less; consult a health care provider before using it if you are pregnant or nursing.

Conscientious consumer information: To make the active principles milder, the bark must be aged one year or heat treated. Fresh dried bark produces a laxative that's too strong for safe use. It also induces vomiting.

CAT'S CLAW (*UNCARIA TOMENTOSA, U. GUIANENSIS*)

Also called: Una de gato.

Source: South American rain forests; commercial supplies are wild-harvested in Peru and Brazil.

Parts used: Root, stem.

Forms available: Capsules, extracts, tablets, tinctures. Products standardized for total alkaloid content are available.

Uses: South American folk medicine uses cat's claw for intestinal disorders, dysentery, arthritis, wounds, and cancer. Modern research indicates significant immune-stimulating activity and antiviral, cancer-fighting, and antioxidant effects. German and Australian physicians have used cat's claw to stimulate the immune systems of cancer patients. Extracts have been used to treat rheumatoid arthritis, allergies, herpes, gastric ulcers, and side effects of chemotherapy.

Caution: Avoid use in autoimmune diseases, such as tuberculosis, multiple sclerosis, and HIV infection. Safety is not established for children or women who are pregnant or nursing. In Germany and Australia, standardized cat's claw products are not allowed to be combined with hormones, insulin, fresh blood plasma, or certain vaccines. Consult a doctor before using cat's claw.

Cayenne (*Capsicum annuum, C. frutescens*)

Also called: Capsicum, hot pepper, chili pepper.

Source: Native to the tropical Americas and naturalized worldwide.

Part used: Fruit.

Forms available: Spice, tea, capsules, tablets, tinctures. Cayenne's fiery compound, capsaicin, is used in topical creams.

Uses: Internally for antioxidant action, nutrition; topically for osteoarthritis and rheumatoid arthritis, shingles, diabetic neuropathy, at the site of healed infections.

Caution: May interact with anticoagulant drugs; consult your doctor. Excessive internal use may irritate the intestinal tract. Manufactured, topical capsaicin creams can cause a burning sensation. Try a patch test on a small area of skin first. Wash your hands with soap after applying the cream to avoid spreading it to the eyes, nose, or other sensitive tissues.

Chamomile (*Matricaria recutita*)

Also called: German chamomile, Hungarian chamomile, true chamomile.

Source: Hungary, the Czech Republic, Slovakia, Germany, Argentina, Egypt.

Part used: Flower.

Forms available: Tea, salves, tinctures, essential oils; ingredient in bath and body-care products. Some products are standardized to 1.2 percent apigenin/0.5 percent essential oil.

Uses: Indigestion, nausea, insomnia, inflammation, wound healing.

Caution: Persons allergic to the pollen of other members of the aster family, such as ragweed, may be allergic to chamomile. Chamomile is associated with rare contact dermatitis. It also may interact with anticoagulant drugs.

CRANBERRY (*VACCINIUM MACROCARPON*)

Also called: Trailing swamp cranberry.

Source: Bogs from Newfoundland west to Manitoba, south to Virginia, and into the Midwest. Commercial berries are produced in Massachusetts and Wisconsin.

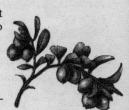

Part used: Fruit (berries).

Forms available: Whole fruit, raw or jellied, juice, fruit concentrate, capsules.

Uses: Prevention and treatment of urinary tract infections, nutrition.

.Cranberry

Caution: No known risks associated with use.

DANDELION (*TARAXACUM OFFICINALE*)

Also called: Lion's tooth, cankerwort, wild endive.

Source: Found nearly everywhere on the planet; grown commercially in the United States and Europe.

Parts used: Root, leaf.

Forms available: Cooking, teas, capsules, liquid extracts, tablets, tinctures.

Uses: Leaves are used for enhancing bile secretion and decreasing water retention and bloating accompanied by flatulence and appetite loss. Roots are used for indigestion, as a diuretic, to promote bile secretion, and to treat rheumatism.

Caution: For use in treating gallstones, German health authorities recommend supervision by a qualified health care practitioner. If you have obstructed bile ducts, don't use it at all. The milky substance in fresh dandelion leaves may cause contact dermatitis. The bitterness in the root may cause hyperacidity. Avoid ingesting dandelion from areas where pesticides have been applied.

DANG GUI (*ANGELICA SINENSIS*)

Also called: Chinese angelica, dong quai, tang kuei.

Source: Cool mountain woods of southern and western China.

Part used: Root.

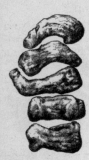

Forms available: Teas, capsules, tablets, tinctures, combination products; common ingredient in Chinese formulations.

Uses: Menstrual cramps, menopausal symptoms, premenstrual syndrome, tonic for liver and female glandular system. In China, the herb is valued as highly as ginseng.

Caution: Avoid during pregnancy or nursing unless monitored by a qualified health care practitioner. May interact with anticoagulant drugs. In Traditional Chinese Medicine, dang gui is not administered to persons with diarrhea because of its mildly laxative action.

Dang gui

ECHINACEA (*ECHINACEA ANGUSTIFOLIA*, *E. PALLIDA*, *E. PURPUREA*)

Also called: Purple coneflower.

Source: *E. angustifolia* and *E. pallida* are native to the prairies of midwestern United States. Over-harvesting in the wild has led to commercial cultivation of both species. *E. purpurea*, the most commonly used species, is also native to the Midwest, but the world supply of this species is cultivated.

Parts used: Root, above-ground parts.

Forms available: Capsules, juice of fresh flowering plant, tablets, tinctures.

Uses: Stimulating the body's defenses against minor viral and bacterial infections such as colds and flu.

Caution: Persons allergic to the pollen of other members of the aster family, such as ragweed, may also be allergic to echinacea. Don't use the herb if you have autoimmune diseases such as tuberculosis, multiple sclerosis, or HIV infection.

Conscientious consumer information: Echinacea is threatened in the wild, so be sure to buy it from reputable sources. Substitute the more commonly cultivated *E. purpurea* for *E. angustifolia* where possible.

ELDERBERRY (*SAMBUCUS CANADENSIS*, *S. NIGRA*)

Also called: American elder, common elderberry, elder flower (*S. canadensis*), European elder, elder flower (*S. nigra*).

Source: American elder grows from British Columbia east to Nova Scotia, south to the mountains of North Carolina, and west to Arizona. European elder grows throughout much of Europe, western Asia, and northern Africa, and is widely cultivated for its fruit.

Parts used: Ripe fruit (berries), flower.

Forms available: Teas, capsules, tablets, tinctures, combination products.

Uses: Preventing and treating colds and flu (fruit); treating colds, fevers, and bronchitis (flowers).

Caution: The dried or cooked fruits and flowers are safe to use. Eating the fresh flowers or raw and unripe fruit can cause adverse reactions.

ELECAMPANE (*INULA HELENIUM*)

Also called: Scabwort, alant, horseheal, yellow starwort.

Source: Native to Europe and temperate Asia; cultivated in Europe and China; naturalized in the eastern United States.

Part used: Root.

Forms available: Teas, tincture, dried root.

Uses: Eases respiration and promotes expectoration in chronic bronchial coughs, asthma, emphysema, and tuberculosis. Modern research supports its use for pulmonary diseases. Elecampane has also been shown to contain powerful antibacterial properties.

Caution: Large doses cause vomiting, diarrhea, spasms, and symptoms of paralysis. Avoid during pregnancy. Use only under the supervision of a qualified health care practitioner.

EPHEDRA (*EPHEDRA SINICA*, *E. INTERMEDIA*, *E. EQUISETINA*)

Also called: Ma-huang, Chinese jointfir (*E. sinica*), Chinese ephedra (*E. sinica*).

Source: Native to the steppes of north and northwestern China.

Part used: Stem.

Forms available: Capsules, tablets, teas, tinctures. Some products are standardized to 6 to 8 percent ephedrine/pseudoephedrine.

Uses: Mild seasonal or chronic asthma, nasal congestion, sinusitis.

Caution: Don't use ephedra—or products that contain it—if you have high blood pressure, heart disease, thyroid disease, diabetes, anorexia, bulimia, or glaucoma. The herb may interact with MAO inhibitors, cardiac glycoside drugs, and pharmaceuticals, so consult your doctor if you have questions.

Avoid during pregnancy or while nursing unless under medical supervision. Numerous side effects of ephedra include insomnia, nervousness, tremors, and loss of appetite. Discontinue use if your symptoms worsen or do not abate in an hour. Keep out of children's reach.

EVENING PRIMROSE (*OENOTHERA BIENNIS*)

Source: Native to eastern North America and widely naturalized in Europe and western North America; most seeds for oil production are grown commercially.

Part used: Seed oil.

Forms available: Capsules, expressed oil, in skin preparations and cosmetics.

Uses: Atopic eczema, fatty acid deficiencies (especially gamma-linolenic acid or GLA), premenstrual syndrome.

Caution: In clinical studies, fewer than 2 percent of people taking the herb for long periods noted side effects such as nausea, abdominal discomfort, and headache.

FENNEL (*FOENICULUM VULGARE*)

Source: Native to the Mediterranean and widely naturalized throughout the world; common to California.

Part used: Fruit ("seeds").

Forms available: Teas, capsules, tinctures, lozenges.

Uses: Bloating, flatulence, mild digestive spasms, catarrh, coughs; has antimicrobial, antispasmodic, and anti-inflammatory properties.

Caution: Rare allergic skin and respiratory tract reactions have been reported. Fennel is a potential source of synthetic estrogen, and should be avoided during pregnancy.

FENUGREEK (*TRIGONELLA FOENUM-GRAECUM*)

Source: Ancient herb native to southern Europe and southwest Asia; cultivated in warm regions throughout the world.

Part used: Seed.

Forms available: Capsules, tablets, seeds for cooking, powdered seeds for poultices.

Uses: Approved in Germany as an internal treatment for gastritis and loss of appetite, and as a poultice for inflammations. Used traditionally to stimulate flow of breast milk. Shows promise in lowering cholesterol and blood sugar.

Caution: May interfere with certain drugs for diabetes. Therapeutic dosages of fenugreek should be avoided during pregnancy, but use in cooking is okay. In clinical trials, some patients have reported intestinal gas and diarrhea. High in mucilage, the seeds may coat the stomach and block absorption of other drugs.

FEVERFEW (*TANACETUM PARTHENIUM*)

Source: Naturalized in Europe and North and South America.

Part used: Leaf.

Forms available: Fresh or dried leaves, capsules, tablets, tinctures. Parthenolide and other related constituents may be responsible for the herb's action; some products are standardized to 2.6 percent parthenolides.

Uses: Migraine prevention and treatment, fever, arthritis.

Caution: May interact with anticoagulant drugs. Avoid during pregnancy. Some people who chewed the fresh leaves reported experiencing mouth ulcers, tongue inflammation, lip swelling, and occasional loss of taste.

FLAXSEED (*LINUM USITATISSIMUM*)

Source: Among the world's oldest cultivated plants; commercial supplies imported from North Africa, Argentina, Turkey, and Canada.

Part used: Seed.

Forms available: Whole seed; expressed oil of seed in bottles or capsules.

Uses: Constipation, irritable bowel syndrome, source of omega-3 fatty acids. May benefit women with ovarian dysfunction and reduce risk of breast and colon cancer.

Caution: Do not take flaxseed if you have a painful bowel condition or if you suspect you may have a bowel obstruction. May interact with anticoagulant drugs. Mucilage from the seeds may affect absorption of other drugs.

Flaxseed

GARLIC (*ALLIUM SATIVUM*)

Source: The bulb is unknown in the wild, having evolved over 5,000 years under cultivation.

Part used: Bulb.

Forms available: Fresh or dried cloves, capsules, tablets, tinctures, aged extracts.

Uses: Stimulating the immune system and fighting cancer. Well-documented health benefits include lowering cholesterol and triglycerides (a type of blood fat), fighting infections, and reducing blood pressure.

Caution: May interact with anticoagulant drugs. Rare cases of allergic reactions are known. Some people experience heartburn or flatulence.

GENTIAN (*GENTIANA LUTEA*)

Source: Native to the mountains of central and southern Europe; it is both cultivated and wild-harvested.

Part used: Root.

Forms available: Teas, capsules, tinctures, liquid extracts, combination products.

Uses: Dyspepsia, appetite loss, flatulence, bloating, digestive tonic.

Caution: Do not use gentian if you have stomach or duodenal ulcers. Some people experience headaches from using gentian.

Conscientious consumer information: May be at risk in the wild but needs further study.

Ginger (*Zingiber officinale*)

Also called: Gingerroot.

Source: Native to the Eastern Hemisphere; cultivated for millennia in China and India; reached the West at least 2,000 years ago.

Part used: Root.

Forms available: Fresh root, teas, capsules, tablets, tinctures, liquid extracts, candied slices.

Uses: Indigestion, nausea, motion sickness; may help reduce cholesterol and narrowing of the arteries.

Caution: May interact with anticoagulant drugs. Do not take therapeutic quantities if you have gallbladder disease. The amounts used in cooking are safe. Despite its blood-thinning qualities, ginger is unlikely to be harmful before or after surgery. Pregnant women who wish to use ginger for morning sickness should first consult their health care practitioner.

Ginkgo (*Ginkgo biloba*)

Also called: Maidenhair tree.

Source: Commercial production takes place mainly in South Carolina, France, China.

Part used: Leaf.

Forms available: Teas, capsules, liquid extracts. Some products are standardized to 24 percent flavone glycosides.

Uses: All forms of cerebral insufficiency, including short-term memory loss, dizziness, Alzheimer's disease, tinnitus, impotence.

Caution: May interact with MAO inhibitors and anticoagulant drugs. Rare cases of gastrointestinal upset and headaches have been reported.

Conscientious consumer information: At risk in the wild but needs further study.

GINSENG (*PANAX GINSENG, P. QUINQUEFOLIUS*)

Also called: Asian ginseng, Korean ginseng, Chinese ginseng, oriental ginseng, ginseng root (*P. ginseng*); American ginseng (*P. quinquefolius*).

Source: Asian ginseng is cultivated in China, Korea, and Japan; American ginseng grows in eastern North America and is wild-harvested.

Part used: Root.

Forms available: For Asian ginseng, teas, capsules, extracts, tablets, tinctures; some products standardized to 5 to 15 percent ginsenosides. For American ginseng, capsules, tinctures.

Uses: Fatigue, mental dullness, convalescence, athletic performance, aphrodisiac, tonic.

Caution: Do not take this herb if you have high blood pressure, heart palpitations, insomnia, asthma, or high fever. May interact with caffeine, other stimulants, and anticoagulant drugs. With high doses or long-term use, some people experience over-stimulation or stomach upset.

GOLDENSEAL (*HYDRASTIS CANADENSIS*)

Also called: Yellow puccoon, orangeroot.

Source: Woods from Vermont to Georgia, west to Alabama and Arkansas, and north to eastern Iowa and Minnesota.

Part used: Root.

Forms available: Capsules, tinctures, salves, ointments, liquid extracts. Some products are standardized to 5 percent hydrastine.

Uses: Antiseptic, cold remedy (for inflamed mucous membranes), stomach infections.

Goldenseal

Caution: May interact with anticoagulant drugs. Safety for pregnant women and children has not been established. The fresh plant may cause skin irritation.

Conscientious consumer information: Goldenseal is increasingly scarce in the wild, but many cultivation projects were launched in the 1990s. Use cultivated goldenseal when possible, or substitute other antimicrobial herbs that are not threatened with extinction, such as Oregon graperoot and barberry.

GOTU KOLA (*CENTELLA ASIATICA*)

Also called: Indian pennywort, tiger grass.

Source: Native to tropical Asia where it is commercially cultivated; also grows in Hawaii and other tropical areas.

Parts used: Whole plant, leaf.

Forms available: Teas, capsules, tinctures, tablets; ingredient in body-care products. Some products are standardized to 10 percent asiaticosides.

Uses: Internally for improving memory, reducing stress; externally to relieve inflammation and help heal wounds. Considered a rejuvenating herb in ancient Ayurvedic tradition.

Caution: No known risks associated with use.

HAWTHORN (*CRATAEGUS* SPP.)

Also called: English hawthorn (*C. laevigata*); oneseed hawthorn (*C. monogyna*).

Source: Found in North America, Europe, East Asia.

Parts used: Fruit, leaf, flower.

Forms available: Teas, capsules, tinctures, extracts. European products are standardized to oligometric procyanidins and flavonoids.

Uses: Angina, coronary insufficiency, early stages of congestive heart failure. Preliminary experiments in China show that preparations of hawthorn berries may help prevent and treat hardening of the arteries.

Caution: May interact with digitalis.

HOREHOUND (*MARRUBIUM VULGARE*)

Also called: White horehound.

Source: Throughout much of Europe; naturalized in North America.

Part used: Whole herb.

Forms available: Teas, cough drops, candies.

Uses: Coughs, catarrh, appetite loss, dyspepsia.

Cautions: No known risks associated with use.

HORSE CHESTNUT (*AESCULUS HIPPOCASTANUM*)

Also called: Buckeye.

Source: Native to central Asia; naturalized in western Europe and the United States. Much of today's medicinal supply is produced in Poland.

Parts used: Bark, seed, leaf.

Forms available: The crude herb may be toxic; therefore, only standardized preparations (typically to 20 percent aescin) are recommended.

Uses: Weak veins, varicose veins, edema, bruises, sprains. Injectable forms are used in Germany to treat severe head injuries and to reduce postsurgical swelling.

Caution: Rarely, people using horse chestnut have reported stomach upset, nausea, and itching.

HORSETAIL (*EQUISETUM* SPP.)

Also called: Scouring rush, Dutch rush, rough horsetail (*E. hyemale*); field horsetail, bottlebrush, shavegrass (*E. arvense*).

Source: Common in North America, but most of the supply comes from Europe and China.

Part used: Whole herb.

Forms available: Teas, capsules, tinctures.

Uses: Internally for water retention; externally for wound healing.

Caution: Do not use horsetail if you have heart or kidney disease, or if you are pregnant or nursing. Not recommended for children. Proper identification is crucial because some Equisetums, such as *E. palustre,* are poisonous. Do not take this herb long-term; data on toxicity are lacking.

Horsetail

KAVA-KAVA (*PIPER METHYSTICUM*)

Also called: Kava, kava pepper.

Source: Exact origin is unknown because of cultivation over centuries. Today the herb is found throughout the South Pacific islands, from Hawaii to New Guinea.

Part used: Root.

Forms available: Capsules, tablets, tinctures, combination formulas. Some products are standardized to 30 to 40 percent kavalactones.

Uses: Anxiety, stress, insomnia.

Caution: Do not use during pregnancy or nursing. Do not use if you've been diagnosed with depression. May increase the effects of alcohol and other substances that act on the central nervous system. Exercise caution when driving or operating machinery. Do not exceed the recommended dose, and limit use to one to three months. Excessive or long-term consumption can cause a scaly yellowing of the skin, which goes away when treatment is discontinued.

Conscientious consumer information: Threatened in the wild; purchase from reputable sources.

LICORICE (*GLYCYRRHIZA GLABRA*)

Also called: Gan cao.

Source: Native to and commercially cultivated in Europe and Asia. It also grows in North and South America and Australia.

Part used: Root.

Forms available: Teas, capsules, tinctures, extracts, tablets, candy. Used in many traditional Chinese formulas; some products are standardized to 12 percent glycyrrhizin.

Uses: Stomach or duodenal ulcers, premenstrual syndrome, congestion of the upper respiratory tract, coughs, low adrenal function.

Caution: Do not use licorice if you have high blood pressure, heart disease or liver disease, or diabetes. May interact with diuretics or digitalis. Do not use during pregnancy. Do not exceed recommended dose; discontinue use after six weeks.

Linden (*Tilia* spp.)

Also called: Large-leaved linden, lime tree flowers, linden flowers.

Source: Throughout northern temperate regions.

Part used: Flower.

Forms available: Teas, tincture.

Uses: Nervous tension, headaches, feverish colds, and flu. Used since the late Middle Ages to promote perspiration and for nervous conditions, diarrhea, and indigestion. Scientific studies confirm the herb's ability to promote perspiration.

Caution: Overuse of linden-flower tea may cause heart damage. If you have heart problems, consult your doctor before using.

Marshmallow (*Althaea officinalis*)

Source: England, Europe from Denmark and central Russia south to the Mediterranean, and the United States in salt marshes from Massachusetts to Virginia and in the western mountains.

Parts used: Root, leaf.

Forms available: Teas, capsules, tablets, tinctures.

Uses: Sore throats and dry coughs, upset stomach, lung congestion; soothes and softens irritated mucous membranes. Traditionally, the root has been used in poultices for bruises, inflammation, insect bites, minor injuries, and burns.

Caution: The herb's main active ingredient, mucilagin, may delay the absorption of other drugs in the digestive tract.

Motherwort (*Leonurus cardiaca*)

Also called: Common motherwort.

Source: Grows throughout much of Europe and has become naturalized in the United States. For the U.S. market, motherwort flower is imported from Europe.

Parts used: Flower, whole herb, seed.

Forms available: Teas, tinctures. Chinese formulations contain both herb and seeds.

Uses: Heart disease, high blood pressure, muscle cramps, irregular menstruation, excessive menstrual bleeding, kidney disease; also recommended for improving circulation.

Caution: May interact with blood-thinning medications. Avoid use if you're pregnant or nursing.

MULLEIN (*VERBASCUM THAPSUS*)

Also called: Great mullein, Aaron's rod, velvet dock, lungwort.

Source: Widely grown in Europe and Asia and naturalized throughout North America. Commercially harvested in Europe and the United States.

Parts used: Leaf, flower.

Forms available: Teas, flowers in olive oil (for ear ailments), tinctures, tablets; also an ingredient in numerous European cough and bronchial medicines.

Uses: Respiratory catarrh, earache.

Caution: No known risks associated with use.

OATS (*AVENA SATIVA*)

Also called: Oatstraw, common oat.

Source: Native to the Mediterranean region; cultivated in cool temperate regions worldwide.

Part used: Tops.

Forms available: Teas, tinctures, tablets, capsules, dried tops, bath products.

Uses: Cooked oats have traditionally been used to regulate the digestive system and calm nerves. It's now known that eating oat bran reduces cholesterol. Added to baths, oats are a folk remedy for skin disorders, arthritis, and rheumatism. German health authorities have approved oats as a treatment to soothe inflamed, itchy skin.

Caution: No known risks are associated with use.

PEPPERMINT (*MENTHA × PIPERITA*)

Also called: Brandy mint, lamb mint, American mint.

Source: Native to Europe; commercially grown in Indiana, Wisconsin, Oregon, Washington, and Idaho.

Part used: Leaf.

Forms available: Teas, tinctures, essential oil, enteric-coated capsules of peppermint oil, chewing gum, mints.

Uses: Indigestion, gastrointestinal spasms, flatulence, irritable bowel syndrome, nausea, respiratory congestion.

Caution: Do not take this herb if you have insufficient hydrochloric acid in the stomach, gallbladder or bile-duct obstruction, inflammation, or related conditions. Do not give any form of peppermint to infants. Exercise caution when giving peppermint tea to children because the menthol in the herb may make them choke. Do not apply the essential oil directly to mucous membranes; use the oil topically with care, dilute it in vegetable oils as directed. Do not add more than the directed amount to bath water.

PLANTAIN (*PLANTAGO MAJOR, P. LANCEOLATA*)

Also called: Hoary plantain, English plantain, greater plantain.

Source: Native to Eurasia and widely naturalized in North America.

Part used: Leaf.

Forms available: Teas, capsules, tablets.

Uses: Catarrh, bronchitis, skin irritations. German health authorities have found plantain to be safe and effective for soothing mucous membranes and as an astringent and antibacterial.

Caution: Do not use plantain if you're taking a bulk laxative containing psyllium seed, which comes from other *Plantago* species. Otherwise, plantain is generally safe. Instances of toxicity have resulted from misidentification or contamination with the leaves of *Digitalis lanata*.

PSYLLIUM (*PLANTAGO SPP.*)

Also called: Blond psyllium, ispaghula (*P. ovata*), black psyllium (*P. indica*).

Source: Blond psyllium is native to the Mediterranean, North Africa, and western Asia, and is grown commercially in India and Pakistan. Black psyllium is native to the Mediterranean.

Parts used: Seed, seed husk.

Forms available: Capsules, powders, an ingredient in bulk laxatives.

Uses: Constipation, hemorrhoids, lowering cholesterol.

Caution: Do not use psyllium if you have intestinal obstruction. Consult your doctor before taking it if you have insulin-dependent diabetes; preparations of psyllium often contain sugar. Do not use if you are also taking plantain.

RED CLOVER (*TRIFOLIUM PRATENSE*)

Also called: Purple clover, cleaver grass, cow grass, trefoil.

Source: Native to Europe and naturalized throughout the United States.

Part used: Flowering tops.

Forms available: Teas, capsules, tinctures.

Uses: Folk remedy for blood purification, bronchitis, whooping cough, asthma, skin conditions, and cancer; also a rich source of phyto-estrogen isoflavones, which may help prevent cancer.

Caution: Avoid during pregnancy unless monitored by a qualified health care practitioner.

RED RASPBERRY (*RUBUS IDAEUS*)

Source: Grows throughout Eurasia and North America; most of the commercial supply comes from Europe.

Part used: Leaf.

Forms available: Teas, capsules, tablets, tinctures.

Uses: Popular as a folk remedy for painful and profuse menstruation and as a tonic during pregnancy. Also valued traditionally as an astringent treatment for diarrhea, stomach ailments, colds, mouth sores, and inflamed mucous membranes of the throat.

Caution: Red raspberry is a mild uterine stimulant. Pregnant women should consult a qualified health care practitioner before using it.

REISHI (*GANODERMA LUCIDUM*)

Also called: Ling-zhi, ling chih, ling chi mushroom.

Source: Reishi mushroom grows wild on plum trees in Japan; it is commercially cultivated in China, Japan, and the United States.

Part used: Fruiting body.

Forms available: Capsules, tablets, tinctures, extracts.

Uses: Recommended as an immune stimulant and general tonic;

also to treat anxiety, high blood pressure, hepatitis, bronchitis, and asthma.

Caution: Though rare, side effects including dry throat, nosebleeds, stomach upset, and bloody stools have been reported after three to six months of continuous use.

ROSEMARY (*ROSMARINUS OFFICINALIS*)

Source: Native to the Mediterranean, from Spain and Portugal south to Morocco and Tunisia, where it is also commercially grown. Some rosemary is commercially produced in the United States.

Part used: Leaf.

Forms available: Teas, tinctures, extracts, essential oil; dried leaves for cooking; also an ingredient in bath and body-care products.

Uses: Upset stomach, flatulence, rheumatism, apathy, stimulating the appetite, enhancing coronary blood flow; traditionally thought to improve memory.

Caution: Rosemary and its essential oil can harm the uterus or fetus when taken in therapeutic amounts during pregnancy; amounts used in cooking are generally considered safe.

SAW PALMETTO (*SERENOA REPENS*)

Also called: Sabal.

Source: Native to the southeastern United States; most of the supply is wild-harvested in Florida.

Part used: Fruit.

Forms available: Capsules, tinctures. Some products are standardized to 90 percent free fatty acids.

Uses: Prostate enlargement (benign prostatic hyperplasia, or BPH).

Caution: Rarely, people taking the herb experience cases of stomach upset. More important, before you take saw palmetto, consult your doctor for a diagnosis; prostate cancer has symptoms similar to BPH.

SCHISANDRA (*SCHISANDRA CHINENSIS*)

Also called: Magnolia vine.

Source: All species of the genus Schisandra are native to East Asia except *S. coccinea,* which is native to the southeastern United

States. Most of the commercial supply is grown in China, but some comes from eastern Europe and Russia.

Part used: Fruit.

Forms available: Teas, capsules, tinctures, combination products. Some products are standardized to 2.6 to 4 percent schisandrins.

Uses: Hepatitis, liver protection tonic. Laboratory studies in conjunction with clinical trials indicate that schisandra helps normalize blood pressure, improve brain efficiency, increase endurance, build strength, and is strongly antioxidant.

Caution: In rare cases, appetite loss and stomach upset have been reported by people taking schisandra.

SIBERIAN GINSENG (*ELEUTHERO SENTICOSUS*)

Also called: Eleuthero, Ussurian thorny pepperbush.

Source: Grows in thickets in northeast China, eastern Russia, Korea, Hokkaido (Japan's northern island), and eastern Europe.

Parts used: Root, stem.

Forms available: Capsules, tinctures, tablets.

Uses: A tonic for fatigue, convalescence, stress, mental weakness, and decreased work output.

Caution: Increases the effectiveness (and side effects) of some antibiotics. German health authorities caution persons with high blood pressure not to use the herb, but no solid clinical proof supports this warning.

SKULLCAP (*SCUTELLARIA LATERIFLORA*)

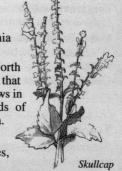

Also called: Mad-dog skullcap, Virginia skullcap.

Source: Found in the woods of eastern North America. *S. baicalensis*, a popular species that has been the subject of recent research, grows in southwestern China and the sandy fields of northeastern China and neighboring Russia.

Part used: Whole herb.

Forms available: Capsules, teas, tinctures, combination products.

Skullcap

Uses: Nerve tonic, sedative.

Conscientious consumer information: Some bulk supplies of skullcap were found in the past to be contaminated with germander (*Teucrium* spp.), a plant that has been linked to liver damage. If you buy skullcap in bulk, purchase it from a reputable source.

ST.-JOHN'S-WORT (*HYPERICUM PERFORATUM*)

Source: Native to Europe and naturalized in Asia, Africa, North America, South America, and Australia. Commercially cultivated and wild-harvested in Chile, the United States, and Europe.

Part used: Flowering tops.

Forms available: Teas, capsules, tablets, tinctures. Some products are standardized to 0.3 to 0.5 percent hypericin. Another compound, hyperforin, is also thought to combat depression.

Uses: Internally for mild to moderate depression; externally for cuts, burns, abrasions.

Caution: May intensify the effect of narcotics and some antidepressants; may cause increased skin reactions to sun exposure. Worsens the side effects of sun-sensitizing drugs, alcohol, and supplemental melatonin.

TEA TREE (*MELALEUCA ALTERNIFOLIA*)

Source: Moist areas on the northern coast of New South Wales and southern Queensland, Australia.

Part used: Essential oil.

Forms available: Essential oil, vaginal suppositories, an ingredient in deodorants and other body-care products.

Uses: Candida, fungal infections, acne, sore throat (diluted and used as a gargle). Used traditionally by the aborigines as a local antiseptic.

Caution: Do not take the essential oil internally; if using as a gargle, spit out and rinse the mouth.

TURMERIC (*CURCUMA LONGA, C. DOMESTICA*)

Also called: Jiang huang, curcuma.

Source: Most of the supply is imported from tropical Asia.

Part used: Root.

Forms available: Capsules, tinctures, powder for cooking. Some products are standardized up to 95 percent curcumin.

Uses: Peptic ulcers, hardening of the arteries, indigestion, liver problems. Curcumin, the yellow pigment in turmeric, has been shown to possess antioxidant, anti-inflammatory, cholesterol-reducing, and cancer-fighting properties.

Caution: Do not take this herb if you have gallstones or obstruction of the bile ducts. May interact with anticoagulant drugs.

VALERIAN (*VALERIANA OFFICINALIS*)

Also called: Garden valerian.

Source: Native to North America and Europe; grown commercially in the United States, Europe, and elsewhere.

Part used: Root.

Forms available: Teas, capsules, tablets, tinctures, extracts, sleep-inducing preparations. Products are sometimes standardized to 0.8 to 1 percent valeric acid.

Uses: Mild sedation in the relief of insomnia and anxiety. Preliminary studies indicate that valerian also relieves muscle spasms.

Caution: Though rare, minor side effects—including headaches, excitability, and insomnia—may occur with continual use.

VITEX (*VITEX AGNUS-CASTUS*)

Also called: Chaste tree.

Source: Native to west Asia and southwestern Europe; naturalized in the southeastern United States; grown commercially in Europe.

Part used: Fruit (berries).

Forms available: Teas, capsules, tinctures, tablets, combination products.

Uses: Premenstrual syndrome, heavy or frequent menstruation, spotting, impaired menstrual flow, swelling and tenderness of the breasts, infertility, menopausal symptoms, and other female conditions requiring hormone regulation.

Caution: Do not use vitex if you are taking hormone replacement therapy or birth control pills. Generally not recommended for use during pregnancy; however, in cases of progesterone deficiency, vitex has been administered under medical supervision to prevent miscarriages in the first trimester. Occasional minor skin irritations have been reported.

RESOURCES

HERBS AND HERBAL PRODUCTS FOR BUYING

HERBAL AND NATURAL MEDICINE ASSOCIATIONS

AMERICAN ASSOCIATION OF NATUROPATHIC PHYSICIANS (AANP)
601 Valley Street, Suite 105
Seattle, WA 98109

AMERICAN BOTANICAL COUNCIL
PO Box 201660
Austin, TX 78720

AMERICAN HERB PRODUCTS ASSOCIATION
4733 Bethesda Avenue
Bethesda, MD 20814

AMERICAN HERBALISTS GUILD
PO Box 70
Roosevelt, UT 84066
www.healthy.net/herbalists

AMERICAN HOLISTIC HEALTH ASSOCIATION
PO Box 17400
Anaheim, CA 92817-7400
www.healthy.net/pan/chg/ahha
e-mail: ahha@healthy.net

HERB RESEARCH FOUNDATION
1007 Pearl Street, Suite 200
Boulder, CO 80302
www.herbs.org

HERBAL PRODUCTS

AVENA BOTANICALS
219 Mill Street
Rockport, ME 04856

CHERYL'S HERBS
836 Hanley Industrial Court
St. Louis, MO 63144

ECLECTIC INSTITUTE, INC.
14385 Southeast Lusted Road
Sandy, OR 97055-9549

FRONTIER HERB CO-OP
PO Box 299
Norway, IA 532218
(800) 669-3275

GAIA HERBS
108 Island Ford Road
Brevard, NC 28712

GREEN TERRESTRIAL
328 Lake Avenue
Greenwich, CT 06830

HERB PHARM
PO Box 116
Williams, OR 97544

HERBALIST & ALCHEMIST
PO Box 553
Broadway, NJ 08808

HORIZON HERBS
PO Box 69
Williams, OR 97544

JEAN'S GREENS
119 Sulphur Spring Road
Newport, NY 13416
(888) 845-8327

LONGHERB HEALTH PRODUCTS
307 E. Washington Ave.
Fairfield, IA 52556-3148
(Smoker's Aroma smoking
cessation product)

MOUNTAIN ROSE HERBS
20818 High Street North
North San Juan, CA 95960
(800) 879-3337

PACIFIC BOTANICALS
4350 Fish Hatchery Road
Grants Pass, OR 97527

RAINBOW LIGHT
207 McPherson
Santa Cruz, CA 95060
(800) 635-1233
(800) 227-0555 (in California)

WAY OF LIFE
1210 41st Avenue
Capitola, CA 95010

WISE WOMEN HERBALS
PO Box 279
Creswell, OR 97426
(800) 532-5219

VITALITY WORKS
134 Quincy Street
Albuquerque, NM 87108

ZAND HERBAL FORMULAS
1722 14th Street, Suite 230
Boulder, CO 80302
www.zand.com

CHINESE HERBS
AND PRODUCTS

MAYWAY CORPORATION
1338 Mandela Parkway
Oakland, CA 94607
(800) 262-9929

TASHI/MIN TONG HERBS
5221 Central Avenue, Suite 105
Oakland, CA 94804
(800) 538-1333

ESSENTIAL OILS

AROMA VERA
5901 Rodeo Road
Los Angeles, CA 90016-4312

AVENA BOTANICALS
219 Mill Street
Rockport, ME 04856

**ORIGINAL SWISS
AROMATICS**
Pacific Institute of Aromatherapy
PO Box 6723
San Rafael, CA 94903

SIMPLER'S BOTANICALS
PO Box 2534
Sebastopol, CA 95473
(800) 652-7646

PUBLICATIONS

HERBS FOR HEALTH
Herb Companion Press, LLC
201 East Fourth Street
Loveland, CO 80537-5655
www.interweave.com
For subscriptions:
PO Box 7714
Red Oak, IA 51591
(800) 456-6018

HERBALGRAM
American Botanical Council
PO Box 144345
Austin, TX 78714-4345
(800) 373-7105
www.herbalgram.org
e-mail: custserv@herbgram.org

AMERICAN HERB ASSOCIATION NEWSLETTER
PO Box 1673
Nevada City, CA 95959

MEDICAL HERBALISM
PO Box 20512
Boulder, CO 80308

MENO TIMES
1108 Irwin Street
San Rafael, CA 94901
(newsletter)

WOMEN'S HEALTH CONNECTION
PO Box 6338
Madison, WI 53716
(800) 366-6632
(newsletter)

MOTHERING
PO Box 1690
Santa Fe, NM 87504
www.mothering.com
e-mail: mother@ni.net

MEDICAL HERBALIST MAGAZINE
PO Box 20512
Boulder, CO 80308
www.medherb.com

ASSOCIATIONS AND SUPPORT GROUPS

AMERICAN PARKINSON'S DISEASE ASSOCIATION
116 John Street
New York, NY 10038

AMERICAN SLEEP DISORDERS ASSOCIATION
1610 14th Street NW
Suite 300
Rochester, MN 55901

ASHA RESOURCE CENTER
PO Box 13827
Research Triangle Park, NC 27709
(800) 230-6039
(national herpes hotline)

ENDOMETRIOSIS ASSOCIATION
8585 North 76th Place
Milwaukee, WI 53223
(800) 992-ENDO
(800) 426-ENDO (Canada)

MULTIPLE SCLEROSIS FOUNDATION
6350 North Andrews Avenue
Fort Lauderdale, FL 33309
(800) 441-7055

**NATIONAL OSTEOPOROSIS
FOUNDATION**
Department MQ
PO Box 96616
Washington, DC 20077-7456

**NATIONAL SLEEP
FOUNDATION**
1522 K Street, NW, Suite 500
Washington, DC 20005
www.sleepfoundation.org

**THE NORTH AMERICAN
MENOPAUSE SOCIETY**
PO Box 94527
Cleveland, OH 44101
e-mail: nams@apk.net

CONTRIBUTING WRITERS

D. Paul Barney, M.D., is a family-practice and emergency room physician in Layton, Utah. He is also an adjunct professor at Weber State University and author of *The Doctor's Guide to Natural Medicine* (Woodland, 1998).

Michael Castleman is one of the nation's top health writers. He is the author of 10 consumer health books, including *Blended Medicine* (Rodale, 2000). His book on herbal medicine, *The Healing Herbs* (Bantam, 1996) is one of the best-selling herbals of all time. Castleman's work has appeared in *Herbs for Health, The Herb Companion, The Herb Quarterly, Reader's Digest, Prevention, Redbook, Self, Family Circle, Glamour, American Health for Women,* and many other publications.

Logan Chamberlain, Ph.D., is president of Herb Companion Press and publisher of *Herbs for Health* magazine. He is the author of *What the Labels Won't Tell You* (Interweave Press). He also hosts a weekly nationally syndicated radio program, *Herbs and Your Health,* and serves on the board of the Education Committee of the National Nutritional Foods Association. He received his Ph.D. in Human Resource Development from Colorado State University.

Christopher Hobbs, L.Ac., is a fourth-generation herbalist and licensed acupuncturist. Author of *Women's Herbs, Women's Health* (Interweave Press, 1998) and *Herbal Remedies for Dummies* (IDG Books, 1999), Hobbs writes and lectures internationally on herbal remedies. He is a member of the advisory board for *Herbs for Health* magazine, and practices as a clinical herbalist in Santa Cruz, California.

Lois C. Johnson, M.D., is a holistic physician in private practice in Sebastopol, California. She is board-certified in Internal Medicine. She teaches classes in advanced clinical herbalism, and her articles have appeared in *Herbs for Health, The European Journal of Herbal Medicine,* and other publications.

Cindy L.A. Jones, Ph.D., is a biomedical writer, reasearcher, consultant, and educator with a Ph.D. in biochemistry and molecular biology. Her most recent book is *Alternatives to Antibiotics.* She was a contributor to *The Gale Encyclopedia of Medicine, The Medical Disability Advisor, The World Book Health & Medical Annual,* and the *Grolier Encyclopedia Yearbook.* She is a frequent contributor to *Herbs for Health, Nutrition Science News,* and other periodicals.

Erika Lenz is editor-in-chief of *Herbs for Health,* the leading consumer magazine about medicinal herbs. She has an M.F.A. in creative writing from Arizona State University and a B.A. in English literature from Colorado State University. Her writing has appeared in *Natural Home, Utne Reader, Art in Arizona,* and *The Yearbook of Contemporary Literary Criticism.*

Robert Rountree, M.D., received his medical degree from the University of North Carolina School of Medicine at Chapel Hill in 1980. He subsequently completed a three-year residency in family and community medicine at the Milton S. Hershey Medical Center in Hershey, Pennsylvania, after which he was certified by the American Board of Family Practice. He is a coauthor of *Smart Medicine for a Healthier Child* (Avery, 1994) and *A Parent's Guide to Medical Emergencies* (Avery, 1997). He is an assistant clinical professor in the Department of Family Medicine at the University of Colorado School of Medicine.

Victor Zeines, D.D.S., has been practicing holistic dentistry for the past 25 years. He received his degree from New York University College of Dentistry in 1970 and completed an internship at the Eastman Dental Center in Rochester, New York. In 1980, he received a Master's in Science (nutrition) from the University of Bridgeport, Bridgeport, Connecticut. Dr. Zeines is the author of *The Natural Dentist* (Kensington, 1999). He has also taught nutrition at Ulster County Community College, New York.

INDEX